D1246002

Collision Sports: Injury and Repair

Collision Sports
Injury and Repair

David Fevre MCSP SRP
Senior Physiotherapist, Manchester United Football Club

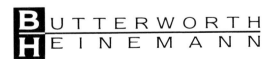

BUTTERWORTH
HEINEMANN

OXFORD   BOSTON   JOHANNESBURG   MELBOURNE   NEW DELHI   SINGAPORE

Butterworth-Heinemann
Linacre House, Jordan Hill, Oxford OX2 8DP
225 Wildwood Avenue, Woburn, MA 01801-2041
A division of Reed Educational and Professional Publishing Ltd

A member of the Reed Elsevier plc group

First published 1998

© Reed Educational and Professional Publishing Ltd 1998

All rights reserved. No part of this publication may be reproduced in
any material form (including photocopying or storing in any medium by
electronic means and whether or not transiently or incidentally to some
other use of this publication) without written permission of the
copyright holder except in accordance with the provisions of the Copyright,
Designs and Patents Act 1988 or under the terms of a licence issued by the
Copyright Licensing Agency Ltd, 90 Tottenham Court Road, London,
England W1P 9HE. Applications for the copyright holder's written
Permission to reproduce any part of this publication sould be addressed
to the publishers

British Library Cataloguing in Publication Data

A catalogue record for this book is available from the British Library

Library of Congress Cataloguing in Publication Data

A catalogue record for this book is available from the Library of Congress

ISBN 0 7506 3142 2

Composition by Genesis Typesetting, Laser Quay, Rochester, Kent
Printed and bound in Great Britain by The Bath Press

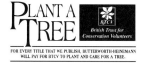

FOR EVERY TITLE THAT WE PUBLISH, BUTTERWORTH-HEINEMANN
WILL PAY FOR BTCV TO PLANT AND CARE FOR A TREE.

Contents

The therapist

'As the trainer has to spend many hours with a player after injury, teaching him therapeutic exercises, during this period they must develop a close bond of respect. The trainer will be asked questions way beyond those concerned with the injury; social, domestic, financial and emotional problems will be discussed. Often it is the trainer who first finds the seeds of discontent which may lead to a transfer request later; and in the case of very serious injuries, the player will draw on the trainer's knowledge of other players who have sustained similar troubles and whether they ever returned to the game'.

Harold Sheperdson MBE

Physiotherapist, Middlesbrough and England Football Teams, 1960/1970s.

The player

'A rugby player must be hard because he is expected to play against hard men and he must make contact with hardness. A player will experience bumps and jolts and he will fall or be flung to the ground like a rag. Players will fall on him and even tread on him. Elbows, knees or even hard heads will strike him without pity and if the player has a faint heart these things will hurt him and even frighten him'.

Crawford

Springbok Rugby Union coach, 1978.

Preface

Sport is often divided into two categories, contact and noncontact. If this division is correct, then any sport in which contact with another player is made can be included in the former group – even ballroom dancing!

'Collision' gives a more precise title to many of the more popular sports played by amateur or professional, male or female, young or old sportspersons. Coupled to the enjoyment factor, the speed and collision aspect of these activities is often the reason why so many people participate in such sports, which carry a higher than average risk of injury.

Thanks to the profession I took up after leaving school, my career has enabled me to work with many of these individuals. Having been a collision sportsman myself, it has been very rewarding to continue in this field as my career started to overtake the playing aspect of my life. The important thing to remember as a physiotherapist, however, is that at no time are you still a player or even a coach. You are involved as the physiotherapist and your sole responsibility is to provide the best professional care you can for your players. Good results on the pitch are nice, but it should be more important to you that good results are occurring in the treatment room.

To be in the medical team involved with such players is comparable to working in the Casualty department of a busy general hospital. The 'buzz' which accompanies every fresh injury scenario as you wait on the touchline produces identical adrenaline releases to those in the medical staff awaiting the next emergency ambulance, never sure what will happen next. How you handle each situation, both physically and mentally, will often determine the outcome of the player's condition.

Textbooks on sports medicine, however, tend to be very academic, and I often wonder how many of the authors have actually got their hands dirty where it really counts . . . in the dressing room. The only way to learn the basics is to start at the bottom, create a good foundation, and if fortune does smile on you with bigger and better opportunities, never forget those early lessons learnt when working with the enthusiastic social players of the local pub team.

This book has been written to give both clinical and practical advice to those wishing to get involved with sports medicine. I have tried to produce an informal yet factual script which should provide reading material for both coaching and teaching staff, as well as basic grade and senior physiotherapists. It provides basic fundamentals for care of the acute injury and gives pointers as to the appropriate form of treatment in the more chronic injury problem. These rules of the treatment room are applied regardless of the level of competitor being cared for. The chapters which cover the first aid and acute injury phase have been written to help the individual make an instant yet accurate decision as to which appropriate steps need to be taken quickly. Other chapters have been written with more of a discussion-type emphasis, to help the physiotherapist take a more balanced view when planning the short- and long-term treatment programme. Case studies have been included to give more reality to situations that many therapists have only been able to read about in academic texts. This book has been written to be used and to become dog-eared from its use. It must be kept off the bookshelves and in your clinic or treatment room, as it has an allergy to dust!!!

Finally, in writing this text I have consulted many leading medical experts, who have been actively involved in sports medicine at all levels of competition. In particular I would like to thank Mr J. Noble, Mr I. MacLennan, Mr S. McLoughlin, Mr J. B. Williamson and Mr J. Haines, who all provided surgeons' views on spinal, upper and lower limb injury; Dr M. Stone for his help on the role of the general practitioner in sports medicine; my professional colleagues, the chartered physiotherapists from all the various specialities of the job, not just those involved with sports medicine; the many coaches and players from different sports who I have worked with; photographers John Peters and Andrew Varley for their visual contributions to the book; the staff at Butterworth-Heinemann, especially Caroline Makepiece for all her help and advice in the three years it has taken to create this book; and the most important team in my life, my family – Sue, Paul, Suzanne, John, Lauren, mum, dad and my mother- and father-in-law, who could all probably write a book of case studies on being related to a chartered physiotherapist involved in sports medicine!

1

Medical team structure

Every club, whatever the contact sport, whether it be school, amateur or professional, has an obligation to provide good, sound, basic medical facilities at every match and training session, no matter the level of competition or standard of play. Injured players are not 'pieces of meat' to be cast aside when unavailable for team selection. They need to be given sound advice and appropriate care in terms of initially trying to prevent injury. If they do get injured, they need help immediately and then right up until they return to the team. Many young players have had poor advice and treatment after being injured early in their careers, and then never quite reached the heights expected of them.

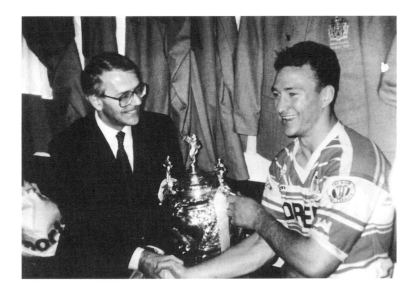

Figure 1.1 Team success is the priority for the manager, but is it for the physiotherapist?

Several years ago, a colleague of mine took up a post as physiotherapist to a professional football club, which shall remain nameless. The team manager would only allow him to treat the 42 players who would make up the first team. He said these were the players who would gain the team promotion, and not the remaining 22 apprentices on the club's books. All injured apprentices had to go in the gymnasium with no supervision and return to training when the injury had corrected itself in time. The chartered

Case study

physiotherapist who worked at the club was in a no-win situation here. Professionally he felt obliged to look after any injured player at the club, yet if caught treating the youngsters he ran the risk of losing his job. Success of the first team is paramount for many team managers, and achieving it is their job. Unfortunately, the development of young players in many sports is often neglected, which in the long term benefits nobody. Thankfully, I have never worked with any club or individuals with such ideals.

Medical network

Every club within its infrastructure should have its own network to provide optimal medical cover for the players. This will involve not only the medical personnel responsible for the players, but also members of the coaching and administrative staff. In turn, the players play a key role in the efficiency of this system and need to be both cooperative and disciplined. The full extent of the personnel involved is shown in Figure 1.2.

From this diagram, it is seen that two-way communication (as illustrated by the two-directional arrows) is necessary for the basic management infrastructure to function successfully. In many cases it is necessary for the physiotherapist to maintain a full-time post away from the club, as the financial rewards in many sports-related jobs are insufficient to maintain a reasonable standard of living. In the ideal situation this extra job responsibility, which can have a detrimental effect on the role of the physiotherapist within the club, will not arise.

Following on from Figure 1.2, the medical network needed to provide a complete service for the players and the team needs to be examined in more detail (Figure 1.3).

Several of the relationships in these figures need to be discussed in order to understand the importance of each team member.

The most important links in the chain are those between each member of the medical team – consultant, club doctor and physiotherapist. These members must link closely together otherwise other individuals in the system may be only too happy to create a split. A player may test this by asking an opinion of one the medical team about an injury they have. If they are not happy with the diagnosis made, they may then approach a different member of the group and be given a different opinion. A potentially volatile situation then exists and this needs to be avoided. Regular meetings where all medical team members can give their opinions within the four walls of the treatment room office help to avoid

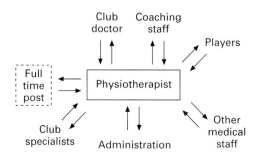

Figure 1.2 Personnel network related to medical care of the injured athlete.

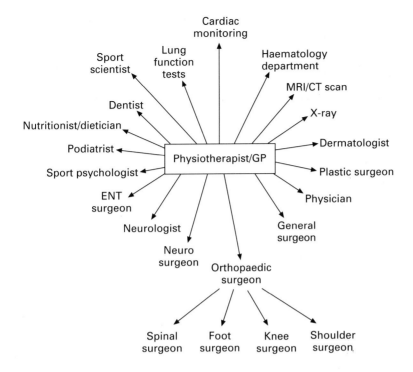

Figure 1.3 Medical personnel involved in the medical care of the injured athlete.

this situation and a uniform diagnosis and prognosis can then be given to the player. Teamwork and communication are vital to prevent such a split.

The relationship between physiotherapist and team coach is also a very important one. Many physiotherapists feel that they should have the final say as to the fitness of a player and his selection for the team. Realistically, the coach, player and physiotherapist should all contribute to the final decision. As the physiotherapist, you should give a concise and factual report to the coach from your assessment of the player's fitness, both clinical and functional. Coaches do not want to hear 'He may be fit'; they want 'Yes' or 'No'. Players need to be involved in the decision, as many have high pain thresholds and will want to play if it is at all possible. For some players, playing sport may be their only means of earning a living, an external factor irrelevant to the medical facts. In the end, once you have given your professional opinion with regard to the injury, it is up to the coach and the player either to act on this information or to ignore it. If the player does then suffer a recurrence of the injury, having played against your advice, that is not the time to gloat. There may be times when your decision is incorrect. Learn from the experience and use it accordingly.

As physiotherapist to a team, the hardest relationship to establish is that between player and physiotherapist, yet it is probably the most important. Initially, common factors such as personal fitness level, age, social and sporting interests help to develop the relationship. From this initial meeting phase, the physiotherapist should always consider the mental as well as the physical approach of the player to the different stages of rehabilitation. The physiotherapist should recognize the level of the player's understanding of the injury, and the response to not competing. An injured player's attitude will fluctuate throughout rehabilitation and the physiotherapist has to be able to adapt to each different situation to get the best out of the individual. This is often the reason why many chartered physiotherapists are unable to work successfully with sportspersons, whose attitude to injury is so different to that of the normal hospital patient even though the physical signs are identical. At the same time it is important to keep taking stock of the situation and maintain the clinical patient/physiotherapist relationship. Friends, like relatives, are more difficult to treat and clinical judgements tend to be affected by too close a relationship with the patient.

Case study

When I first became involved in professional football, I was given two pieces of advice by a senior coach which I have never forgotten to this day. First, 'Players will take the milk out of your tea if you let them'. From experience, even though most collision sports are team games, players have to be selfish to ensure they are in the first team every week. Secondly, 'Always remember you are a physiotherapist and not a coach. You are responsible for the medical care of the players and not the development of their footballing talent'. Never lose track of your role within the club. At the same time, some physiotherapists who work in sport may suggest that the coach should remember that he is not the physiotherapist!

The final important relationship is not shown on either of these two diagrams, and that is the one between you as an individual and you as a chartered physiotherapist. First of all, recognize that your job description in sport is different to the one you may have working in a hospital environment. Figure 1.4 shows that the basic foundation is the same, but many supplementary skills are required to perform the job adequately.

Table 1.1 demonstrates that the hours of work and rewards to be gained differ between employment in the hospital and sporting environments.

In the sporting environment, the work may provide little variety and often involves making important decisions with little or no medical backup. First, stop and think. Is this really what YOU want from a job? To label yourself as a chartered physiotherapist with a speciality in sports medicine is currently a

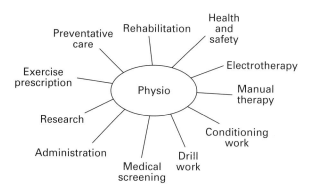

Figure 1.4 Job description of the chartered physiotherapist in sport.

Hospital	Sport
Fixed number of working hours	Flexible number of working hours
Fixed salary	Negotiated salary
Internal promotion	No internal promotion
Limited fringe benefits	Possible larger number of fringe benefits
Work with other medical staff	Often work individually
Limited course opportunities	Limited course opportunities
Standard annual paid leave	Little annual/weekend leave
Large number of treatment units	Large number of treatment units
Job to gain experience	Experience required
Variety of work	No variety of work
Written contract of employment	Often verbal contract – little job security

Table 1.1 *Differences and similarities in the job profile of the chartered physiotherapist in the hospital and sporting environments*

fashionable title. If you are happy just to go through the motions and do a good job in your own eyes, then your professional standing with the team will suffer. Get involved immediately, watch other professionals at work, both coaching and medical staff and learn and absorb. Then push yourself to improve your own professional ability and maintain that drive for the job until the day comes when the enthusiasm disappears. Then it is time to pack it all in. Avoid being the physiotherapist who is happy to wear blazers and tracksuits from the teams looked after just for an afternoon. Instead, continue to apply yourself, and become a better physiotherapist. That should be the attraction in taking up such a career in the first place.

Medical team

At this stage it is important to comment on the role of the individuals who make up the medical team. Various specialities need to be covered in order to provide as complete a system as possible.

1. Club doctor

A local general practitioner who is qualified in sports injury care would be the optimal person to fill this role. This in the real world is obviously not possible due to the number of teams competing in different sports. Many who work in this field have an interest in the sport, and give up their professional time for the love of the game. As with the team physiotherapist, a good doctor is a vital member of any medical team whose experience and wide ranging knowledge of many non-sports-related illnesses is very useful with the variety of conditions of which players will complain. The doctor provides an ideal person with whom to discuss injury problems, often placing a different slant on the situation. Clinically, the doctor's main role is the same as in a general practice-treating the acute injuries as they occur, prescribing medication and referring players for diagnostic tests or specialists' opinions. An up-to-date knowledge of accident and emergency procedures is vital.

2. Orthopaedic surgeon

Injuries that require the skills of the orthopaedic surgeon are obviously very common in collision sports. Many surgeons are nowadays tending to specialize in one particular area, and again ideally it would be nice for the club doctor to be able to refer an injured player to an orthopaedic surgeon who specializes in that particular problem. Due to the volume of players and shortage of such specialists, this is not a realistic possibility for the majority of injured sports people.

3. General surgeon

Abdominal injuries are common problems in collision sports. Whether it be the goalkicker who develops a gradual pain in the abdominal area on the side of his kicking leg, or a player who suffers acute trauma to the thorax covering the vital internal organs, the skill of such a surgeon is required. Ideally a specialist who has an interest in sporting injuries would be the obvious first choice, but the services of such individuals are not readily available to the average sportsperson.

4. Doctor of medicine

Many players often develop or inherit chest conditions which can affect physical performance. Asthma is obviously the most common example and can be a greater problem in countries that have high levels of pollution or damp weather. A knowledge and understanding of the demands of the sport and the legal pharmological aids permitted are important requirements for the consultant involved.

5. Ear, nose and throat (ENT) consultant

The aforementioned specialist is associated with the ENT surgeon. Traumatic or inherited medical conditions may require a referral to an ENT consultant, with the use of surgery as and when required.

6. Dentist

Close links with a local dentist who offers emergency facilities are important when working in any collision sport. Most players think they have the looks of a Hollywood film star and see this as a service vital to their wellbeing. Preventative measures such as the manufacture of protective gumshields are necessary, as well as treatment for the other common dental problems produced by trauma, decay or infection.

7. Radiology department

In many of the acute injury situations that arise in collision sports, the million dollar question 'Is it broken?' regularly crops up. The only accurate way of answering this question is by taking X-rays and treating accordingly. Similarly, with chronic injuries, radiological pictures are very useful in answering some of the questions that arise. Variations such as stress X-rays, stork views, bone scans, arthrograms, tomography, CT (computerized tomography) and MRI (magnetic resonance imaging) scans are also very useful diagnostic services provided by such a unit.

8. *Dietician*

In obtaining an ideal playing weight and recommending the correct foods to eat for competing, the services of a dietician are very important. Fashionable foods for optimal performance are constantly changing as different research is produced, so the team dietician needs to be constantly updating ideas and keeping pace. With injured players, body fat can very easily increase due to the reduction in physical activity. The rehabilitation programme provided by the physiotherapist therefore needs to be linked to professional dietetic advice and monitoring of the situation with regular body fat measurements.

9. *Podiatrist*

All players in collision sports run and perform functional skills involving the lower limb. The tools of the trade – the feet – ideally require the professional services of a chiropodist or podiatrist. Genetic conditions and trauma in the lower limb produce various abnormalities that can be assisted by a combination of orthotic control, exercises and, occasionally, surgery. Preventative measures may be necessary in some adolescent conditions in order to reduce the chances of developing greater complications.

10. *Sports scientist*

Baseline measurements and regular reassessment of the physiological makeup of the player are now important factors to both the physiotherapist and coach. Individual and group comparisons can be made and appropriate training measures used if a problem arises. Qualified sports scientists are able to use the most accurate measures available and then recommend appropriate remedies to try and rectify any physiological problems.

11. *Sports psychologist*

This field of sports science continues to be called upon more frequently as teams and players look for that extra edge in improving performance. In injury terms, the player with a long term injury may benefit from such help, as the mental and physical roundabout of the situation changes over time. Stress counselling is often necessary for high profile players with external problems, to good effect.

Occasionally other specialists such as a neurosurgeon or rheumatologist, for example, may be required. Often there is a need for consultation with any number of the specialists listed in order to give a better overall picture of the injury being investigated.

Medical structure

The facilities that are available to the everyday medical team are largely determined by the financial aspects of the club and its interest in providing good facilities for the players. Many clubs will obviously have limited financial resources, but adequate care should not be beyond the means of all. It may be that a medical room has to be shared by numerous teams who are playing at the same facility, in order to care for the acute injuries that occur in training or whilst playing. In many cases, for the local Sunday league team no such facility may be available at all, so a well stocked medical bag and an individual with first aid experience is essential.

Ideally, the acute care medical room should be positioned with easy access to and from the playing and training facilities. Consideration should be given to accessibility for players who may enter or leave the room on stretchers, with crutches or in wheelchairs. The room itself should have a sink with a hot and cold water supply and an area designated for administrative duties. The age of the mobile phone has made outside communication a lot easier for the medical staff working in such facilities. Lockable cupboards are a necessity if any kinds of drugs are to be kept on the premises, and a power supply will be needed if any form of electrotherapy treatment is to be used. Units are available which can be charged up and used in most places – whilst travelling, or where a power supply is not available. A plinth, on which to examine and treat the players is essential, and these are available as collapsible units so they can be taken wherever desired.

During the game, access to the room will be required by the medical services available for emergencies. If suturing is to be conducted on the premises, then adequate lighting will be required by the doctor. Other facilities which would be useful include:

Stretcher
Axillary and elbow crutches
Refridgerator for drug storage and supply of ice
Chairs and table to assess minor upper limb injuries
Towels and blankets
Sterilizing units for medical instruments and drinking bottles
Disposable sharps box
Litter bin
Storage cupboards for medical stock.

Hygiene is obviously very important, and there can be no excuse if this area is neglected in such an environment.

After the game, minor injuries can be assessed and treated accordingly. Records must be kept of all assessments and treatment modalities used. Unfortunately, 'compensationitis' is one of the biggest growth industries in sport today, and accurate record keeping is the only defence the medical team has in such a situation. At higher levels of competition, the medical room will often become the designated drug testing area. A strict code of practice is needed with these tests, so it is important to be familiar with the procedures before the situation arises.

Medical equipment

The facilities which have already been mentioned are basic requirements for collision team sports. When the team plays away games, rather than having to rely on the home team, try to have enough equipment and the resources to cater for your own players' needs. Emergency contact numbers, access to a telephone system and a notepad for important memos are essential nonmedical items.

Medically, divide your luggage into the following sections for the days' forthcoming events:

1. Pre-match medical bag
2. Pitch side medical bag
   (a) Emergency
   (b) Routine
3. Post-match medical bag.

This allows easy retrieval of the items required during the different stages of a normal match day. More bulky items which are only required occasionally, such as elbow crutches, can be left in the boot of the car.

In the dressing room before the game, the physical and mental preparation begins. Each player will have his own routine and requirements, and the physiotherapist needs to be prepared for all the many idiosyncrasies that exist. The essential items include:

Pre-match bag

Elastic adhesive bandages (all sizes)
Zinc oxide tape (all sizes)
Blister prevention tape (Sleek)
Underwrap
Insulation tape
Disposable razors
Scissors
Nail clippers
Adhesive glue
Heat sprays and creams
Vapour rub
Smelling salts
Massage oil
Petroleum jelly
Adhesive felt (various types and densities)
Elasticated stockinette (Tubigrip)
Tie ups (to prevent socks rolling down).

It is also important to have a small supply of basic drugs, especially if any of the players suffer from such conditions as asthma or diabetes. These will have been prescribed by the player's own general practitioner or the team physician. Essential items should include:

Prescribed inhalers (asthma)
Prescribed antibiotics (infection)
Prescribed anti-inflammatories (soft tissue injury)
Paracetamol (pain)
Electrolyte powder (diarrhoea)
Throat lozenges
Antihistamines (hay fever/insect bites)
Travel sickness pills

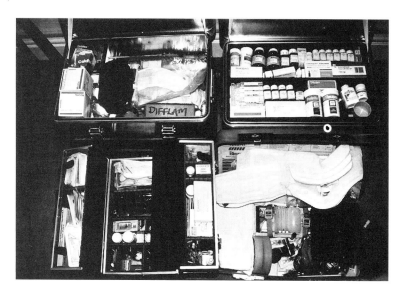

Figure 1.5 Extensive medical supplies required for any emergency.

Each item should be checked regularly to ensure the expiry date has not lapsed, and that any change to the banned substance lists produced by each sport's governing body does not concern any of the drugs used by the medical team. Knowledge of the contraindications or allergic reactions to drugs is important.

Pitch side bag

1. *Emergency*
Ideally, this part of the physiotherapist's kit is only used in cases of emergency, so it is very important to ensure that each piece of equipment is working adequately and that all members of the medical team are familiar with how each item is used.

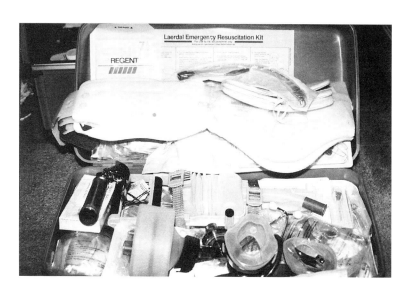

Figure 1.6 Emergency resuscitation equipment.

Lost seconds running back to the dugout may prolong an injured players agony, so organization of the match bag is vital. Important items include:

Airway
Disposable mouthpiece
Rigid cervical collar, that can be altered in size
Splints for upper and lower limbs
Ankle braces (right and left)
Wrist supports (right and left)
Scissors
Slings for upper limb injuries.

2. Routine
In most instances, the physiotherapist is called onto the field of play to assess any injuries that occur. Fortunately the majority are soft tissue injuries, and an instant decision needs to be made as to whether it is safe and functionally possible for the player to continue playing. Occasionally a player may only need a minor adjustment to pre-match strapping, so it is important to be prepared for all situations. Items necessary for this section of the bag include:

Elastic adhesive tape (various sizes)
Zinc oxide tape (various sizes)
Insulation tape
Sterile dressings for external bleeding
Nasal plugs for nose bleeds
Scissors
Dry towel/piece of cliniband to help reduce interphalangeal dislocations
Petroleum jelly
Spare tie ups
Plastic bags to dispose of soiled dressings and to make ice packs
Disposable gloves
Cold sponge
Ice
Wraps with Velcro fastenings to hold ice packs in place
Inhalers*
Glucose tablets*
Spare contact lenses and fluid*.

(*If required by individual team members.)

A colleague of mine tells a story about the time he was offered a financial bonus (about £10!!) if he was to run onto the pitch during a televised game carrying a particular company's first aid bag with their logo on the side. He explained to the salesman that it would be unethical of him to accept this 'bribe', but that he would be glad to do so if the money could be donated to his favourite charity. The salesman agreed on the understanding that this donation would only be made if the aforementioned bag appeared on the television, when treating an injured player on the field of play.   Case study

Unfortunately, my colleague never entered the field of play in the first half, so during the break he made an agreement with one of the players to go down and feign injury five minutes from the end if he had not been on the pitch by this time. As in the first half nobody got injured, and so with five minutes left the aforementioned player fell to the ground and my colleague entered the field of play. He carefully positioned the bag on the ground, 'treated' the player and left the field. After the game, he met up with the sponsor only to be told that he had placed the first aid bag the wrong way round, with the logo facing in the opposite direction to the camera! Having said that, the company still made the donation.

Post-match bag

When the game has finished, all injuries can be thoroughly assessed and treated accordingly. Appropriate first aid is applied with basic home advice, before reassessment at the earliest possible time. Some players are unforthcoming with information on their injuries, so it is important to approach each player individually and ensure no minor injury has been missed. Items that may be necessary here include:

Crepe bandages (various sizes)
Elastic cohesive bandages (various sizes)
Dressing packs
Disinfectant
Plasters
Steristrips
Sterile dressings
Adhesive felt
Plaster remover
Cotton buds
Mouthwash
Eyewash
Friars balsam
Cotton wool
Gamgee
Forceps
Blade cutters
Needles
Syringes
Scissors
Nail clippers
Ice
Plastic bags
Wraps with velcro fastenings
Slings for upper limb injuries
Elbow/axillary crutches.

To obtain every item listed can be very expensive to many clubs, so prioritize the main articles. At the same time, careful management can provide many of the commodities required.

Medical stock can be very expensive for many clubs, even at the highest level. In the 1993/94 season, it cost a rugby team I was looking after £86 per game for taping requirements alone. When one considers this club ran three teams and played in total 130 matches per season, this becomes quite a substantial figure.

Medical facilities

Very few amateur teams will be able to run their own treatment rooms and rehabilitation facilities for injured players. In the United Kingdom only a minority of hospitals provide a basic unit for injured sportspersons, and a more thorough system is necessary if ideal backup is going to be available for these non-professional players. Teams and individual players who can afford to pay for treatment will find more facilities available in the private sector of the medical profession. At professional level all soccer and rugby clubs provide at least a qualified doctor, with many having a full complement of qualified medical personnel.

Ideally the medical centre should have several subdivisions which cover different areas of rehabilitation.

Treatment room

Here the players can be reassessed after an injury has occurred in training or during a match. Both first aid facilities and treatment units should be available to help progress the stages of rehabilitation. Most common items present would include:

Variable height plinths
Ice
Hot and cold water supply
Short wave diathermy
Pulsed short wave interferential ultrasound

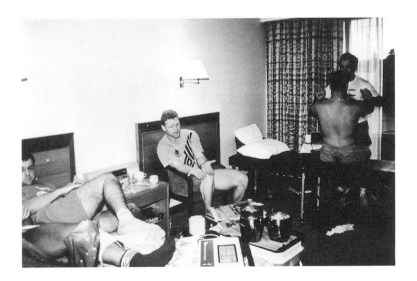

Figure 1.7 The treatment room on tour, all necessities provided.

Laser
Cervical and lumbar traction
Intermittent pressure unit (Flowtron)
Trophic muscle stimulator
Portable EMG unit
Infrared
Sterilizing unit
Refridgerator.

The physiotherapist will have their own preferential combination of these units, although space available and funding is bound to have a large part to play in this choice. As already mentioned, many of the units are now available in a more portable form, often with a rechargeable battery supply, so they can be used in any desired location. This is definitely a facility that should be considered by the physiotherapist who works with a team involved in a lot of travelling.

Gymnasium   Finance and available space will determine the availability of such a facility to the injured players of any team. Often a more logical step is to use a suitable local gymnasium or health club, though this will limit the amount of input the physiotherapist can have on the rehabilitation programme of any injured player.

Apparatus to consider in creating a rehabilitation gym should include:

Isokinetic assessment unit
Free weights
Individual cam weight stations with range of movement limiters
Free standing units for isolated muscle work, i.e. abdominals
Cycle ergometers
Rowing ergometers

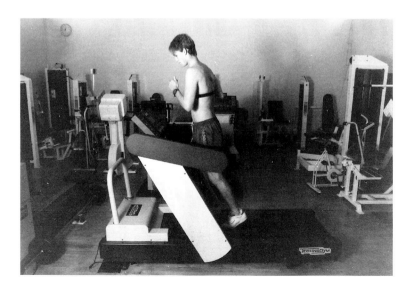

Figure 1.8 Gymnasium facilities, an important rehabilitation requirement.

Step machine
Treadmill
Trampets
Rocker boards (wobbleboard)
Variable height benches
Gym mats
Selection of cones/markers
Wall bars
Springs
Frame suspension
Punchbag/speed ball/pads/mittens
Pulsemeters/watches
Medicine balls (various weights)
Weight boot
Gymnastic balls (various sizes)
Mirror (assess for symmetry)
Resistance tubing (Cliniband)
Sports-related equipment (balls, tackle bags, shields)
Safety equipment (weight belts and gloves).

Office

An area is required for administrative work, a necessity where any form of treatment is taking place. Records must be kept of all appropriate treatments, a player's past medical history and immunization records. A telephone link is important in any area where an emergency may take place. Computerization now allows a greater freedom for the busy physiotherapist in compiling and maintaining medical records.

Indoor/outdoor area

Functional work is a vital part of any player's recovery from injury. Aerobic and anaerobic levels need to be improved and individual sports skills need to be assessed and practised before recovery is complete. An open area of space is therefore necessary, and can be adapted by the physiotherapist to particular needs with regard to the types of exercise regimes and drills required.

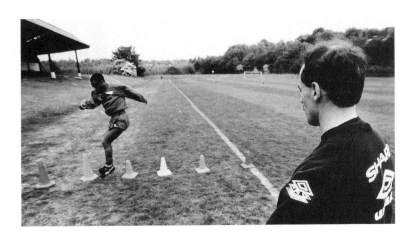

Figure 1.9 Functional outdoor rehabilitation.

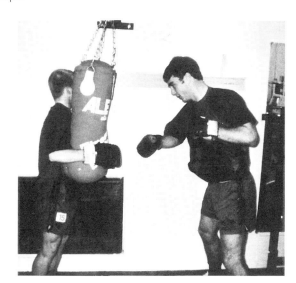

Figure 1.10 Functional indoor rehabilitation.

Use of other sports and the desired skills are a very useful tool in the rehabilitation of any injured player. Physically and mentally, various selected skills can be used from other disciplines and provide a more interesting and functional rehabilitation programme. With this in mind, basketball and volleyball courts, for example, can be marked out within the aforementioned area and used in advanced stages of rehabilitation.

Hydrotherapy pool

Throughout the entire rehabilitation programme, use of a hydrotherapy or swimming pool can be very beneficial. Progressive resistance exercises and early weightbearing activities can be started much sooner due to the buoyancy provided by the pool. In the more advanced stages, a full swimming training programme can be incorporated into a player's schedule to maintain and improve the anaerobic and aerobic state of fitness. Accessories which are useful include:

Arm and leg floats
Hand paddles
Running jackets
Running belts
Weighted objects
Flippers
Functional equipment.

Figure 1.11 contains a typical routine I have used with professional soccer players.

All players use pulse monitors, and the training information can be downloaded onto the computer to assess the intensity of the session. Any weak swimmers are allowed to use the relevant swimming aids to allow them to keep up with the time schedules set along with the more advanced swimmer.

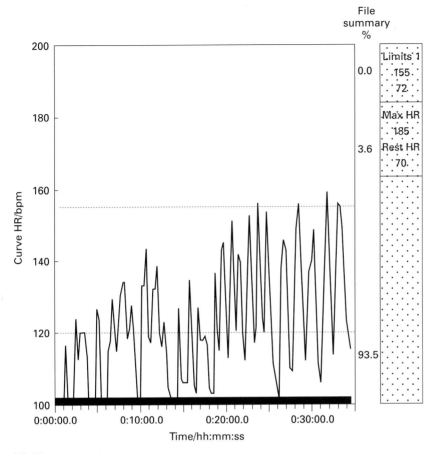

HR: 79
Time: 0:00:00.0

Person		Date	13/03/1997	Average	120 bpm	Recovery - 36 bpm
Exercise	1997/03/13 9:44:18	Time	9:44:18.0	Duration of exercise: 0:34:40.6		
Note				Selected period: 0:00:00.0 - 0:34:30.0 (0:34)		

Figure 1.11 Aerobic swimming rehabilitation programme as monitored by a heart rate monitor.

In order to incorporate a non-weightbearing running programme into the rehabilitation programme, consideration must be given to the depth of the pool and the distance available. Cost is a limiting factor to many clubs having their own pool; arrangements with local facilities can often provide the answer.

Screening of the players' posture, flexibility and physiological state is a very important part of any sports physiotherapist's job in helping to prevent injury and gain a benchmark of the level of fitness of each player. There are many devices and tests available to meet this end, and a relevant programme can soon be devised for the particular sportspersons concerned.

Assessment area

Class area

In some injury situations group work can be more beneficial than individual care. Exercise classes provide competition and variation from one-to-one care. An open gymnasium allows classwork to be used in the rehabilitation programme of many injuries, and often requires only the minimum of equipment.

A lot of time and effort and a degree of finance is needed to provide ideal facilities. To produce such a facility is not on the training curriculum of the physiotherapist, and it is therefore based on experience and the willingness to continue to improve the services provided for the injured personnel and the team.

2

Avoid injury if possible

Prevention of injury is an important part of the team physiotherapist's job, particularly in collision sports where traumatic injury is very common. Table 2.1 demonstrates the comparative rate of injury for several collision sports.

Collision sport	Injury rate per 1000 player hours
Rugby league (UK/Winter)	34 (Stephenson *et al.*, 1996)
Rugby league (UK/Summer)	53.9 (Gissane *et al.*, 1997)
Rugby league (Australia)	44.9 (Gibbs, 1993)
Australian rules football	33.5 (Brukner *et al.*, 1991)
Rugby union	52.5 (Addley and Farren, 1988)
Ice hockey	78.4 (Lorentzon *et al.*, 1988)
Outdoor soccer	16.9 (Ekstrand, 1982)

Table 2.1 *Injury rate (per 1000 player hours) in various collision sports*

Many variations on these statistics exist because inconsistencies occur in defining the degree of injury, and in calculating the incidence of injury. The statistics used have very similar methodologies.

There are many factors which can have an effect on injury incidence, but it is the areas where careful planning can be used to avoid such problems, that need to be investigated further.

Staff

The selection of team coach, trainer or conditioner, whatever the job title, is an important factor in the prevention of injury. A fully qualified coach is necessary in order to use conditioning and training methods which improve the fitness and skills of the players and at the same time control the number of injuries produced. The training sessions need to be pre-planned, disciplined throughout and of a desirable time period in order to eliminate injuries that may result from fatigue or inadequate warm up. Regular meetings between the medical and coaching staff allow a joint approach as to how to get the most out of individual players without aggravating or causing unnecessary injury. Coaches can be introduced to and instructed about the medical aspects of the sport, with many of them requiring a basic first aid qualification within their training. This

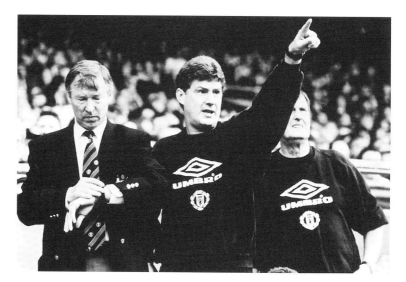

Figure 2.1 The coaching team, vital for success on and off the field.

knowledge can then be carried through to the coaching part of the job where greater emphasis can be placed on the importance of correct techniques, especially in the areas of the game where injuries are most likely to occur. Both parties therefore become better educated as to each other's role in the backroom team, with the players benefitting from this sharing of knowledge.

Level of fitness

When a player returns from injury, it is not unusual to suffer another injury due to loss of anaerobic and aerobic fitness. Players often think that it is possible to store fitness away whilst recovering from injury and then be able to draw upon this as soon as they recover. Preseason conditioning and maintenance of fitness levels whilst injured are important stages in the players' season if they are to make a worthwhile contribution to the team's performance. The physiotherapist will have a large part to play in these particular areas, especially the latter.

Research has shown that in soccer there is a higher incidence of injury in matches compared to training, and in preseason training compared to training in season (Engstrom *et al.*, 1991; Nielson, 1989). Training levels can also have a bearing on incidence of injury, with teams who have a lower level of fitness initially suffering more injuries with increased training (Ekstrand and Gillquist, 1983). It is suggested that this is due to poorer coordination, less oxygen uptake, less strength and a lower skill level. It is also suggested that higher estimated VO_2 max. scores in amateur soccer players can produce a higher number of overuse injuries than those with a lower value. This may be explained by the fitter players undergoing more intensive training routines (Eriksson *et al.*, 1986).

Technical skills

The ability of the player to perform the technical skills of the game correctly can have a great effect on the possibility of avoiding injury.

In both rugby codes, many studies have been produced which show the main phases of the game to produce injuries are the scrum, tackling, being tackled,

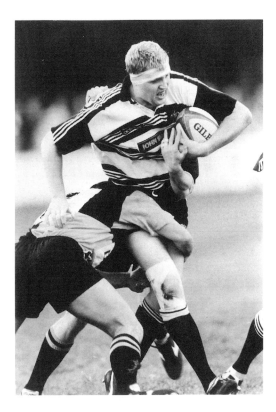

Figure 2.2 The tackle in rugby union.

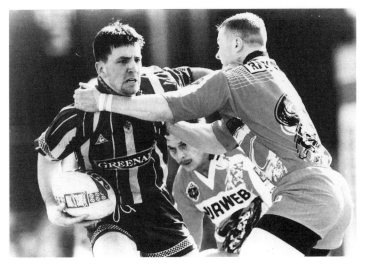

Figure 2.3 The 'higher' tackle in rugby league.

rucking and mauling (Silver and Gill, 1988; Addley and Farren, 1988; Sugerman, 1983). With scrummaging, the rules and how they are applied are the most important factors in attempting to prevent injury. The loose play situations of rucking and mauling again require the understanding of the referee to apply the rules, and education of the players to make them aware of the dangers of blindly charging into such situations. The players who construct a ruck or maul may be exposed to deliberately aggressive charging, jumping and trampling. Also, the ball carrier may experience violence from frustrated opponents, who turn their attention to his head or neck instead of the imprisoned ball. Rugby league, where more tackles are made, produces the greatest proportion of its injuries during this phase of the game with the tackled player being at greater risk than the tackler (Gissane *et al.*, 1993). This is because tackles tend to be a lot higher on the chest than in union in order to prevent a quick release of the ball. 'Spear' tackles (where a tackled player is lifted and thrown head first onto the ground) occur and 'gang' tackles (where more than one tackler is involved) are also part of the modern game. A player must therefore be taught safe methods of tackling, and be shown ways of landing which reduce the risk of injury.

Laws of the game

The rules and regulations laid down by the governing body of each sport need to be enforced and reviewed, where appropriate, to ensure certain injuries are kept to a minimum. In rugby league, situations such as the high tackle and the ball carrier leading with a raised elbow have produced many controversial incidents in the past few seasons. In soccer, problems have arisen when two opposing players have jumped up together to try and head the ball and a stray elbow from one has injured the other. However, with television playing such a major part in sport, the culprits are finding it much harder to avoid detection.

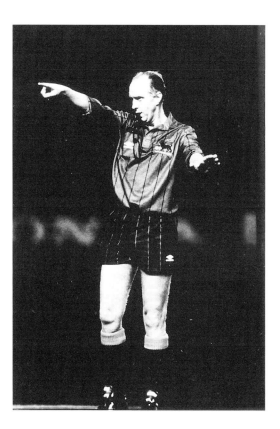

Figure 2.4 The referee – an important individual who can help to prevent injury.

The job of the relevant disciplinary committee is therefore an important one, in order to ensure the punishment fits the crime as well as being a deterrent for other players.

Case study

The decisions made by the law courts in relation to sport are also giving a new dimension to this aspect of injury prevention. In April 1987, an Australian court awarded damages of more than $2 million to a youth who became tetraplegic after a rugby league scrum collapsed. The judge blamed the state government for failing to make known to the player and his coach the fact that players with long necks were much more vulnerable to cervical injury and should not be allowed to play in the front row of a scrum. Since the administration was known to be aware of this fact, it was found to be negligent in not issuing appropriate warnings.

In 1996, an English rugby union player who was paralysed when a scrum collapsed successfully won an action for damages against the match referee. The judge ruled that the referee had 'failed to exercise reasonable care and skill' in preventing scrum collapses. New rules to prevent young players from such injuries had been introduced at the beginning of that particular season, yet the referee concerned was involved in his first under-19 game of the season and his only knowledge of these new rules was based on the written text in the rule book.

Playing surfaces

In both the training and match situation, players are required to perform on numerous different playing surfaces. Whether it is the seasonal changes that affect the playing surfaces, the training requirements of indoor facilities or the use of athletic tracks in preseason training, injuries can very easily arise or be aggravated by a change in the degree of cushioning or friction provided by the training surface.

The general assumption is that the degree of cushioning influences the frequency of injury. The impact forces produced by a hard surface can cause an overload injury to the collagen tissues of the body with single excessive or repeated submaximal impact forces. The degree of force required to produce an injury is dependent on the individual characteristics of each player, such as weight, gait pattern and anatomical site of trauma. The higher incidence of soccer injuries in winter and preseason training may reflect this assumption (Engstrom *et al.*, 1991; Ekstrand *et al.*, 1983b).

A degree of friction is required for a player to run, start, stop and make changes to their pattern of movement. This is dependent on the playing surface and type of shoe worn by the player. In collision sports, injury often arises when a player is tackled with the weightbearing leg fixed to the ground. The degree of rotational friction is thought to have a bearing on the risk of injury in such a situation. Differences have been reported in pattern and mechanisms of injury, for example when playing soccer on grass or on artificial surfaces (Albert, 1983; Renstrom *et al.*, 1977).

Uneven and slippery pitches carry the risk of greater injury to a player. Municipal facilities provided for the recreational player may not be maintained to the highest standards, and injuries may occur due to the poor quality of the playing surface.

Protective equipment

The selection and correct fitting of protective equipment is essential if such items are to assist in reducing the number of injuries in collision sports. Items may include the following:

Head

1. *Scrum caps*
   Worn in rugby league or union to prevent friction over the ears when scrummaging, or to protect a previous head wound.
2. *Helmets*
   Used in American football. These come in three different categories, padded, air and fluid suspension. There should be no movement when external pressure is applied, even if jaw pads are fitted, and a full visual field is vital. The chin strap should be central with equal tension throughout. The face bar should sit forward of the helmet, with good fixation to the shell.

Upper limb

1. *Shoulder pads*
   Can only be worn in American football and either rugby code, after inspection by the referee. The more conventional 'off the shelf' pads are now being replaced by customized pads to suit the body shape of each player. This ensures a better fit as well as giving the player more protection to previous shoulder girdle and upper limb injuries if required.
2. *Shoulder harness*
   This consists of a series of straps and a supporting sling. It is often recommended after a player has suffered a dislocation problem at the glenohumeral joint. The purpose of such a support is to reduce the degree of lateral rotation at the joint, and therefore reduce the chances of further injury.
3. *Forearm pads*
   Forearm pads are used to protect previous injuries in this area, and not to improve the ferocity of a tackle in sports such as American football or rugby league, where they can be worn. They can be made from different foam densities depending on the needs of the player, but must be checked by the match officials before being used in a game to ensure opposing players are not put at risk of injury from them.

Thorax

1. *Chest pads*
   These items can be used in American football and rugby league, and are often incorporated with the shoulder pads. Players in either sport may start using a chest pad following a fracture to the sternum.

Lower limb

1. *Padded shorts*
   Some rugby league players have used such items in order to protect the outer thigh from trauma and reduce their chances of suffering a haematoma to the quadriceps (a 'dead leg'). A problem for the player is that these items tend to be bulky and very rarely stay in place throughout the duration of a game.
2. *Knee braces*
   Functional, prophylactic and rehabilitative knee braces are widely available. In most collision sports, knee braces are classified as being too dangerous to

opposing players and cannot be used in training or playing. In American football, prophylactic braces can be worn, the purpose being to protect the player from a lateral blow to the knee. Theoretically this should then prevent a valgus force to the joint, and reduce the chances of injury to the medial collateral ligament, anterior cruciate ligament or medial meniscus. Appearances can be deceiving and the available literature is still inconclusive (Grace *et al.*, 1988; Teitz *et al.*, 1987).

3. *Shin pads*

These are compulsory in professional soccer, and are used in many other collision sports. The various types of shin pads on the market can provide protection to the malleoli of the ankle as well as to the tibia and fibula – very important after a distal fracture to the lower limb. Also, the various materials available to the manufacturer (such as plastic or polyurethane) can give good protection and yet remain both comfortable and light to wear. Very little research has been done on the protective value of shin pads. It has, however, been shown that shin pads are most effective in preventing abrasion injuries, rather than lower limb fractures (Von Laack, 1985).

4. *Ankle braces*

Various devices are available on the market, but very few are accepted by the majority of players as being comfortable to wear in a match situation. Individuals may find a particular style that suits their injury as well as themselves, but most tend to use a strapping technique to provide any mechanical or proprioceptive support they require.

Ankle braces are often used following reconstruction of ligamentous tissue during rehabilitation, but are no substitute for the support given by the ligaments themselves or the surrounding muscle tissue. Proprioceptively, a brace may reinforce the body's own receptors. Impracticality, discomfort and the tendency for the brace to slip are common problems for the athlete.

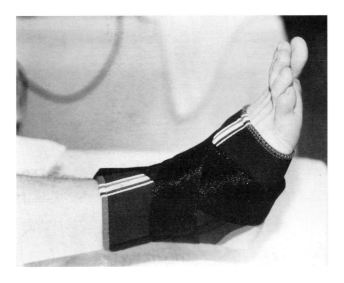

Figure 2.5 Ankle supports – how beneficial are they in functional activity?

General

1. *Thermal supports*

   These are available for most joints and muscular areas of the body and will increase and retain heat during exercise. This will help in improving flexibility, and hopefully reduce the player's chance of suffering a muscle injury. Mechanically, no support is given to weak joints, but proprioception may well be reinforced.

   The choice is dependent on the governing body of the sport, though few make protective gear a condition of competition. Quality items from a reputable manufacturer should be recommended, but due to the financial cost to the player this may not always be possible. Most importantly, no new hazards should be created from the use of protective equipment. In American football, the face guard on the helmet reduces the number of soft tissue injuries or fractures to the face. At the same time, whiplash injuries to the cervical spine have increased, as the tackling player can use the bar as a handle to stop the forward progress of the player.

   Players are often reluctant to use mouthguards (gumshields) as they feel uncomfortable and may find it difficult to maintain a normal breathing pattern. Chapman (1985) stated that 67% of the 1984 Great Britain rugby league team suffered orofacial injuries on the tour to Australia. Only 25% of that squad used a mouthguard regularly. Evidence exists that a mouthguard reduces the transmission of impact forces to the skull, brain and cervical spine (Heywood, 1978; Hickey *et al.*, 1967) and reduces the incidence of fractures to the mandible (Clegg, 1969).

Footwear

In order to reduce the chances of injury from match boots, training boots with moulded studs and training shoes, regular checks as to their condition are necessary. Players are often reluctant to get rid of a pair of boots they have been playing well in, regardless of the present condition. Professional players, who often have their footwear supplied by a sponsor may continue to wear the same shoes until the sponsor sends them a new pair. Unfortunately, a lot of sports shoes are made for the benefit of the manufacturer and their profit margin, and not for the player – a sad fact of life in today's commercial market. The physiotherapist and podiatrist, however, can gain a lot of information from

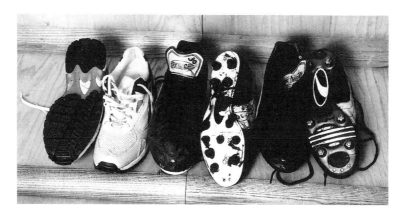

Figure 2.6 Different variations of footwear used by the professional soccer player.

players' footwear with regard to their running style's and biomechanics, which can then be used to educate them and treat any relevant injuries.

When examining any type of sports shoe, whether buying new or when looking for biomechanical clues to help diagnose an injury, there are several areas to look at closely. Different players require different qualities from any type of footwear, so the individual needs, biomechanics and amount of use should be taken into consideration. Often the shoe that a physiotherapist recommends and that is designed to help reduce the chances of injury is not the shoe that gives the player a good grip on a muddy pitch.

In most collision sports, players can vary in weight from 63–126 kg (10–20 stone), and it would be expected that the heavier players need to replace their footwear far more frequently due to the extra weight carried. Lighter players, however, can also experience problems. Imagine a set of car tyres. Fitted correctly on the wheel with correct tracking the wear is even and steady, but if one of the tyres is not in a neutral plane (as is often the case with the human foot) then the tyre will wear quickly and soon become bald on the inner or outer edge. The same can apply to the boots or training shoes of a player. When examining the shoe tread of a training shoe or stud arrangement of a match boot, the physiotherapist will be able to determine if the player is heel, midfoot or forefoot striking in that particular shoe. Always look at the full selection of shoes a player uses, both for playing and everyday life, in order to get a full understanding of their gait pattern in different circumstances.

Excessive pronation and supination of the foot will produce rapid wear along the sides of the shoe and the heel cup will often be distorted when placed on a flat surface. A degree of pronation is necessary for normal movement, but excessive pronators with a distorted heel cup and wear on the outer edge of the heel and under the ball of the foot will need extra help in their choice of footwear, or orthotic control. All footwear should have a firm heel cup. If the cup gives way when pressure is applied by squeezing between thumb and forefinger, then that item needs replacing or should not be purchased, as the quality of material is so poor that no support will be given to the subtalar joint on weightbearing.

Ground reaction forces, dependent on the weight of a player and the surface they are playing on, can have a large bearing on creating or aggravating an injury. The shock absorbency a shoe provides is therefore important in reducing this component. Top quality training shoes use different material densities in the midsole to help reduce this problem, with different combinations for different players' demands. In boots, very little effective cushioning is available, so extra shock absorbency insoles are often used. For a player to use them, they need to be comfortable, light, and of a good fit.

Traction with the ground is provided by the studs on the sole of the boot, or on harder surfaces, players will often wear astroturf boots which have a rigid, dimpled surface. Too much or too little friction can increase the possibility of injury, so correct selection of footwear according to the surface conditions can have a large bearing on the injury incidence.

Anatomically correct positioning of the studs on the sole of a boot is a factor players and manufacturers rarely consider. Players with extra callus growth over old fractures of the foot, or who have hallux valgus or varus of the big toe, can often develop problems over these chronic injury sites due to the extra pressure created by a badly positioned stud. Removal of the offending item or footwear with a more appropriate stud pattern usually gives a quick and easy answer to the problem.

It has also been suggested that the height of a boot can have a bearing on the risk of injury. Rugby players have the choice of high or low cut boots, and research carried out by Garrick and Requa (1973) showed a positive effect (with regard to injury) when high topped boots were used by basketball players in preference to the low cut ones.

Do not, however, fall into the trap of 'moulding' information to fit the injury. Thorough subjective and objective assessment skills are still important to avoid missing the real cause of an injury.

Case study	*During preseason training, a player came into the medical room complaining of bilateral shin soreness which had developed during a particular training session. Subjectively, he could not think of any training variable which may have brought on his symptoms, and objectively there was nothing to find from a biomechanical or mobility aspect. When I asked him to show me his boots, he said he had left them back at his flat and had borrowed a pair for training that day. The problem was that he had used the boots of a player who was already injured, as they were the only spare ones available. On examination, the boots were both grossly distorted at the heel cup and forefoot, so it was easy to see why the acute symptoms of this particular player had arisen. The original owner of the boots had not trained for five weeks as he had developed bilateral compartment syndrome in both shins, and had thrown the boots into a corner of the dressing room after showing them to the medical staff when he first presented with his particular symptoms.*

Taping
Many taping techniques exist which, it is suggested, play a role in the prevention of injuries. Most of the scientific literature on taping is virtually limited to its effect on the ankle joint, the most commonly taped area in sport. This is probably related to the fact that the ankle, and in particular the lateral ligament, is the most commonly injured area in the athlete (Smith and Reischl, 1986; Garrick, 1977). Studies involving basketball players (Garrick and Requa, 1973) and footballers (Ekstrand and Tropp, 1990; Ekstrand et al., 1983a) have shown a reduction in the number of injuries by applying taping techniques to this area.

Theoretically, the aim of taping is to stabilize the ankle joint externally, without interfering with the normal mechanics of movement. Evidence suggests that, after application, movement restriction predominantly occurs in plantar-flexion, plantarflexion/inversion and inversion in neutral, which are the movements that taping is supposed to restrict to prevent injury (Fumich et al., 1981). This initial restriction was up to 30% of the normal directly after the application of the tape (Fumich et al., 1981; Myburgh et al., 1984). During exercise, this restriction gradually reduced. Other research with taping and passive movements suggests that the supporting force is reduced by as much as 40% after 10 minutes of vigorous exercise (Rarick et al., 1962); more recently, taping and active movement research gives statistics of 18% after 15 minutes

(Laughman *et al.*, 1980). If exercise continues for longer than one hour, all mechanical restriction is lost (Fumich *et al.*, 1981). To add to these statistics, the physiotherapist must also consider how much force is required to injure the lateral ligaments of the ankle. It will almost certainly be far greater than the passive movement or active exercise used in the bulk of the existing research, particularly in such collision sports as rugby or American football. With the techniques and materials available, mechanical support is therefore limited to the extreme ranges of movement with a limited time span of functional effectiveness.

The other mechanism by which taping helps to reduce the incidence of injury is proprioception. This acts to stimulate the action of the normal neuromuscular mechanisms that protect against injury, which in the case of the ankle joint involves the peroneal muscle group. In active movement, taping peroneus brevis has been shown to stimulate the action of correcting the position of inversion prior to the heel strike phase of movement, and thus to stabilize the ankle and foot (Glick *et al.*, 1976). Peroneal reaction time has also been shown to shorten with taping application (Karlsson and Andreasson, 1992).

Taping to produce a dragging effect on the skin can occasionally be used to remind a player in the subacute stages of injury of the problem. In the appropriate player, this secondary warning device may help guard against further injury once the acute pain and loss of function stage has disappeared. Player compliance and understanding of the irritation produced by this technique is necessary if this is to help the injury.

Warm-up

In order to prepare for training or play in a match, it is suggested that a rise in muscle temperature and an increase in the range of movement of both the joints and muscle tendon units is desirable in order to prevent injury (Zarins and Ciullo, 1983).

A warm-up routine prior to exercise will raise body core temperature by 2–3°C and improves the metabolic efficiency of muscle action by 10% or more per 1°C. The heating effect that is produced comes about due to the heat of activation from elastic energy, from the thermoelastic heat that is produced after any muscular contraction ends, and from the opening of intramuscular blood vessels. This effect can last for up to half an hour after the contraction (Hill, 1950).

The biochemical changes produced in the muscle following any warm-up stretches the musculotendinous unit and results in an increased length at a given load. With less tension produced at the musculotendinous junction, one of the most common sites of injury or strain in the muscle unit (Safran *et al.*, 1988; McMaster, 1933), a reduction in the incidence of injury at this site has been reported (Safran *et al.*, 1988).

Physiologically, both an active (jogging, applied skills at a slow pace, flexibility exercises) and passive (massage) warm-up will produce an increase in enzyme and metabolic activity, an increase in blood flow and oxygen levels and a decrease in contraction and reflex times of the muscle. All of these factors help to raise tissue temperature and improve functional coordination, which help to reduce the possibility of injury. An active warm-up is more beneficial, as the passive warm-up is less likely to have an effect on the deep muscle tissue and could be counterproductive, as the greater proportion of the blood is diverted to the skin rather than to the muscle tissue (Anderson *et al.*, 1984).

Flexibility

During the warm-up and warm-down phases of a player's training and playing routine, flexibility work is included in order to:

1. *Reduce muscle soreness*

   Delayed onset muscle soreness (DOMS) has been experienced by every sportsperson after vigorous or unaccustomed exercise. Subjectively, the player complains of a constant dull, aching pain in the musculotendinous junctions and muscle bellies of the affected tissues. Objectively, the signs and symptoms may include reduced muscle strength, oedema, and an elevated serum creatine kinase – a common marker of exercise-induced skeletal muscle damage. Pain is first felt later in the day after a particularly intense training session, and may last for up to four or five days. It is most common in the muscles that play a large part in the eccentric phases of movement (Newham *et al.*, 1983).

   Various studies provide conflicting evidence as to the benefits of stretching DOMS affected muscle tissue. Abraham (1977) and DeVries (1966) suggest flexibility work is beneficial in reducing the acute soreness produced in this condition, whereas McGlynn *et al.* (1979) and Buroker and Schwane (1989) found no effect on acute or chronically affected muscles. The important fact to come out of these studies, however, is that the type of stretching programme used and the player's perception of the severity of the symptoms are vital to any benefit gained from any such work.

Treatment notes

Various other treatment and exercise modalities have been suggested as being effective with players suffering from DOMS. These include:

Anti-inflammatory medications
Submaximal concentric exercise
Cryotherapy
Transcutaneous nerve stimulation
Massage
Topical creams, i.e. trolamine salicylate cream
Continuous and pulsed ultrasound
Herbal remedies, i.e. *Arnica montana*.

Research covering the effectiveness of these various approaches is contradictory and limited (Gulick and Kimura, 1996) for a problem that is difficult to avoid due to the eccentric component of functional physical activity.

2. *Prevent injury*

   Flexibility work is commonly used by players during their warm-up programme in the belief that certain injuries can be prevented in the more intense activities of training or playing. It is also suggested that the increase in muscle temperature produced by a thorough warm-up prior to a flexibility session makes stretching safer and more productive (Sapega *et al.*, 1981).

Research has shown a positive correlation between muscle strain and muscle tightness of the lower extremity in amateur soccer players (Ekstrand *et al.*, 1983). Players with adductor strains and tendinitis showed a decreased range of movement in hip abduction than players without adductor injuries.

3. *Improve performance*

Maximum range of movement around the performing joints is necessary in order to produce the best technical results. In most collision sports, however, the majority of players only require an average range of movement in order to produce the desired performance, unlike sports such as gymnastics or any of the martial arts which place a much greater emphasis on flexibility. In soccer, the goalkeeper needs to have some of the characteristics of a gymnast in terms of flexibility and plyometrics, so more specific work in these areas is necessary for such individuals. For the majority of players, however, symmetry of movement is of far greater importance in both improving performance and preventing injury.

Several methods of stretching exist, each with various advantages and disadvantages. These include:

Treatment notes

1. *Static (passive)*

Passive, static stretching involves a player requiring the assistance of another individual, usually the physiotherapist. When stretching the soft tissues passively, feedback from the player is essential. This tells the physiotherapist how far the soft tissues can be stretched safely.

2. *Static (active)*

This involves an active, relaxed and sustained stretch on the noncontractile elements of the muscle tissue. An excellent description on how to stretch actively is outlined by Anderson (1987). This breaks the stretch phase into three areas (Figure 2.7):

(a) Simple stretch

This level starts from a position of no stretch and ends once a mild tension is felt in the muscle tissue by the player. This type of stretch is specifically used in the early stages of rehabilitation following injury to a

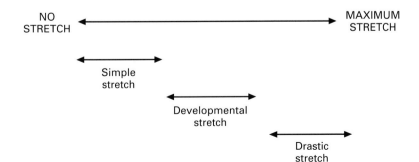

Figure 2.7 Application and understanding of flexibility exercise.

muscular area, so will rarely be used by fully fit players. The position of stretch should be held for 10–30 seconds, and the mild tension should disappear after five seconds.

(b) Developmental stretch

During any flexibility session, the old adage 'no pain, no gain' is not one to recommend to any player. This stage starts at the end of the simple stretch and finishes at the point where muscular tension fails to disappear in the fully stretched position. The player should be instructed to apply the stretch over a full range of motion, and muscular tension should disappear after 15 seconds, otherwise they are moving into the final stage, the drastic stretch. A developmental stretch should be held for 30 seconds.

Understanding of the difference between tension, which eases after a short period of time, and constant pain, which is harmful, is vital for this method of stretching. The physiotherapist must therefore spend time to explain everything fully and get constant feedback from the players to assess whether they have understood the correct stretch technique.

(c) Drastic stretch

This final stage should be avoided, but is the one a lot of players associate with improvement. The constant feeling of pain reassures them that only this degree of stretching work will benefit them. Many will not appreciate that to stretch in the drastic stage will increase their chances of injury.

Muscle tissue is protected by a mechanism called the stretch reflex. Stretch receptors in the muscle spindle and Golgi tendon organs in the muscle tendon respond to changes in the length of the muscle, pain, and excess tension by sending signals along the afferent nerve supply to the brain. This then sends information along the efferent nerve supply to muscle tissue, instructing the protective muscles to contract to eliminate this painful sensation. These tend to be the flexor withdrawal muscle groups. The player can override these messages, though, and the defence mechanism of the body is ignored. This harmful method of stretching will therefore continue to produce pain, as well as physical damage, due to micro trauma in the muscle tissue, and formation of scar tissue, with a gradual loss of elasticity.

3. *Ballistic*

This involves taking the limb to the end of its range of movement and adding repeated bouncing movements. It may be argued that this type of stretching is more realistic in terms of the physical demands placed on the player during a match situation, but it is less popular nowadays. It has been suggested that injury may be more prevalent using this technique (Etnyre and Lee, 1987).

4. *Proprioceptive neuromuscular facilitation (PNF)*

This technique can be used to strengthen as well as stretch the various muscle groups involved. The action is determined by the type of technique applied. In the situation of improving flexibility, the PNF patterns used are contract, relax; slow reversal hold, relax and hold, relax (Tanigawa, 1972). Each technique uses a combination of alternating an isometric or isotonic 'pushing phase' with subsequent relaxation of both the agonist and antagonist muscles.

Such techniques are best performed with the physiotherapist, as application of appropriate resistance and positioning of hands to stimulate contraction are important components of each pattern. If this is not possible, resistance can be applied using a wall or piece of elasticated tubing.

Strength

In the majority of rehabilitation and injury prevention programmes designed for players, strengthening ligamentous and relative muscle groups has become an important component in order to reduce the risk of primary or secondary injury to the area concerned. In terms of recovery times of muscle atrophy after injury and the necessary immobilization period, several studies have been performed which suggest that the physiological responses, the biochemical and contractile properties of the muscle, can virtually be restored by the appropriate rehabilitation (Grimby *et al.*, 1980; Houston *et al.*, 1979). The time period for this to happen is often underestimated, and is dependent on the duration of immobilization, age of player, sex, rehabilitation programme, fibre composition of the affected muscles and the condition of the muscles prior to immobilization.

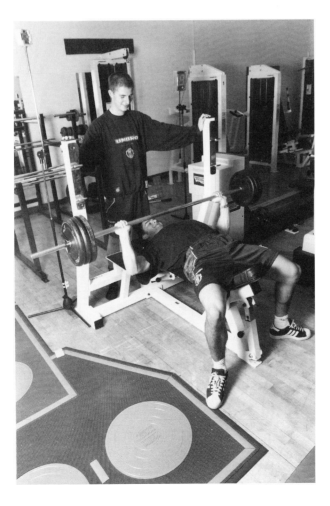

Figure 2.8 Strength work in rehabilitation. Note the use of a second person – 'a spotter' – for safety reasons.

Strength work is also vitally important following previous injury in order to reduce the possibility of the acute injury becoming chronic. Giove (1983) showed this using a rehabilitation programme with an emphasis on hamstring strengthening in individuals with anterior cruciate ligament deficient knees. A higher level of sports participation was achieved by those with hamstring strength equal to or greater than their quadriceps strength. This suggests that overstrengthening the hamstrings may compensate for the loss of the cruciate ligament.

Knowledge of the biomechanics of motion at each joint and understanding of the relationship with strengthening work is very important in designing rehabilitation programmes.

Treatment notes

Quadriceps strength is critical in collision sports for function and athletic use of the lower extremity. In individuals who have had anterior cruciate ligament (ACL) reconstruction, a 'paradox of exercise' exists in terms of rehabilitation of this particular muscle group. The quadriceps can be exercised isometrically at knee flexion angles of 60–90° without causing undue strain on the ACL graft (Renstrom *et al.*, 1986; Arms *et al.*, 1984). A common complication of ACL reconstruction is patellofemoral pain which is exacerbated when performing quadriceps exercises in greater than 30° of knee flexion (Hungerford and Barry, 1979). This therefore suggests that strength work in the 60–90° range should be avoided. Patellofemoral pain may be prevented and treated by strengthening the quadriceps in the 0–30° range (Bourne *et al.*, 1988), but this is the range which places maximal strain on the ACL graft if the only muscle contracting is the agonist (Zavatsky *et al.*, 1994) so a dilemma exists if isolated quadriceps work is used at the wrong stages of recovery after such a surgical procedure.

It has also been demonstrated that the possibility of patellofemoral pain can be greatly reduced by ensuring full hyperextension of the knee is regained as soon as possible following ACL reconstruction surgery (Shelbourne and Trumper, 1997). Conventional rehabilitation protocols tend to avoid an urgency to regain full hyperextension for fear of placing excessive stress on the new graft and producing long term instability. It is now thought that restoration of symmetrical hyperextension encourages a better fit of the new graft into the intercondylar notch and prevents the formation of scar tissue.

Warm-down

Similar to the warm-up, a warm-down is recommended after playing and training. Realistically though, once a game has finished it is difficult to convince tired players that further exercise is going to be of benefit to them, so unless it becomes compulsory for the whole team only the disciplined players tend to participate.

The warm-down should be in the form of light exercise which will give a gradual decrease in body core and muscular temperature. Certain individuals have been known to work harder in the warm down than in the training session or match itself!

Screening of players in the many aspects of their health and physical fitness is an important tool in the prevention of injury. Pre-sport medical examination is very valuable in identifying players with cardiorespiratory conditions which may predispose to their chances of sudden death. Age is not a restriction in this problem, as a screening programme presently exists in English soccer for all youth training scheme players (16–18 year olds) with professional clubs to try and identify individuals who may have hereditary heart conditions such as hypertrophic cardiomyopathy or arrhythmogenic right ventricular cardiomyopathy, which may precipate an abrupt and fatal end to the sporting career of a young player. In Italy a similar programme exists, but is compulsory from the age of 12 years.

An appropriate medical screening programme for new players is therefore very useful in providing information on the medical state and fitness level of each player. Categories should include:

1. *An orthopaedic assessment*
   A full medical, surgical and family history; orthopaedic assessment of neck, thorax, lower back, shoulder, elbow, forearm, wrist, hand, abdomen, pelvis, hip, groin, calf, feet and toes.
2. *A general practitioners (GP) assessment*
   Date of birth, registered GP, previous clubs, brief medical history, general appearance, weight, height, blood pressure, urine test (albumen and sugar), vision.

Medical screening

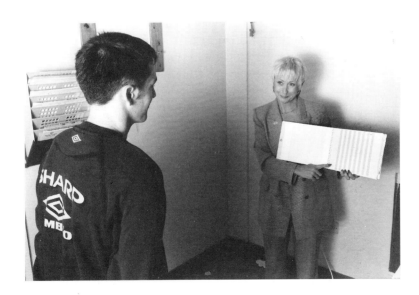

Figure 2.9 In depth vision assessment.

3. *A physiotherapy assessment*
   Postural assessment of shoulder, scapula, spine, pelvis, hip, patella, foot; flexibility measurements of thoracic and lumbar spine, hamstrings, quadriceps hip, calf; isokinetic testing of relevant joints.

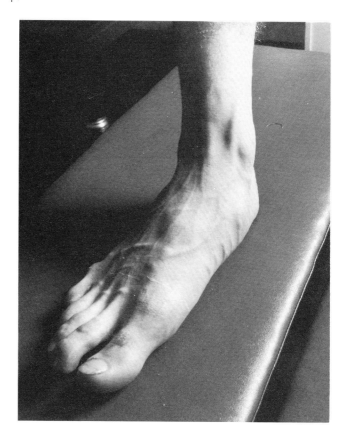

Figure 2.10 Podiatric assessment for the tools of the trade – 'the feet' – in weightbearing sport.

4. *Podiatric assessment*

   Gait analysis; pedobaragraph pressure analysis; biomechanical examination.

5. *Nutritional assessment*

   Body weight; % body fat, using skinfold calipers; assessment of a previously recorded food diary.

6. *Sport science assessment*

   Standard field tests for anaerobic and aerobic fitness come in various formats and should relate to the various physical demands of the sport. Use of cycle ergometry tests for rugby players is not ideal as the test is not directly related to the mode of locomotion in that particular sport.

   Anaerobic tests relate to explosive power and include:

Sargent jump
Margaria–Kalmen power test
Timed 40 m sprint.

Aerobic fitness can be measured directly or indirectly. Maximal oxygen consumption testing is the most valid form of testing, yet it is often difficult to perform, exhausting and occasionally hazardous. Predicting the maximum volume of oxygen consumed per minute (VO_2) using submaximal tests is not as accurate, but avoids any of the aforementioned complications.

Direct methods include:
(a) Treadmill Tests
   Mitchell, Sproule, Chapman (Mitchell *et al.*, 1957)
   Saltin–Astrand (Saltin and Astrand, 1967)
   Ohio State (Camaione, 1969; Fox, 1975).
(b) Cycle tests
   Discontinuous loading
   Continuous loading (McCardle *et al.*, 1973).

Indirect methods include:
(a) Astrand–Astrand nomogram (Astrand *et al.*, 1954)
(b) Fox equation (Fox, 1973).
7. *Cardiac screening*
   Subjective family history, resting and exercising ECG; two-dimensional echocardiogram. Other noninvasive tests may be necessary if any anomalies are found.
8. *Relevant investigative procedures*
   X-ray
   Magnetic resonance (MRI) scan
   Computerized tomography (CT) scan
   Blood profiles – blood glucose, cholesterol, triglycerides, white and red blood cell count.

Please note diagnostic radiology is controlled by the *Protection of Persons Against Ionising Radiations Regulations (1985)* and the *Ionising Radiation (Protection of Persons Undergoing Medical Examination or Treatment) Regulations (1988)*, which were introduced to bring the United Kingdom into line with other EEC countries and to improve awareness of the risks of radiation. These laws basically allow X-rays to be taken in cases of trauma or injury, or when the player has other symptoms referrable to a particular area. However, the use of radiographs for screening procedures in fit, healthy, sportspersons is difficult to justify and a medical reason is needed for taking any particular X-ray film. From this information, players can be counselled on any anomalies found and any preventative measures taken. In order to insure professional players, HIV tests are compulsory. Counselling is necessary prior to such testing.

Foreign travel

Before travelling abroad, all personnel should obtain the necessary inoculations relevant to that particular part of the world. Precise clinical records for each individual should be kept of all relevant dates to ensure that boosters or repeat injections are administered at the appropriate time intervals. The most common injections include:

Tetanus
Typhoid
Cholera
Hepatitis
Yellow fever.

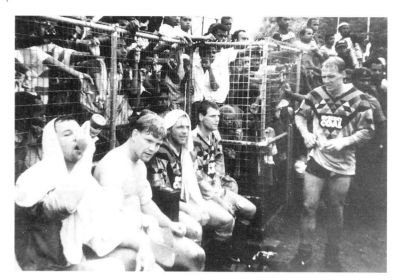

Figure 2.11 Climatic conditions in foreign countries can have a large bearing on sports performance.

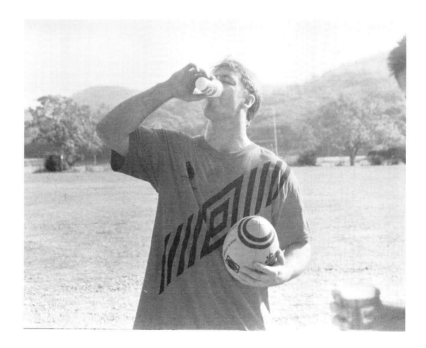

Figure 2.12 Avoid dehydration.

In the case of malaria, antimalarial tablets must be taken prior to, during and on return from visiting any country which comes within the malarial zone of the world. Other preventative measures such as appropriate clothing to cover open skin, creams and sprays should be administered liberally during the time spent abroad.

If players are unaccustomed to training or playing in hot countries, overexposure to sunlight should be avoided by gradually increasing the time spent in the open climate. Suncreams with relevant factor protection for the skin type of the player should be used at all times to prevent sunburn.

Dehydration must be avoided by the regular intake of fluid, especially clean water, before, during and after training or playing. Be aware of the numerous systemic symptoms which may develop in such a situation. These include:

Reduction in volume of urine excreted
Increased urine concentration
Renal tract complications
Constipation
Muscular cramp
Fatigue.

Alcohol should be kept to minimum quantities, as this will only enhance any state of dehydration.

Other aspects of foreign travel and the medical care of individuals needs careful planning. Information prior to departure concerning suitable medical facilities and supplies in the areas of travel and competition can save a lot of aggravation on arrival. Dietary intake, both food and fluid, needs to be considered prior to departure, as various supplies may need to be prepacked along with other medical items to ensure any minimal changes have a negligible effect on performance.

References

Abraham, W. M. (1977). Factors in delayed muscle soreness. *Med. Sci. Sports*, **9(1)**, 11–20.

Addley, K. and Farren, J. (1988). Irish rugby union survey: Dungannon Football Club (1986–87). *Brit. J. Sports Med.*, **22(1)**, 22–24.

Albert, M. (1983). Descriptive three year data study of outdoor and indoor professional soccer injuries. *Ath. Tr.*, **18**, 218–220.

Anderson, B. (1987). *Stretching*, pp. 12–13. Pelham Books.

Anderson, B., Beaulieu, J. E., Cornelius, W. L. *et al.* (1984). Roundtable: Flexibility. *Nat. Str. Cond. Assoc.*, **6**, 10–22, 71–73.

Arms, S. W., Pope, M. H. and Johnson, R. J. (1984). The biomechanics of anterior cruciate rehabilitation and reconstruction. *Am. J. Sports Med.*, **12(1)**, 8–18.

Astrand, P. and Rhyming, I. (1954). A nomogram for calculation of aerobic capacity (physical fitness) from pulse rate during submaximal work. *J. Appl. Physiol.*, **7**, 218–221.

Bourne, M. H., Hazel, W. A. and Scott, S. G. (1988). Anterior knee pain. *Mayo Clin. Proc.*, **63(42)**, 491.

Brukner, P., Miran-Khan, K. and Carlisle, J. (1991). Comparison of significant injuries in AFL players and umpires. *Aust. J. Sports Med.*, **3**, 21–23.

Buroker, K. C. and Schwane, J. A. (1989) Does post-exercise static stretching alleviate delayed onset muscle soreness? *Phys. Sportsmed.*, **17(6)**, 65–83.

Camaione, D. N. (1969). A comparison among three tests for measuring maximal oxygen consumption. Doctoral Dissertation, The Ohio State University, Colombus, Ohio.

Chapman, P. J. (1985). Orofacial injuries and the use of mouthguards by the 1984 Great Britain rugby league touring team. *Br. J. Sports Med.*, **19(1)**, 34–36.

Clegg, J. H. (1969). Mouth protection for the rugby football player. *Br. Dent. J.*, **127**, 341–343.

DeVries, H. A. (1966). Quantitative electromyographic investigation of the spasm theory of muscle pain. *Am. J. Phys. Med.*, **45**, 119–134.

Ekstrand, J. (1982). Soccer injuries and their prevention. Thesis, Linkoping University, Linkoping, Sweden. Linkoping University Medical Dissertations No. 130.

Ekstrand, J. and Gillquist, J. (1983). The avoidability of soccer injuries. *Int. J. Sports Med.*, **4**, 124–128.

Ekstrand, J., Gillquist, J. and Liljedahl, S. (1983a). Prevention of soccer injuries. *Am. J. Sports Med.*, **11**, 116–120.

Ekstrand, J., Gillquist, J. and Moller, M. (1983b). Incidence of soccer injuries and their relation to training and team success. *Am. J. Sports Med.*, **11**, 63–67.

Ekstrand, J. and Tropp. H. (1990) The incidence of ankle sprains in soccer *Foot Ankle*, **11**, 41–44.

Engstrom, B., Johannson, C. and Tornkvist, H. (1991). Soccer injuries among elite female players. *Am. J. Sports Med.*, **19**, 273–275.

Eriksson, L. I., Jorfeldt, L. and Ekstrand, J. (1986). Overuse and distortion soccer injuries related to the players estimated maximal aerobic work capacity. *Int. J. Sports Med.*, **7**, 214–216.

Etnyre, B. R. and Lee. E. J. (1987). Comments on proprioceptive neuromuscular facilitation stretching. *Res. Quart. Ex. Sport*, **58(2)**, 184–188.

Fox, E. (1975). Differences in metabolic alterations with sprint versus endurance interval training. In *Metabolic Adaption to Prolonged Physical Exercise* (H. Howard and J. Poortmans, eds). pp. 119–126. Basel: Birkhauser Verlag.

Fox, E. (1973). A simple accurate technique for predicting maximal aerobic power. *J. Appl. Physiol.*, **35(6)**, 914–916.

Fumich, R. M., Ellison, A. E., Geurin, G. J. *et al.* (1981). The measured effect of taping on combined foot and ankle motion before and after exercise. *Am. J. Sports Med.*, **9**, 165–170.

Garrick, J. G. and Requa, R. K. (1977). The frequency of injury, mechanism of injury and epidemology of ankle sprains. *Am. J. Sports Med.*, **5**, 241–242.

Garrick, J. G. (1973). Role of external support in the prevention of ankle sprains. *Med. Sci. Sports*, **5**, 200–203.

Gibbs, N. (1993). Injuries in professional rugby league. *Am. J. Sports Med.*, **21(5)**, 696–700.

Giove, T. P., Miller, S. J., Kent, B. E. *et al.* (1983) Non operative treatment of the torn anterior cruciate ligament *J. Bone Jt. Surg.*, **65A**, 184–192.

Gissane, C., Jennings, D. C. and Standing, P. (1993). Incidence of injury in rugby league football. *Physiotherapy*, **79(5)**, 305–308.

Gissane, C., Phillips, L. H., Jennings, D. *et al.* (1997). Injury in rugby league football: the new super league. *Br. J. Sports Med.*, **31**, 84–87.

Glick, J. M., Gordon, R. B. and Nishimoto, D. (1976). The prevention and treatment of ankle injuries. *Am. J. Sports Med.*, **4**, 13–14.

Grace, T. G., Skipper, B. J., Newberry, J. C. *et al.* (1988). Prophlactic knee braces and injury to the lower extremity. *Am. J. Bone Joint Surg.*, **70(3)**, 422–427.

Grimby, G., Gustaffson, E., Peterson, L. *et al.* (1980). Quadriceps function and training after knee ligament surgery. *Med. Sci. Sports Ex.*, **12**, 70–75.

Gulick, D. T. and Kimura, I. F. (1996). Delayed onset muscle soreness: what is it and how do we treat it. *J. Sports Rehab.*, **5**, 234–243.

Heywood, J. R. (1978). Recent advances in the management of facial fractures. *Int. J. Oral Surg.*, **1**, 263–264.

Hickey, J. C., Morris, A. L., Carlson, L. D. *et al.* (1967). Relation of mouth protectors to cranial pressure and deformation. *J. Aust. Dental Assoc.*, **74**, 735–740.

Hill, A. V. (1950). The dimensions of animals and their muscular dynamics. *Sci. Progr.*, **38**, 209–230.

Houston, M. E., Bentzen, H. and Larsen, H. (1979). Interrelationships between skeletal muscle adaptions and performance as studied by detraining and retraining. *Acta Physiol. Scand.*, **105**, 163–170.

Hungerford, D. S. and Barry, M. (1979). Biomechanics of the patellofemoral joint. *Clin. Orthop.*, **144**, 9–15.

Karlsson, J. and Andreasson, G. O. (1992). The effect of external ankle support in chronic lateral ankle joint instability. *Am. J. Sports Med.*, **20(3)**, 257–261.

Laughman, R. K., Carr, T. A., Chao, E. Y. *et al.* (1980). Three dimensional kinematics of the taped ankle before and after exercise. *Am. J. Sports Med.*, **66**, 425–431.

Lorentzon, R., Wedren, H. and Pietila, T. (1988). Incidence, nature and causes of ice hockey injuries. A three year prospective study of a Swedish elite ice hockey team. *Am. J. Sports Med.*, **16**, 392–396.

McArdle, W., Katch, F. and Pechar, G. (1973). Comparison of continuous and discontinuous treadmill and bicycle tests for max VO_2. *Med. Sci. Sports.*, **5(3)**, 156–160.

McGlynn, G. H., Laughlin, N. T. and Rowe, V. (1979). Effect of electromyographic feedback and static stretching on artificially induced muscle soreness. *Am. J. Phys. Med.*, **58(3)**, 139–148.

McMaster, P. E. (1933) Tendon and muscle ruptures – clinical and experimental studies on the causes and location of subcutaneous ruptures *J. Bone Jt. Surg.*, **15**, 705–722.

Mitchell, J., Sproule, B. and Chapman, C. (1957). The physiological meaning of the maximal oxygen intake test. *J. Clin. Invest.*, **37**, 538–547.

Myburgh, K. H., Baughan, C. L. and Issacs, S. K. (1984). The effects of ankle guards and taping on joint motion before, during and after a squash match. *Am. J. Sports Med.*, **12**, 441–446.

Newham, D. J., McPhail, G. and Mills, K. R. (1983). Ultrastructural changes after concentric and eccentric contractions of human muscle. *J. Neurol. Sci.*, **61(6)**, 109–122.

Nielson, A. B. Y. de J. (1989). Epidemiology and traumatology of injuries in soccer. *Am. J. Sports Med.*, **17**, 803–807.

Rarick, G. L., Bigley, G., Karst, R. *et al.* (1962). The measureable support of the ankle joint by convential methods of taping. *J. Bone Joint Surg.*, **44**, 1183–1190.

Renstrom, P., Petterson, L. and Edberg, B. (1977). *Valhalla Artificial Pitch at Gothenburg 1975–1977. A Two Year Evaluation.* Gothenburg: Rapport Naturvardsverket.

Renstrom, P., Stanwyck, T. S., Johnson, R. J. et al. (1986). Strain within the anterior cruciate ligament during a hamstring and quadriceps activity. *Am. J. Sports Med.*, **14(1)**, 83–87.

Safran, M. R., Garrett, W. E., Seaber, A. V. et al. (1988). The role of warm up in muscular injury prevention. *Am. J. Sports Med.*, **16(2)**, 123–129.

Saltin, B. and Astrand, P. (1967). Maximal oxygen uptake in athletes. *J. Appl. Physiol.*, **23**, 353–358.

Sapega, A. A., Quendenfeld, T. C., Moyer, R. A. et al. (1981). Biophysical factors in range of motion exercise. *Phys. Sports Med.*, **9(12)**, 57–65, 106.

Shelbourne, K. D. and Trumper, R. V. (1997). Preventing anterior knee pain after anterior cruciate ligament reconstruction. *Am. J. Sports Med.*, **25(1)**, 41–47.

Silver, J. R. and Gill. S. (1988). Injuries of the spine sustained during rugby. *Sports Med.*, **5**, 328–334.

Smith, R. W. and Reischl, S. F. (1986). Treatment of ankle sprains in young athletes. *Am. J. Sports Med.*, **14**, 465–471.

Stephenson, S., Gissane, C. and Jennings, D. (1996). Injury in rugby league: a four year prospective survey. *Br. J. Sports Med.*, **30**, 331–334.

Sugerman, S. (1983). Injuries in an Australian schools rugby union season. *Aust. J. Sports Med. Ex. Sci.*, **15(1)**, 5–9.

Tanigawa, M. C. (1972). Comparison of the hold relax procedure and passive mobilisation on increasing muscle length. *Phys. Ther.*, **52**, 725.

Teitz, C. C., Hermanson, B. K. and Kronmal, R. A. (1987). Evaluation of the use of braces to prevent injury to the knee in collegiate football players. *Am. J. Bone Joint Surg.*, **69(1)**, 2–9.

Von Laack, W. (1985). Untersuchungen uber die Druckverteilung durch Schienbeinschoner im Fussballsport. *Dtsch. Zeitschr. Sportmed.*, **7**, 203–208

Zarins, B. Ciullo, J. V. (1983). Acute muscle tendon injuries in athletes. *Clin. Sports Med.*, **2(1)**, 167–182.

Zavatsky, A. B., Beard, D. J. and O'Connor, J. J. (1994). Cruciate ligament loading during isometric muscle contractions. *Am. J. Sports Med.*, **22(3)**, 418–423.

3

Down man on the field

In any traumatic incident which happens in a game, rapid evaluation and management are necessary and usually have a large bearing on the outcome of the incident. Suitably qualified medical personnel are required for this role, and they are an essential part of the pitch side management team. If a chartered physiotherapist is not available, a suitably qualified first aider will do an adequate job in an emergency. Revision of first aid techniques is vital to even the most qualified medical individual. Never be afraid to learn from other groups of people who work in acute trauma such as paramedics or casualty staff because they are constantly in contact with many of the injuries that the sporting medical personnel see only occasionally and are aware of any new techniques or apparatus which might help in such situations. The three recognized voluntary aid societies in the United Kingdom – St John Ambulance, St Andrew's Ambulance Association and the British Red Cross – all run first aid courses, and further details can be obtained by contacting the local branches in your area.

A club doctor is again an ideal person to have on the touchline, but at least ensure that you have some form of telephone communication readily available and the appropriate numbers for the local ambulance/hospital/casualty department.

Many incidents which happen on the pitch have a funny side to them, but this should not take away the need for switching onto and recognizing a serious situation. All necessary emergency equipment, particularly those articles listed in the previous section for the therapist and doctors bag, should be in a good operating and clean condition and all medical team members must be trained in how to use such items. Larger items such as stretchers should be readily available and in full working order, with accessibility to medical rooms possible from any part of the playing area.

At the very end of a rugby league game I was involved with, one of our players dislocated his elbow. Due to the severity of the injury, he very quickly went into shock and had to be stretchered off immediately. The stretcher team had to manoeuvre through the departing crowd before reaching the building where the medical room was situated. We then had to climb a flight of stairs before reaching the medical room, which was situated at right angles to our point of entry. Very quickly it was obvious that there was no way the laden stretcher could be lifted into

Case study

the room, so the player, who was clearly in a lot of pain, had to be placed on the floor whilst we waited for the ambulance to arrive. This meant blocking a stairway – there was no option due to the layout of the building. Having seen the situation, one of the directors of the opposition approached us and said 'You can't place him there, it's blocking the entrance to the players' bar and we will lose money. There are a lot of thirsty people waiting to get in!' As you can imagine, my answer was short and to the point. The room that was designated the medical room was obviously a room that nobody else wanted. Accessibility for medical equipment such as stretchers had clearly never been considered an important priority when planning the layout of the building.

Constant updating of old and new first aid techniques is essential for both medical and coaching staff. Many courses are available, most of which are practically based and involve working through various injury scenarios. A good personal reference library is also very helpful in theoretical terms to support any hands-on experience.

Assessment

Even though a player is not in the ideal treatment room situation, an immediate assessment of the injury is necessary whilst on the pitch. This process begins by realizing that you are on the touchline not as a spectator but as the medical employee of the team. On many occasions you will miss exciting moments in the game because you are watching a previous collision that has occurred to see if the players concerned pick themselves up and get on with the game. If they stay down, show signs of limping or appear to be in distress, your work commences. Watch them carefully over the next minute or two, and enter the field of play as the rules of the game allow. In soccer this is at the discretion of the referee, whereas in rugby league it is at your own discretion. Both these situations have pluses and minuses for different reasons, and it does take several matches to adapt to the different rules. Once you are called onto the field of play, the assessment procedure begins in your head, first recalling the incident involved in case it gives you any help with regard to the damage that may have been done. The basic principles of all first aid are:

1. Preservation of life
2. Prevention of further injury
3. Promotion of recovery of the injury.

With this list in mind, the following injury scenarios are discussed in the same order. In terms of frequency, the life threatening situations thankfully only occur very occasionally.

Head injury

Head injuries in collision sports are unfortunately very common, yet with correct management and quick, accurate assessment they become bread and butter work to any therapist who works with a team. Between 1931 and 1961, head injuries in American football accounted for 2.6 deaths per 100 000 football players. From the peak of 3.4 deaths per 100 000 players in 1968, there has been a steady decline to the figure of 0.5 per 100 000 players

(Mueller and Schindler, 1987). To this end, many collision sports have brought in a special code of practice to deal with such injuries.

Case study

My preference for head injury protocol is that recommended by both the Australian Sports Medicine Federation and the Great Britain Rugby Football League. This form classifies the head injury as grade one, two or three (mild, moderate or severe), and then states the action that should follow for the player. A completed copy of the form is sent to the governing body, one copy is kept by the club doctor or physiotherapist, one copy is kept by the club and the last copy is given to the player. This I feel has been an excellent idea, so much so that I have had similar forms produced for all the medical staff to use at Manchester United Football Club (Figure 3.1). Although it does not reduce the number of head injuries, it does recommend to the coaching staff and the injured player certain time periods before they should be allowed to train or play a competitive match. It also stipulates the signs and symptoms to look out for over the next 24 hours in case a problem develops. Some coaches would argue that there are certain players who get 'knocked out' each week, and after two minutes and a wipe of the magic sponge they are up and playing again as normal. What individuals forget is that it is not just the acute symptoms, but the effect repeated trauma has on the brain that can cause damage. Several other variations exist on this particular format, i.e. the Glasgow coma scale, which is discussed later in this chapter (see 'Concussion'). The scarcity of scientific evidence makes practical decisions on the safe return of an athlete to competition very awkward (Roos, 1996). The difficulty in reaching a consensus of opinion amongst the experts provides more confusion for any inexperienced medical team member. The best advice is to pick one set of suggested guidelines and use them carefully for several years whilst developing your own on-field decision making skills.

When any trauma to the head occurs, approach the player and look for any signs of movement; if there are no obvious signs, grab hold of the shoulder to see if this stimulates any reaction. Verbal stimulation may provoke a response. If not, it is time to place the individual in the correct position so further steps can be taken to prevent problems. The player should be placed supine for further assessment and treatment. If lying face down, the player should be turned over using the log roll procedure. If you are the most qualified member of the initial entourage, you must take control of both the players head and the situation. Your commands need to be crisp and concise, using other individuals where possible to help at this critical time. Ideally three extra people are needed, and they should be positioned at the shoulders, hips and knees whilst you maintain the head position in line with the body. On your command, the player is then rolled into the supine position.

Problem	An unconscious state or injury above the clavicle may give an associated cervical spine injury which could have major consequences if not handled correctly.
Solution	Maintain the head in a neutral position with in line traction wherever possible.
Danger	Use of smelling salts may cause a sudden awakening and movement could cause further injury.

MANCHESTER UNITED FOOTBALL CLUB
OLD TRAFFORD, MANCHESTER M16 0RA

HEAD INJURY FORM
PLEASE READ CAREFULLY

ONE COPY OF THIS FORM TO BE KEPT BY CLUB PHYSIO AND PLACED IN THE MEDICAL RECORDS AND ONE COPY GIVEN TO PLAYER OR TO AN ACCOMPANYING PERSON.

Name of Player .... Age ....

Sustained .... concussion
Doctor or Physiotherapist to insert severity (see below)

Time of Injury .... Date ....

EMERGENCY NUMBERS

Physiotherapist ....

Doctor ....

Hospital ....

IMPORTANT WARNING

He should be taken to a hospital to be seen by a doctor or consultant immediately if:
- He vomits
- Headache develops or increases
- He becomes restless or irritable
- He becomes dizzy, drowsy or cannot be roused
- He has a fit (convulsion)
- Or anything else unusual occurs.

FOR THE REST OF TODAY HE SHOULD:
- Rest quietly
- Not consume alcohol
- Not drive a vehicle.

TO DETERMINE THE SEVERITY OF CONCUSSION

Note the time from when the injury occurs to when the player responds normally to verbal commands.

SEVERITY OF CONCUSION	ACTION
MILD: no loss of consciousness (L.O.C.) (i) Full memory of event	can usually continue playing (after being checked).
(ii) Memory deficit of event	must cease playing: no training or playing for 48 hours, and only after a medical check by the Club Doctor.
MODERATE: L.O.C. of up to 2 minutes	must cease playing: no playing or training for 15 days and only after a medical check by the Club Doctor.
SEVERE: (i) L.O.C. of up to 3 minutes	must cease playing: no playing or training for 22 days and only after a medical check by the Club Doctor.
(ii) L.O.C. of over 3 minutes	must cease playing and be admitted to hospital for observation: no playing or training for 29 days and only after a medical check by the Club Doctor.

All cases of SEVERE concussion should have X-rays taken of the skull and cervical spine.

Details of the incident and concussion must be entered in the Accident Book at the club and details of the concussion must be entered in the players Medical Record Card.

If the concussed player's Club Doctor is not available, this form must be completed by the Duty Doctor or the opposing Team Doctor.

Doctor/Physiotherapist Name .... Date ....
(Please underline your title)   (Block letters please)

Figure 3.1
Head injury form.

NOW FOLLOW THE STEPS FROM THE MNEMONIC 'ABCDE'

AIRWAY   Establish access to the airway by tilting the casualty's head back and lifting the chin to open the airway (Figure 3.2).

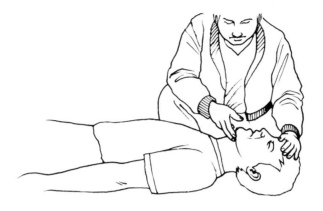

Figure 3.2 Maintain the airway.

Problem   The airway is blocked by a foreign body, i.e. gumshield, tongue.

Solution   Quickly clear the cavity using your finger. Use an airway only if the patient is unconscious, as it can stimulate vomiting in the conscious patient.

Problem   A fracture to the larynx with or without associated oedema may be obstructing the airway.

Solution   The medical team leader must perform an emergency cricothyrotomy or directly insert an endotracheal tube into a gaping wound created in the trachea to maintain the patency of the airway. Transfer immediately to hospital.

BREATHE   If the player is not breathing, you can breathe for them and thus oxygenate the blood by giving artificial respiration. With the player lying supine, place the side of your face just above the nose and mouth whilst looking down the length of the ribcage. Any air flow coming from the player's mouth or nasal passages can then be felt on your face whilst you are observing to see if there is any rise or fall of the thorax, suggesting air entry in that area (Figure 3.3). Once you

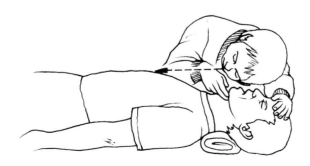

Figure 3.3 Look, listen and feel for any sensation of respiration.

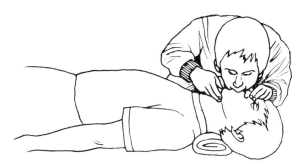

Figure 3.4 Artificial respiration.

have ascertained that breathing is absent, then artificial respiration is required (Figure 3.4). An open airway must be maintained, so tilt the head backwards with one hand under the chin of the individual and the other cupping the skull. Close the airway of the nasal passages by pinching the nose with the index finger and thumb of the upper hand. Take a full breath and place your lips around the player's mouth to make a good seal. Various disposable mouthpieces are available to prevent the tongue from occluding the larynx, and in most instances utilize a one-way valve to stop the passage of saliva to the physiotherapist. Blow into the mouth of the player until you see the chest rise, which takes about two seconds.

Problem   Chest does not rise.
Solution   Check that the head is tilted back sufficiently, that you have a firm seal around the mouth, the nostrils are completely closed and the airway is not obstructed by vomit or a foreign body. If this last instance is the case, sweep a finger inside the mouth.

Problem   Chest still fails to rise.
Solution   Turn the player onto one side and give four to five blows between the shoulder blades. If this fails to resolve the situation, turn the player back into the supine position, kneel astride the casualty and place one hand below the ribcage, cover it with the other and press inwards and upwards five times. This technique is described as an abdominal thrust (Figure 3.5).

Problem   Asymmetry or laboured respiration, cyanosed. Suspected tension or open pneumothorax.
Solution   A large-bore needle needs to be inserted into the second rib space with a chest drain to follow. This procedure is to be carried out by a doctor or paramedic, unless neither is available.

Problem   Reduced breath sounds, shock (paleness, sweating, rapid pulse) and dullness to percussion on chest examination suggests a haemothorax.
Solution   Ventilation via a chest drain inserted by the doctor.

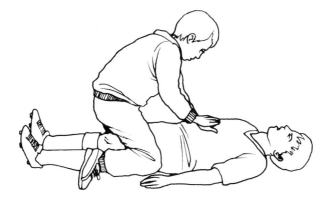

Figure 3.5 Abdominal thrust.

Problem	Asymmetry of the chest wall may be associated with multiple rib fractures – a flail chest.
Solution	Establish ventilation. Assist the affected side manually or by placing sandbags to maintain support.
Danger	Beware the asthmatic. Know your players and the relevant inhalers they may require. Also be well-versed in how they work. The players often are not!!

Case study

Whilst working in rugby league, I would often have to carry up to six different type of inhalers. Once a try had been scored I would position myself on the half way line and give out the appropriate inhalers to the asthmatic players. As soccer is more of a stop/start game this procedure is not as necessary, but timing of drug intake is very important to gain maximum effect.

Choking

In this situation the player has difficulty in speaking or breathing, often with associated cyanosis of the skin. Constant reassurance is required. Position the player in a sitting but flexed posture, and give five sharp blows to the back. If this fails, five abdominal thrusts may be necessary. Continue with this routine until the throat clears. If an unconscious player begins to choke follow the same procedure, with the individual in a lying position, until a normal breathing pattern returns.

CIRCULATION Now check the carotid pulse in the neck to assess the systolic blood pressure, noting the quality, rate and regularity (Figure 3.6).

Problem	No pulse.
Solution	Begin chest compressions at the point where the rib margins meet the sternum, placing the back of one hand on the sternum of the player reinforced by the other hand on top (Figure 3.7). Keeping your arms straight, press down on the sternum, then follow with a release of pressure. Repeat the compressions, aiming for a speed of approximately 80 per minute. In the untrained or inexperienced

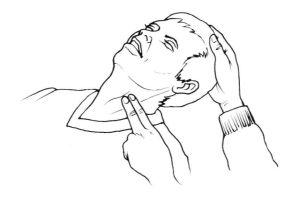

Figure 3.6 Maintaining the head in a tilted position, palpate the contour of the larynx – 'the Adam's apple'. Slide your fingers into the gap between the this and the strap muscles of the neck to palpate the carotid pulse.

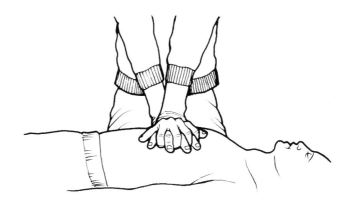

Figure 3.7 Chest compressions.

individual the tendency is to be too gentle; a movement of four to five centimetres is normal. This will help send blood to the brain, but the supply must contain oxygen to be effective. This technique therefore needs to be combined with artificial respiration. If working alone, the accepted ratio is two breaths to 15 chest compressions. Check the pulse after 10 breaths.

If there are two of you at the incident, one should summon help whilst the other begins cardiopulmonary resuscitation. On the return of your partner, one of you gives chest compressions whilst the other gives mouth to mouth resuscitation. The ratio in this case is one breath to five compressions. When the pulse returns and the player begins to breathe alone, place in the recovery position and check the breathing pattern and pulse every three minutes.

Recovery position

The recovery position is achieved by:

1. Placing the arm nearest to you at right angles to the body, elbow bent with palm uppermost (Figure 3.8).

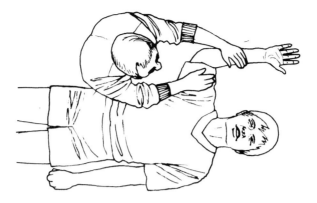

Figure 3.8 Recovery position (a).

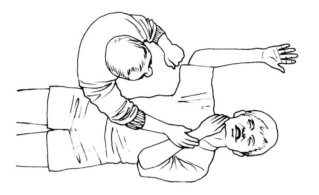

Figure 3.9 Recovery position (b).

2. Bringing the arm furthest away from you across the chest, placing your hand against the casualty's cheek (Figure 3.9).
3. Keeping this hand against the player's cheek and using your other hand to pull the thigh or knee furthest from you, thus roll the player towards you (Figure 3.10).
4. Keeping the head tilted back, continually monitor that the airway remains clear.
5. Adjust the upper leg if required so that both hip and knee are bent at right angles (Figure 3.11).

The player will now need to be lifted and transferred onto a stretcher. This again requires you to take firm charge with precise commands, using up to five individuals if available. If you are the most qualified person present, then you should take control of the most important area, the head. Place the stretcher alongside the player. Use one of the helpers to stand on the opposite side of the stretcher and place the others at the shoulder, hip (usually the strongest one), knee and ankle. Before lifting and transferring, make sure any suspected fractures have been immobilized. On YOUR count of three, everybody lifts together and places the player on the stretcher in the recovery position. Before lifting the

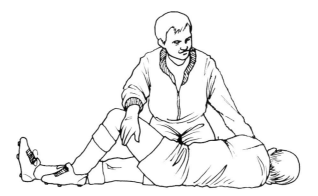

Figure 3.10 Recovery position (c).

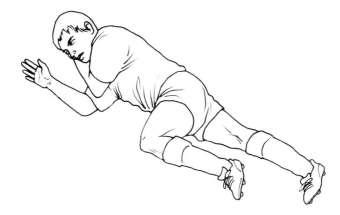

Figure 3.11 Final recovery position.

stretcher, ensure that one of the helpers is at each corner, and again pick up on your count. Make sure all four helpers know the direction they are heading towards, with you monitoring any changes in the conscious state of the player.

Case study	*Some collision sports, such as soccer, now have regulations for the use of stretchers to remove injured players from the field of play. If players require any form of treatment, they must leave the field of play once an assessment has been made of the injury. Stretchers with fixation straps and head immobilizers are recommended for use, and all stretcher bearers must be trained in the handling of injured players under the supervision of the club's medical staff.*

In one such injury scenario, an injured player was lifted onto a stretcher by his club's medical team and newly trained stretcher bearers. The stretcher was then lifted by these four individuals under the command of the team's physiotherapist, and everything seemed to be going to plan as it had done in the previous practice sessions. Unfortunately, when it came to walking off with the stretcher two of the bearers were facing in one direction and the other two in the opposite direction, so they ended up pulling against each other. Thankfully, the player remained on the stretcher.

DISABILITY At this stage only a limited neurological examination is possible, assessing the level of consciousness, size of pupil and reaction to light, and motor response. Appropriate action can be taken once diagnosis and assessment have been made.

Concussion is obviously the most common sign seen in a head injury and is graded according to the degree of severity. Just how bad is the level of concussion? A practical way of determining this state is by using the scoring system of the Glasgow coma scale, which is based on eye opening, motor and verbal responses (Table 3.1).

Concussion

Table 3.1 *Glasgow coma scale*

Glasgow coma scale		
Indication	*Response*	*Score*
Eyes open	Spontaneously	4
	To verbal command	3
	To pain	2
	No response	1
Motor response		
Verbal command	Obeys	6
Pain stimulus	Localizes pain	5
	Flexion – withdraws	4
	Flexion – abnormal	3
	Extension	2
	No response	1
Verbal response		
Arouse player with painful stimulus if necessary	Orientated and converses	5
	Disorientated and converses	4
	Inappropriate words	3
	Incomprehensible sounds	2
	No response	1
Total		*3–15*

Friedman (1983).

Responsiveness of the patient is expressed by summation of the figures. The lowest score is three, the highest is 15. A score of seven or less indicates unconsciousness.

Other symptoms of concussion include headache, dizziness, distorted vision and poor concentration. In collision sports, convulsions may also occur within seconds of the head injury occuring. These have been assumed to be due to a form of post traumatic epileptic seizure secondary to underlying brain injury (Gowers, 1907). However, recent studies with Australian rules and rugby league players have shown that these episodes cease spontaneously within 150 seconds, with symptoms indistinguishable from mild concussion (McCrory *et al.*, 1997). These studies were also able to show that the convulsions are a non-epileptic phenomenon with no structural brain injury, and treatment was based purely on the degree of associated concussion with most players returning to playing in a matter of several weeks.

Obviously any player who suffers a moderate (2) or severe (3) head injury needs to be assessed using the ABCDE mnemonic before being transferred onto a stretcher, maintaining the recovery position throughout. With mild (1) head injuries, constant reassessment over the next 24 hours is necessary, looking for any deterioration in the level of response after the apparent recovery. Information regarding such symptoms and important contact phone numbers are provided on the head injury sheet illustrated for other members of the player's family. The player should be advised not to drink alcohol or drive over the next 24 hours, and be placed in the care of a responsible family member.

Spinal injuries

These injuries usually result in severe disablement rather than fatality, and are among the most serious of sports injuries. Thankfully such injuries only occur very occasionally, as the spine is relatively flexible and uses its hydraulic properties to absorb shock from external forces. If handled improperly, an unstable lesion at any level of the spine can produce an immediate paralysis which may be temporary or permanent. Of all the collision sports, rugby tends to have the highest incidence of spinal cord injuries (Scher, 1981).

Follow 'ABCDE' as normal for any such suspected injury. Preserving life is obviously paramount in such a situation. Now perform a quick but comprehensive neurological examination of both the individual and the upper and lower limbs. This should include level of consciousness, pupillary size and reaction to light, and motor responses of both upper and lower limbs. Then you must assess the spinal column itself. Do not move the player, but gently

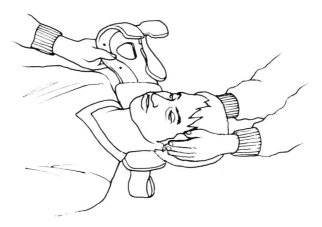

Figure 3.12 Apply manual immobilization along with a properly fitted semi-rigid cervical collar.

palpate the area of the spine involved, feeling for a twist or a step in the normal curve of the spine. Pain and tenderness to palpation are two other signs to note.

Care is needed in the transfer of the player onto a stretcher or preferably a spinal board. **DO NO FURTHER DAMAGE.** Immobilize the cervical spine by applying a properly fitted semi rigid cervical collar and apply manual immobilization (Figure 3.12). As the physiotherapist take control of other personnel available, positioning them in the ideal position whilst maintaining in line stabilization of the most important structure, the skull. A minimum of three other personnel are required to 'log roll' the player, with one to position the spinal board underneath the player on your command. The player is then placed back into the supine position on the board and further immobilization is applied using the head supports and body straps. The player can then be removed from the field of play, with manual in-line stabilization being maintained throughout the transfer before immediate referral to hospital.

Problem	Player develops breathing difficulties.
Solution	The player needs to be carefully turned onto their back and all 'ABCDE' techniques need to be repeated. Maintain head and trunk alignment when putting into the recovery position.
EXPOSE	Exposure involves looking for internal and external bleeding, fractures and dislocations in any part of the body.

Abdominal trauma

Due to the contact nature of all collision sports, abdominal trauma is a very common problem. In the main this is caused by a blunt force, but can occasionally be due to a penetrating object.

Case study

The only time I have seen such an injury in a collision sport caused by a sharp object was when a rugby league winger tried to take on his opponent and went outside him, running adjacent to the touchline. As his opponent tackled him, he was pushed into the temporary advertising boards, which snapped under his weight. Unfortunately for the player, the boards were supported by a metal frame with protruding arms and one of these pierced the left side of his abdomen. Fortunately the damage was only superficial.

This type of problem can have fatal consequences because it is not a common injury and it can often go unrecognized or be poorly treated. As already mentioned, the injury is often caused by blunt abdominal trauma. External signs of damage are limited, and pain will be the initial symptom. Muscular haematomas to this area are very common, and pain is localized to the site of trauma. Should the pain start to spread to other areas of the abdomen, then suspect a more serious problem. Developing signs of abdominal rigidity, muscle spasm, referred pain and loss of mobility suggest an intraperitoneal problem. The onset of shock and all relevant signs and symptoms must be continually monitored in the post-injury stage. These include:

Rapid pulse
Profuse sweating

Low blood pressure
Pale expression
Weakness
Thirst
Rapid shallow breathing.

As the oxygen supply to the brain lessens the player becomes more anxious and aggressive than normal, starts to yawn and gasps for air. Unconsciousness starts and then . . . shock occurs because insufficient oxygen is reaching the arteries due to internal bleeding. The average adult has 4.5–5 litres of blood present in the circulatory system. To lose half a litre is no great problem to the body's system, but as this figure approaches 2–3 litres then these signs start to develop as the hormone adrenalin is released into the system.

The organs which can be damaged are listed below in order of injury frequency, the first being the most common. Figure 3.13 gives a visual reminder of the anatomical site of these structures.

1. Spleen – trauma to the left upper abdominal quadrant, often with associated damage to the tenth, eleventh and twelfth ribs.
2. Liver – trauma to the upper or mid abdomen and right lower chest. Again often associated with damage to the tenth, eleventh and twelfth ribs.

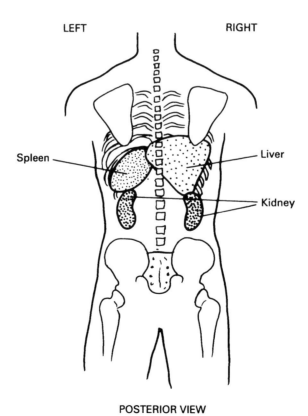

Figure 3.13 Diagrammatic representation of the major internal organs.

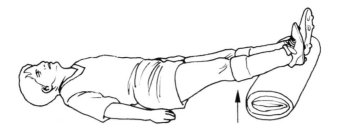

Figure 3.14 The recovery position following the onset of shock.

3. Kidney – trauma to the posterior right or left lower ribcage.
4. Pancreas – trauma to the upper mid abdomen.
5. Duodenum, small intestine, colon.
6. Bladder – associated with pelvic fractures.

If shock does occur, do not let the player drink or smoke or leave him unattended. Position casualty in the supine position, raise the lower limbs above the level of the heart (Figure 3.14), loosen any tightfitting clothing and keep them warm with blankets. Transfer to hospital as quickly as possible.

External bleeding

This is obviously a common problem in any collision sport, and of major concern with regard to such medical conditions as hepatitis and AIDS. Collision sports such as rugby league have introduced the 'blood bin', which allows the injured player to be removed from the field of play. The doctor and physiotherapist then have 15 minutes to repair the laceration, whilst a free substitution is allowed during this time. Also remember that it is important to protect yourself from transmission of body fluids from players who suffer such injuries. Always wear sterile gloves and cover any open wounds where necessary.

Depending on which type of blood vessel is damaged – artery, vein or capillary – the type of bleeding can be categorized. Arterial damage, with its bright red colour, often produces a jet of blood as the injury occurs and is usually the most dramatic. Venous bleeding is darker in colour yet potentially more serious. The initial aim for any wound, regardless of associated problems, is to control the bleeding, minimize the risk of infection and prevent the onset of other complications. Apply direct pressure over the wound with a sterile dressing and maintain this pressure either manually or by covering with a bandage until the wound can be repaired. Wounds which are very narrow in diameter yet deep, e.g. stud wounds, are often left open to allow any foreign bodies to be removed at a later date. Antibiotic protection is necessary for all wounds.

Head wounds often produce large amounts of blood, but once the external blood has been wiped away the cut itself may be quite small. Some of these wounds can be patched up on the pitch, e.g. above the eyebrow, with the use of a sterile pad and elastic adhesive strapping. Petroleum jelly can be applied to minor cuts to seal the area and prevent dirt from entering the wound. Beware of any underlying fractures, which may be hidden by the copious amount of blood which is present initially.

Nose bleeds are common problems, again associated with fractures to the nasal bone. Sit the player down with the head tipped well forward. Ask the casualty to breathe through the mouth, pinching the nose just below the bridge and using disposable cotton swabs to clean up the area. Bleeding should stop after approximately 10 minutes. If this follows a head injury and the fluid is thin and watery, suspect the leakage of cerebrospinal fluid (CSF) from around the brain. Be prepared for the player to suffer from a period of unconsciousness and summon ambulance help immediately.

Problem   Nose bleed persists for longer than 30 minutes.
Solution   Refer to hospital casualty department.

Avoid applying the dressing too tightly otherwise the blood flow will cease altogether with serious consequences. Once in the treatment room the area can be cleansed and sutured if required.

Always ensure the tetanus vaccination programme of each player is up to date. In adults, injections are recommended every 10 years. If such a foreign organism enters an open wound then a dangerous situation can arise. These organisms are present in soil and carried by air and if they enter the body, the toxins produced can cause muscle spasms and paralysis.

Fractures

These need to be divided into two types:

1. *Open fractures*
   This type of injury requires two forms of immediate care:
   (a) Cover the wound with a sterile dressing and prevent further blood loss.
   (b) Splint the fracture without pulling the exposed bone back into the soft tissue. Pad any protruding bone before bandaging the area to immobilize. Do not let the player have anything to eat or drink.
2. *Closed fractures*
   This section can be subdivided into the relevant anatomical area:
   (a) Face
   Swelling and bruising often develop rapidly with an associated open wound inside the highly vascular area of the gums and mouth. This requires X-ray and assessment by the appropriate consultant as soon as possible, in case reduction in theatre is necessary. Apply a cold compress to the area for short term relief.
   (b) Jaw
   The pain is usually intense, with associated trauma to the teeth and gums. At all times maintain the airway before hospitalization. If conscious, encourage the player to support the area with a hand, using a soft pad to reinforce this action.
   (c) Upper limb (shoulder, shoulder girdle and elbow)
   Immobilize the area in a full sling, checking the circulatory and neurological supply constantly and using soft padding wherever necessary.
   (d) Upper limb (forearm, wrist and hand)
   Immobilize and elevate the hand, with padding for compression in the soft tissue areas.

A sling will be necessary to maintain elevation in all four situations before transportation to hospital.

(e) Rib cage

This is recognized by a sharp pain at the site of fracture, particularly on attempting a deep breath. There will also be reduced air entry over the affected area, often due to the pain, but be aware of the possibility of a pneumo- or haemothorax. If the player does become unconscious, or the breathing pattern changes drastically, place in the recovery position with the uninjured side uppermost.

Do NOT strap the area as this will tend to reduce active air entry even more. Transportation is required as soon as possible to assess the full extent of the damage. Painkillers will be necessary to give the player some chance of a good nights sleep. Radiographs will confirm or deny the presence of a displaced fracture.

(f) Pelvis, hip, thigh, shin and ankle

Immobilize the limb using either the other limb as support, an appropriate inflatable splint, or a back slab with padding between the knees, calves and ankles, before transporting the individual to hospital for further investigations.

Most common areas for dislocation are the jaw, shoulder, elbow and small joints of the hand.

Dislocation

1. *Jaw*

Follow the same procedure as for a suspected fracture

2. *Shoulder and elbow*

These two areas need to be immobilized and the player removed from the field of play immediately. Radiographs and reduction under anaesthetic are often needed, so hospitalization is required. Before any transfer to hospital can take place, keep monitoring any symptoms distal to the injury site, as circulatory or neurological complications can very quickly develop.

3. *Thumb*

Often occurs with an associated fracture. This needs immediate immobilization and transfer to hospital as the saddle shape of the articular surfaces requires reducing under anaesthetic.

4. *Interphalangeal joints*

These can often be reduced on the field of play and then taped to the next finger to allow the individual to play on. This obviously depends on the player's position in the team – a goalkeeper in soccer would clearly struggle to continue. After the game, a thorough examination of the surrounding soft tissue structures is necessary to ensure there has been no damage which could produce a flexion, extension or instability deformity. Refer to an orthopaedic consultant if any soft tissue or neurological damage is suspected. As a standard procedure, an X-ray is necessary to assess for any damage to the bony tissue.

All players who suffer suspected fractures and/or dislocations should not be given any food or drink until it has been determined by the hospital that the injury does not require any form of anaesthetic to reduce or fix the fracture.

Common variables

Numerous other vital anatomical areas and medical conditions can be injured in the match scenario and need to be treated accordingly.

Cramp

This is a very painful muscle spasm which tends to occur as a player becomes fatigued during a game or heavy training session. It is most common in the calf and thigh, and is thought to be due to the loss of excess body fluids through profuse sweating. To relieve the symptoms, elevate the affected area and passively move the joints controlled by the affected muscle through their full range. Continue until symptoms ease.

Diabetes

Diabetics are encouraged to take exercise as any normal individual would. If a diabetic is a member of the team, fast-acting sugar foods (e.g. chocolate, sugary drinks) are an important part of their pre match and half time diet. If the sugar level drops too low a hypoglycaemic state of unconsciousness can develop. Symptoms include trembling, excess sweating, irritability and an apparent state of dumbness or confusion. The player will often state they feel dizzy. Glucose tablets are a handy source of sugar for the medical bag in such a situation. Once given to the player, further food such as bread or a sugary drink helps to raise the blood sugar level. Hypostop is a glucose gel which can be administered in an advanced state of unconsciousness by squirting into the side of the player's mouth. If this fails to work then an injection of glucagon is necessary.

If an unconscious state does develop, follow the normal 'ABCDE' procedure. Do not panic, as this not a life-threatening state because the body will release its own glucagon if these external sources fail to work and the player will regain consciousness in a matter of time.

Treatment notes

During a game, a known diabetic collapses to the floor. Is it a hypoglycaemic reaction or a grade 2/3 concussion? A glucometer, to measure the blood sugar level of the player, is a very useful device in this situation. A pinprick of blood is sufficient to give an almost immediate answer. A normative score of 4–7 mmol/L points to a concussive state not related to the blood sugar level. A score of 1–2 mmol/L suggests a possible hypoglycaemic state, and hypostop should be administered immediately to the inside of the mouth. A glucagon injection may be needed in more serious cases.

Ear injuries

The very obvious signs of a throbbing, painful and swollen ear signify the classical rugby players 'cauliflower ear'. This is due to a haematoma, and in severe cases sterile aspiration is required. Recurrence is not uncommon.

Epilepsy

Knowledge of the medical history of the player is imperative, particularly if such an individual has suffered from this condition in the past. A minor (petit mal) or major (grand mal) epileptic attack produces different degrees of seizures and consciousness. The main aims in such a situation are to prevent injury during the fit and to provide care once consciousness has been regained. Once the rigid or tonic phase has passed, breathing may cease or be very noisy before settling into a more normal state. When the aggressive state has passed, place the player into the recovery position and provide constant reassurance, as the casualty may complain of feeling dazed and have no memory of the attack. Emergency help is necessary in most cases.

The severity of injury needs to be assessed immediately in order to follow the correct course of action. The most important factor is to be able to distinguish the difference between a trivial injury and a serious problem. If the latter is suspected, then the player needs to be removed from the field of play and be assessed accurately and rapidly by the relevant medical personnel.

Eye injuries

Assessment pointers include:

1. Blurred vision that does not clear with blinking
2. Disturbance of the visual field
3. Type of pain – sharp or dull
4. Presence of swelling or haematoma
5. Presence of a foreign object
6. Abnormal pupil size
7. Laceration of the eyeball or eyelid
8. Blood between the cornea and the iris.

If any of these symptoms are present, the player needs to shut the eye lightly and a sterile eye pad be placed over the area before transporting the player to the nearest casualty department or doctor with ophthalmological experience. If in the rare situation a penetrating injury to the eyeball has occurred, it is essential that any pressure is avoided. With severe injuries the temptation to give the player a drink should be avoided in case immediate surgery is necessary.

This severe abdominal pain is caused by muscle spasm to the main respiratory muscle, the diaphragm. This is due to fatigue of the muscle or lack of oxygen to the area, so it can occur very early or late in the game. To settle the problem, encourage diaphragmatic breathing by placing two fingers underneath the distal point of the sternum, with plenty of verbal encouragement.

Stitch

In collision sports, a blow to the upper abdomen is not uncommon. Players may struggle to catch their breath temporarily due to the fact that the nerve supply to the diaphragm has been stunned by the blow. Encourage players to relax and stimulate lateral costal breathing by pressure to the lower third of the rib cage.

Winding

Thankfully, the majority of injuries which happen in the match situation are simple, straightforward soft tissue injuries. Immediate and accurate assessment of these injuries is necessary in order to follow the correct first aid procedure. The following mnemonic, SALTAPS, is a very useful step by step procedure to follow.

See
Ask the player
Look at the injury
Touch and palpate the injured area
Active movements from the injured player
Passive movement by the medical personnel
Strength using manual resistance tests.

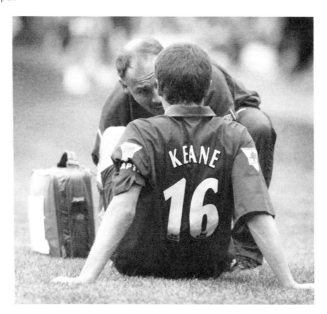

Figure 3.15 Evaluate the injury immediately using SALTAPS.

If the injury is severe enough to affect normal functional movement, the player will need to be substituted. This decision is helped by the physiotherapist's experience of both the player and the particular injury. Once the player has been replaced, begin a rehabilitation programme immediately by keeping the area of damage to a minimum in the acute, bleeding stage. Ice, elevate and compress the area, giving appropriate advice on the rest required and the detrimental affects external factors such as heat, alcohol and poor management can have on any acute injury. The club doctor may prescribe anti-inflammatories at this stage. If so, write everything down, to inform the player and keep your own records up to date.

| Case study | *When working with a rugby league team several years ago, one of our prop forwards went down with an injury. I ran straight onto the pitch to attend to the problem, but after a short time I could see the manager shouting at me to go and attend to another one of our injured players. This particular manager was well known for losing his composure once the game had started, so I ignored his screams and carried on attending to the player who I had gone out to treat originally. By the time I had finished treating this player, the second injured player had managed to get up and resumed playing. I thought nothing of this particular incident and there was no mention of it after the game. However, at training a few days later, the manager asked me to see him in his office. After offering me a drink, he said 'Do you remember the incident in the game on Sunday when we had two players injured at the same time, in different areas of the pitch? I shouted to you to go and look at the second player instead of the one that you were treating'. I replied that I did, but as I had only one pair of hands, how could he expect me to be in two places at once? He replied, 'In those situations you must look at the two individuals who are injured. The player you ran on for initially was a prop forward, and the most he is going to run with the ball is ten yards. The second lad, who* |

I wanted you to treat straightaway, was a winger. Now which one of those two is most likely to run the full length of the pitch and win us the game? Certainly not the prop forward!!'.

References

Friedman, W. A. (1983). Head injuries. *CIBA Clinical Symposia*, **35(4)**, 1.

Gowers, W. R. (1907). *The Borderland of Epilepsy. Faints, Vagal Attacks, Vertigo, Migraine, Sleep Symptoms and their Treatment*, pp. 1–17. London: Churchill.

McCrory, P. R, Bladin, P. F. and Berkovic, S. F. (1997). Retrospective study of concussive convulsions in elite Australian rules and rugby league footballers: phenomenology, aetiology and outcome. *Br. Med. J.*, **314**, 171–174.

Mueller, F. O. and Schindler, R. D. (1987). *Annual Survey of Football Injury Research 1931–1986*. American Football Coaches Association, National Colleigate Athletic Association and National Federation of State High School Association.

Roos, R. (1996). Guidelines for managing concussion in sports. *Phys. Sports Med.*, **24(10)**, 67–74.

Scher, A. T. (1981). Diving injuries to the cervical spinal cord, *S. Afr. Med. J.*, **59**, 603–605.

4

Care of the acute soft tissue injury

Soft tissue injuries include a multitude of conditions which in the main tend to be underestimated, as most players can continue their daily activities soon after the injury has occurred. The different body components – muscle, ligament, tendon, nerve, bone, capillary and connective tissue – can all suffer varying degrees of trauma, and appropriate care is required in order to reduce the possibility of complications.

As with all injuries, an initial assessment is required in order to determine which body tissues have been damaged, and to what degree. The basic but vital tests performed on the field of play will give you early clues to solving each

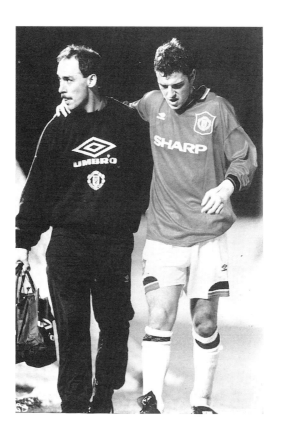

Figure 4.1 Off to the treatment room for a more thorough examination.

particular problem. Now a controlled and more thorough examination can take place in the calm of the treatment room before organizing the next stage in the rehabilitation process, which starts as soon as the acute injury has occurred.

This is no different to other physiotherapy assessments and is based upon a subjective and objective examination as used in both Cyriax (1982) and Maitland (1991) techniques.

Assessment

The initial interview with the player is probably the most important 15 minutes of the entire rehabilitation programme. Communication, in the form of limited questioning and attentive listening, will help to make or break the therapist/player relationship. With experience, the therapist can draw information which will establish mental goals to go alongside the physical progression which is needed to produce the correct end result.

Subjective assessment

The initial priority is the injury and its limitations. The mechanics of the injury are a vital clue to the final diagnosis. This is a good starting point, before making notes on the individual's home address, telephone number and how many dogs are kept!! Even if the injury has had an insidious onset, lay seeds of thought in the mind of the player as to possible causes of the problem. A knowledge of relevant sporting terminology is imperative, and in this age of 24-hour satellite sports channels, there is no excuse for any physiotherapist not to have a basic knowledge of rugby and football or gymnastics and netball. Both the therapist and the player need to become relaxed in each other's company. This will allow the remainder of the subjective examination to flow smoothly, covering other aspects of the injury and the lifestyle of the individual. Key questions, phrases and words are vital to extract the desired information, and do not be encouraged to presume a player's answer. The important factor is to be able to communicate on one another's wavelength without interference from outside parties; this is particularly important when working with the sporting child or adolescent.

The initial priority for most players is the degree of pain produced by the injury. This needs to be investigated as thoroughly as possible in terms of site,

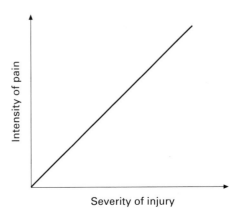

Figure 4.2 The Stimulus–Response (S-R) model of pain experience.

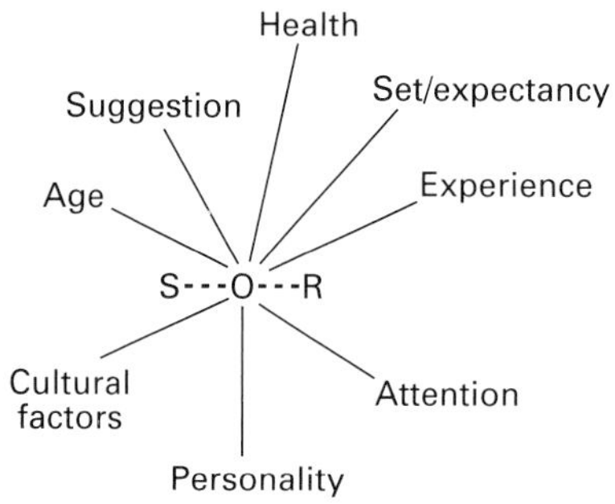

Figure 4.3 A cognitive model of pain experience.

depth, intensity, frequency and effect on functional movement. Pain thresholds between players vary, and personality is an important factor in the perception of and tolerance to pain (Figure 4.2). The supposed linear relationship between severity of injury and intensity of pain, called the stimulus response (S-R) model, is not now fully accepted and modern psychology tends to postulate a state which is governed by many variables other than the severity of injury (S-O-R mode) (Figure 4.3). It is determined in terms of a three-dimensional model with sensory, cognitive and affective assessment as the dominant components (Melzack, 1986). Physical factors have also been thought to be relevant. LeBlanc (1975) claimed pain is highly individual, and is due to three main components:

1. Size and shape of the body
2. Percentage of subcutaneous fat
3. Physical fitness level.

Other works by Beecher (1959) and Melzack (1973) support these views.
    A more general guide to the relevant topics of questioning are listed below:

1. Mechanics of injury
2. Sport
    Level of competition
    Years in the sport
    Weekly training programme
    Position
3. Previous medical history, directly or indirectly related
4. Effects of symptoms on everyday life and in the sporting environment
5. Medical path taken with regard to the injury, if the assessment is some time after the injury (Figure 4.4)
6. Occupational and personal details.

Assessment notes   Social factors often have an effect on the physical recovery rate of an injured player. These variables must always be considered by the physiotherapist in the

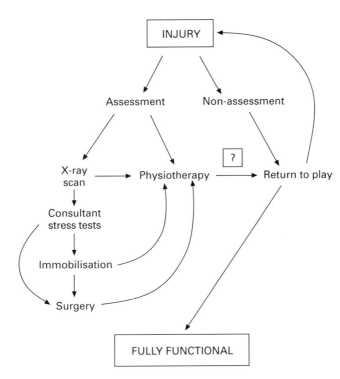

Figure 4.4 The medical pathway relevant to the subjective assessment of the sports injury.

treatment programme and where possible used to assist in the recovery process. Such factors to be considered include:

Facilities available to the injured player
Finance
Family
Ethnic culture
Age
Sex
Occupation
Level of motivation.

Track and field athletes usually keep a training diary, which provides very useful information when they get injured. A similar record of intensity, frequency, duration and type of training would help the physiotherapist of any injured sportsperson. This is particularly so if the injury has occurred in the preseason period when the training programme can be more intense. Many injuries occur in this particular period of the season due to the poor physiological state of the player after a one to two month close season rest, or due to a badly planned training schedule.

Case study

From the written text which is to follow, this part of the examination would appear to require a great deal of time. Experience and a willingness to learn throughout your career enables this whole process to be speeded up. A thorough

Objective assessment

yet direct approach is required, maintaining professional standards in what may be a less formal environment than that of the hospital outpatient department. Just because the facilities may not be ideal does not mean there should be any let-up in the quality of care provided for any injured player.

Observe

The area that is to be examined needs to be exposed, along with the areas proximal and distal to the site of injury before any objective tests can be performed.

Case study

Any male or female physiotherapist working with adolescents, school age children or a team of the opposite sex must appreciate that potentially embarrassing and possibly professionally damaging situations can arise unless the correct protective steps are taken. Injuries to the abdominal and groin area in such situations must be assessed and treated with the competence of the physiotherapist. Embarrassment to the player (particularly in adolescents and 'non-typical' seniors) or physiotherapist must be overcome quickly by both parties to ensure a good working relationship. At the same time, it is imperative that other individuals such as parents or other staff and players be in the treatment room in case any form of malpractice is suggested at a later date. The number of cases are few and far between, yet it is too late to do anything about it should accusations be made afterwards.

In the same circumstances, consider how the spouses of players might feel if individuals were being treated by a member of the opposite sex for an abdominal or groin injury? Some may find it very difficult to accept, particularly if players are away from home on a foreign trip. Consideration must be given to these and other potentially difficult social problems which can arise in the treatment situation.

If splints or dressings have been applied on the field of play, only remove those that are necessary for a more detailed examination to take place. If an obvious severe soft tissue derangement or fracture has occurred, then leave such items *in situ* until an X-ray has been taken and a more complete diagnosis made. Movement of the site of injury and the effect on the total body function of the individual can be assessed during this initial clinical activity. This will often give a better insight into the severity of the pain during regular everyday activity, as it is not unknown for a different picture to be presented when the more formal tests take place. Clinical pointers to note from observation include:

Muscle spasm
Muscle atrophy
Asymmetrical anatomical sites
Swelling
Redness
Bruising
Bony deformity
Biomechanical asymmetry.

Observational assessment should be performed in both the standing and sitting positions, unless the injury is so severe that the pain is dramatically aggravated by abrupt changes in the examination position.

Also at this stage, encourage the player to re-enact the mechanics of the injury if possible, and observe. Note the description of the movement pattern and degree of trauma involved. This functional movement pattern may be the first physical test that brings on the injury symptoms, so record anything that may be relevant.

General handling of the injury and the surrounding tissues provides information on many aspects of the damage present. This basic assessment opportunity is often neglected in favour of more advanced procedures, yet it is usually a guide as to which relevant, specific tests are required. The players experience contact in a game situation, so do not be afraid to handle the area. Blood, sweat and tears can all be cleaned up later!

General

Before proceeding with movement tests, assess for:

Pain
Muscle spasm
Muscle tension
Bony alignment
Swelling
Sensation
Temperature.

Avoid direct, deep palpation at this stage, as aggravation of the injury site may give false information on more functional testing.

How often in magazines and newspapers are pictures used of a physiotherapist treating a patient using an electrotherapy modality instead of a manual procedure? Physiotherapy is a profession of physical therapy which requires the general public to appreciate we are not merely machine technicians.

Case study

A variety of tests now need to be performed to establish the site and degree of the problem.

Active tests

Initially, ask the player to demonstrate the degree of active movement in the joints peripheral and distal to the site of injury. Record any relevant measurements such as range of movement (degrees) and muscle strength (Oxford scale, Table 4.1).

Similar measurements should be noted when testing the active movement in the directly involved structures. A comment on the willingness of the player to perform such tasks may be useful. Overpressure, which is sports-related in the subjects concerned, may be needed at the end of range to demonstrate any positive symptoms.

Following trauma, the loss of motion within the joint is a major complication which requires immediate and appropriate rehabilitation. This loss of movement can also occur following surgical intervention and has been widely recorded (Renstrom and Konradsen, 1997). A full active and passive range of movement is necessary to ensure a full recovery from injury.

Assessment notes

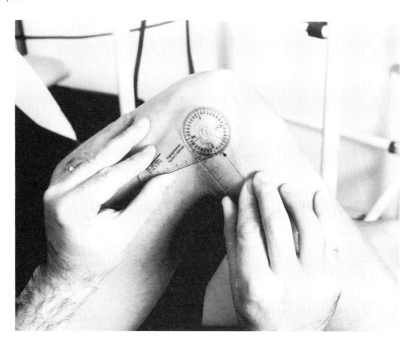

Figure 4.5 Measure and record the range of movement.

Table 4.1 *Oxford classification of manual muscle strength testing*

Grade	Definition
0	No contraction
1	Flicker of contraction
2	Weak. Small movement with gravity counterbalanced
3	Fair. Movement against gravity
4	Good. Movement against gravity and some resistance
5	Normal

Passive tests

These are designed to test the inert structures of the joint, and usually follow the same order of tests as described by Cyriax (1978). The ability of the physiotherapist to 'feel' rather than use a goniometer is required, and the six sensations to monitor include:

1. The 'hard' sensation of **bone to bone** contact. In the joints concerned, does this occur before or at the end of normal range? Note accordingly.
2. The 'hard' sensation of **muscle spasm**.
3. The 'giving' sensation of the **capsular** end of range, which can produce both a normal and abnormal sensation.
4. The 'springing' effect produced at the end of range by a **foreign body**, for example a meniscal tear or loose body in the knee joint.
5. The 'normal' sensation of **tissue compression** and **tissue stretch**, which may limit the range of movement.

6. The 'abnormal' sensation of **pain** which can limit the range of movement at any point, with no definite resistance from the surrounding tissue.

Assessment notes

Confusion often exists between the terms 'instability' and 'laxity', words that both imply a degree of abnormal motion due to ligamentous insufficiency. It is important to differentiate between them in order to appreciate the degree of disability each can have on the injured sportsperson.

Laxity implies a degree of looseness in a static state within the ligamentous tissue, which should be essentially symmetrical for the individual. This can vary slightly from one individual to another, and is graded using the terms mild (1), moderate (2) or severe (3).

Stability and instability define the functional status of the relevant joint. Classification is more complex, but several methods have been proposed. Instability may be one-plane, rotatory or combined (Nicholas, 1978). Hughston *et al.* (1976a and b) classification of knee injuries is based on the functional state of the posterior cruciate ligament (PCL). If the PCL is disrupted, then instability is considered to be in one direction; if the PCL is intact then any instability is considered to be rotational

Resisted tests

Good stabilization is required above and below the affected area to prevent any joint movement and so test for muscle weakness and injury to the contractile tissues. If each test is specific enough to isolate the problem, pain can be produced on the desired isometric action. In practical terms, lightly built physiotherapists may doubt their ability to resist the force exerted by players involved in collision sports. In positioning the player at a mechanical disadvantage and by applying manual resistance at the most distal point possible, raw strength differences between physiotherapist and player can be minimized.

Specific tests

Certain specific tests are unique to each particular joint or contractile tissue which is to be examined, and indicate the level of involvement of that particular area.

Where joint testing is concerned, many of the tests involve assessment of the relevant accessory movements and the degree of laxity present when stressing the joint in a loose packed position. This is the position where the joint and the surrounding tissue structures are under minimal stress, often the most comfortable position when an injury has occurred.

Capsular patterns as suggested by Cyriax (1978) are another means of specific testing, where, as in the passive tests, the 'feel' and limitation of movement are the most important factors to note.

Neural tests

Testing of the nervous system is a vital part of any objective assessment when looking for symptoms involving:

Referred pain
Hypo- and hypersensitivity
Altered temperature control
Muscular weakness
Disturbed reflex response
Adverse neural tension.

It is a well proven fact that referred pain can be caused by compression of the nerve root (Smyth and Wright, 1958) giving referred limb pain, and by other sections of the intervertebral segment which may affect pain sensitive structures such as the nerve root, sleeve or dura (Cloward, 1959; Feinstein *et al.*, 1954). Frequently, the referred pain is often only felt in the distal part of the dermatone, a point often forgotten by many physiotherapists.

Sensory and temperature disturbances are often linked to nerve root involvement, so knowledge of the dermatone supply to the appropriate anatomical areas is very important, particularly in the upper and lower limbs.

Muscular weakness may be due to disturbance of the nerve root pathways and can be tested using specific isometric muscle tests.

Nerve root compression can also be indicated by disturbances in the main reflexes of the upper limb – biceps and triceps – and lower limb – knee and ankle. In chronic sporting injuries, an abnormal physiological and mechanical response may arise when the normal range of movement and stretch capabilities of the nervous system structures are tested using various upper and lower limb tension tests (Butler, 1991). This concept is known as adverse neural tension, a factor which must be considered in the diagnosis and rehabilitation of any injury.

Circulatory tests

Such tests are often necessary to eliminate any circulatory involvement in the injury process. Subjective questioning will determine if there are any genetic links to relevant conditions where circulation to the injury site may be affected, such as diabetes or Raynaud's disease.

Circulatory disturbances can take many forms in relation to injury. Senior players may suffer from vascular claudication, particularly in the lower limb, and this may initially present itself as a neural problem. During exercise, muscle pressure on the blood vessels, particularly in the anterior and posterior compartments of the shin, can produce an inflammatory response in the capillary bed which in turn may alter capillary permeability (Rettig *et al.*, 1988). This is more commonly known as 'shin splints', or compartment syndrome. Supplementary tests such as ultrasound scans, venograms, Doppler testing and/or compartment pressure tests are often required.

In immediate terms, the physiotherapist has to use such manual tests as palpation for temperature change and pulse sites at rest and after exercise, as well as noting the cosmetic appearance of the affected area. Any positive clinical signs noted from these tests may well require further investigation, using the aforementioned supplementary procedures.

Case study

Always be aware of the differential diagnosis. One case I can recall involved a player who exhibited all the classical symptoms of a compartment syndrome in the left shin brought on by playing and training on hard ground, with excessive impact work used in his training schedule. Rest, conventional physiotherapy, orthotics and orthopaedic referral failed to resolve the problem, so the physiotherapist treating the player ended up referring him to a vascular surgeon. After numerous tests and subsequent surgery, it was discovered that the tibial nerve was strangling the vascular blood supply to the calf, and so produced identical symptoms to that of a compartment syndrome.

With regard to rehabilitation, strength is an important ingredient in ensuring a complete and full recovery, particularly in providing a degree of stabilization at a joint or during the repair process of any soft tissue injury. In this assessment stage, a baseline measurement is necessary from which to work, if pre-injury notes are not available from any screening programme. When the individual is reassessed during the rehabilitation programme, these benchmark scores can then be used to monitor progression or regression. The following types of muscular activity need to be considered in relation to their effects on the desired movement patterns of the player and their performance:

Isometric
Isotonic
Isokinetic
Concentric
Eccentric
Synergic.

Obviously in the acute stage of injury these areas of assessment are not priorities, and to quantify the strength parameter the aforementioned Oxford classification of manual strength testing can be used (Table 4.3).

If the assessment is of a more chronic injury, there are various forms of testing available, but these can be very unreliable and may not be specific to sporting activity. Girth measurements, often advocated in that the larger the girth the stronger the muscle, are still used yet can give a very false result. Muscle tissue that is affected by disuse or decreased physical activity may become invaded by connective tissue, particularly as the ageing process occurs in the individual. Also, in certain anatomical areas a decrease in lean muscle mass may be masked by an increase in subcutaneous fat, with little change in the circumference of the area. Therefore girth measurements may not accurately reflect any changes in muscle mass. Delorme and Watkins (1948) devised a routine which involves

Strength tests

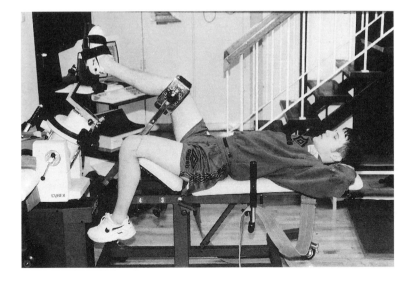

Figure 4.6 Isokinetic testing of the ankle joint. An expensive but informative assessment tool.

recording the maximum weight of one lift (one rep maximum) and ten lifts (10 rep maximum) at natural speed, without rest between lifts. However, this trial and error process to find the maximum weight possible often produces early fatigue and a resultant reduced poundage. Handheld isometric dynamometers give quick, accurate and repeatable scores, yet in many cases provide numerical data not related to sporting activity and only give a measurement at the angle of testing. Isokinetic testing, which is often limited in its use due to the expense and availability of such equipment, can give the most detailed, accurate and functionally related information on the different components of muscle activity already listed. Experience and a willingness to relate the use of the unit to functional demands is absolutely paramount if the maximum potential is to be gained from such testing devices. Far too many isokinetic units are not applied to their full potential in both the hospital and sporting environments.

Case study	*Always remember that different contact sports will produce variations in muscle strength. For example in my experience, using isokinetic testing, several differences occur between the players of two different sports such as rugby and football. This statement can also be extended to other variables such as gender, age, playing position and level of competition.*

Flexibility tests

Flexibility is a vital component in performing certain sports-related skills, so injury will often reduce the capacity of the player in this area. Static flexibility, movement around a joint, can be measured using a flexometer, goniometer or simple tape measure. Many joint-specific tests exist, and isolation of joint movement is vital for accurate results. Dynamic flexibility, the force that opposes such movement, cannot be measured.

Limiting factors to the degree of flexibility other than injury, such as bone, muscle, ligament, tendon and skin, should all be considered at this stage of the assessment.

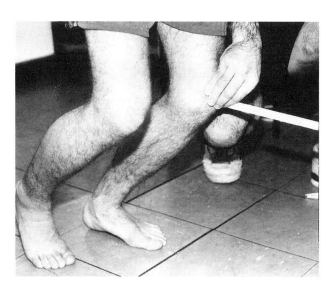

Figure 4.7 Flexibility measurement using a simple tape measure.

Flexibility is often regarded as an important ingredient in any competitor's physical profile in order to assist performance, as well as the suggestion that it may reduce the risk of injury. I will always remember being in attendance at a training weekend for the national junior swimming squad, where all the up and coming youngsters of the time were present. One visual memory has stayed with me from that particular day early in my physiotherapy career. At the side of the pool was a young swimmer, probably about nine or ten years of age with a body weight of about 40 kg, sitting on the pool side with her coach standing behind, pushing her spine into full passive flexion so that her trunk was flat on the floor. He must have weighed 130 kg plus. I just wonder two decades later what condition her cervical and lumbar spine are in!

Always remember that hypermobility can often produce as many problems as hypomobility in both the long- and short-term. Joint laxity and rigidity obviously produce ranges of movement at the opposite ends of the scale. In the long-term, wear and tear in either of these instances occurs but for different reasons. Hypermobility can produce an unstable joint with laxity in supporting ligamentous, tendon and capsular tissue. Hypomobility reduces the lubricating effects of the flow of synovial fluid between the articular bone surfaces. Both pathologies can therefore produce a long term effect on joint wear and tear. Symmetry and a normative range of motion are the two most important factors in flexibility and its effect on injury prevention.

Proprioceptive tests

Balance in sport is a vital component to any functional recovery from injury. Proprioception relies on sensory information from visual, vestibular and somatosensory receptors. It is hypothesized that injury to the structures that contain these receptors – skin, joint capsules, ligaments and musculotendinous units – can alter motor control and balance.

Testing of this parameter, particularly in the chronic stage of injury, may well be important. The method used is often questioned as to the reliability and sensitivity of the test. Numerous specialist devices have been recommended, such as the Chattecx dynamic balance system (Irrgang and Lephart, 1992) and the digital balance evaluator (Davies, 1992). Many research studies have used functional instability – the number of times the joint 'gives way' – as the tool of measurement, particularly in soccer players where this is often the main complaint of persisting symptoms (Tropp *et al.*, 1984). Other tests combine functional strength with joint stability. The hop test, the distance an individual can hop and land on one leg (Friden *et al.*, 1990), and the figure of eight run (Tegner *et al.*, 1986) have both been used to monitor any functional deficit following injury.

The actual cause of any proprioceptive deficiencies is still undetermined. It has been suggested that alteration in the afferent input from the proprioceptive receptors has an effect on the neuromuscular control. Psychologically, though, it may be due to apprehension and fear of further injury. In order to treat this functional loss appropriately, better understanding of these two areas is required.

Cardiovascular tests

When assessing the chronic injury, measurements of the anaerobic and aerobic capacity are necessary in the active sportsperson. A knowledge of the desirable anaerobic/aerobic balance for the particular sport concerned is necessary. It is

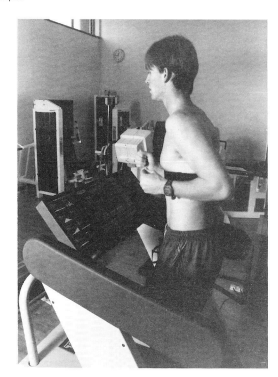

Figure 4.8 Cardiovascular testing using a pulsemeter.

therefore important to be aware of this commodity before performing such tests, otherwise the results produced may look impressive but be totally irrelevant to the sporting demands. The type of test chosen will obviously depend upon the restrictions of the injury. In many cases this may only allow submaximal testing, which is not ideal but still provides a baseline measurement to work from.

Specific palpation

At this final stage of assessment, localized palpation of the injury site should confirm the bulk of the information collected from the subjective and objective assessments. Initially it is important to palpate an area away from the injury site, so the player recognizes the normal sensation that is produced. Most individuals complain of soreness and pain when pressure is applied to a bony prominence or when palpating any tissue deeply, so it is important they can appreciate the differences in sensation.

When palpating, start superficially and move in an organized and anatomically correct pattern to assess the area for variations in:

Temperature
Muscle spasm
Muscle tension
Soft tissue thickening
Swelling
Nodules
Bony abnormality.

Once the site of the injury has been localized, a deeper palpation is often necessary as a final test to confirm the site and diagnosis of the problem. In acute cases be very careful about this final procedure. Players have this theory of 'no pain, no gain' in terms of their training. As physiotherapists, we should perhaps alter this to 'some pain, no gain'. If enough information has been gleaned already in the assessment, there is no need to aggravate the injury by applying deep pressure. In chronic injury cases, however, direct palpation may be necessary as many of the aforementioned objective tests may have produced a negative response. Deep palpation may be one of the few positive signs of the injury lesion.

Having completed the examination process, it is now time to use the information gained to make certain decisions. First priority is, does the player need further investigations or procedures not related to physiotherapy? If access to a club doctor or local general practitioner is possible, the assessment is often a dual procedure and any further tests can be far more easily organized. These may include:

Prognosis

1. Immediate X-rays/blood tests/sutures
2. Consultant referral – orthopaedic, surgical, ENT (ear, nose and throat)
3. MRI scan (magnetic resonance imaging)
4. CT scan (computerized tomography)
5. Appropriate prescribed medication.

In many cases this ideal is not available to the physiotherapist or player. Contact telephone numbers for the local hospital, players and members of the medical network (as detailed in Chapter One) are therefore very important, particularly in the high risk injury sports this book is concerned with.

The great majority of injuries generally tend to require appropriate immediate first aid followed by a thorough treatment and rehabilitation programme. This acute first aid care is an important yet often simple process.

1. Equipment required

Wound care

Cotton wool/buds; dressing packs; dry dressings (various sizes); antiseptic spray/solution (TCP, Savlon Dry); adhesive plasters; elastic cohesive bandages/tubular support bandage (Tubigrip); antibiotic powder; tweezers; disposable gloves.

2. Why?
To prevent infection and promote an ideal environment for regeneration.

3. How?
Apply a mixture of sterile water and antiseptic solution on a cotton bud, cleaning from the centre to the edge of the wound. For larger areas, cotton wool wound around a pair of tweezers may be a better form of application. Only use each cotton ball or bud once, placing all soiled materials in a plastic bag. Remove all dirt from the site of injury, and in the case of small, superficial cuts and grazes apply either a dry iodine spray or antibiotic powder. With larger

wounds it may be an advantage to keep the area moist, using specialized dressings (Compeed, Reflex) which absorb the moisture of the skin to form a white cushion, without the formation of a scab, to protect the damaged tissue. They can also help to provide the optimum healing conditions yet repel water, dirt and bacteria.

Apply an appropriate adhesive plaster or dressing to the area, and support with an elasticated bandage or piece of elasticated tubular support bandage (Tubigrip). A sling may be necessary with an upper limb injury, to ensure that elevation is maintained and thus reduce the possibility of oedema. Essential basic instructions and advice as to the necessary care of the wound over the next 24 hours should be given to the player, before reinspecting the wound the next day. Ensure all waste products are placed in an appropriate plastic bag and destroyed by incineration. Prescription antibiotics may be necessary in certain cases.

Case study

Always inspect every cut regardless of how trivial the player may think it is. Whilst on tour in Papua New Guinea with a squad of rugby league players, cuts and grazes were a common occurrence due to the very hard pitches we had to train and play on. During training one day, myself and the injured players were going through a circuit drill on the half of the pitch that the first team squad were not using. In the warm-up, we went from jogging into a press up position. One of the players then shouted 'Dave, the pitch is moving!' Knowing that he had been out the night before, I ignored him. 'Seriously, Dave, it's moving.' This time I looked through the thick grass and the ground did appear to be moving. As I pushed the grass to one side, the whole of the soil was a mass of moving insects! After every session, each player's cuts and grazes were cleaned and treated accordingly. One player this day suffered a wound which was no bigger than an average-sized coin, yet on initial inspection there was something different about this particular injury. As I started to clean the wound, I realized that several of these local insects had embedded themselves in the flesh! After removing them, the player was immediately put on the appropriate antibiotics, with inspections at very regular intervals to ensure none of the creatures had escaped our initial examination. Imagine the consequences if I had just blindly dressed and sealed the wound!

Suturing

1. *Equipment required*
Needle and thread (various types and sizes); scissors; dressing pack; medical staple gun.

2. *Why?*
To pull the edges of a wound together and promote the healing process.

3. *How?*
This procedure is in the main performed by the GP or Doctor. Physiotherapists are only allowed to perform such a procedure in emergencies. It is essential to ensure that the wound is thoroughly cleaned out before closing it up. Antibiotics and tetanus injections may be necessary to reduce the risk of possible infection. Some deep 'gunshot' type wounds may be better left open to ensure any foreign tissue can drain away. The decision to leave open or to close the wound comes with experience.

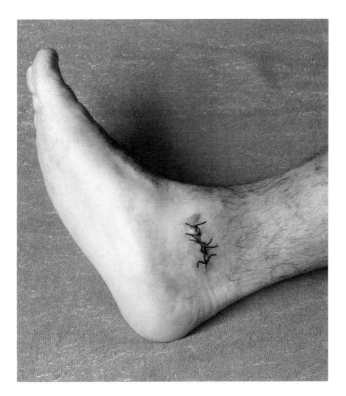

Figure 4.9 Suturing of an open wound.

Medical staple guns can be used for superficial wounds, particularly those on the top of the skull. To remove the staples, the recommended instrument from the manufacturer must be used.

Danger

In many collision sports, lacerations with varying degrees of bleeding are very common. It is important that every member of the medical team takes the appropriate steps to deal with the acute problem, whilst at the same time reducing the possibility of transference of any blood disorder to themselves or other individuals.

It is estimated that in 1996, around 21 900 individuals living in England and Wales were infected with HIV (Human Immunodeficiency Virus), with approximately 1800–2300 new cases expected in 1997 (Sheen and Green, 1997). The risk of transmission following blood or body fluid exposure has been reported to be less than 1% (Cowan and Johnson, 1993). With advancing surgical procedures, consideration must be given to the transmission of HIV. The advent of connective tissue allograft operative procedures, particularly involving the knee joint, provides a potential risk of disease transmission. To minimize this problem, many tissue banks use irradiation as secondary sterilization.

Hepatitis B (HBV) and C (HCV) can also be accidently transmitted through mucosal and cutaneous routes, across breaks in the skin or mucous membrane. Incubation periods of 75 days for HBV and 63 days for HCV have been suggested (Dusheiko, 1994).

In order to reduce the possibility of transmission of such diseases through accidental transfer of blood or body fluids, certain universal precautions should be taken. These include:

Use of surgical gloves
Standardization of wound cleansing procedures
Appropriate disposal of soiled dressings
Sharps boxes for used needles.

The management of accidental exposure to blood or body fluids should also follow a standard procedure and be familiar to all members of the medical team. Immediately following any exposure, the contaminated area should be washed with copious amounts of water and percutaneous injuries encouraged to bleed. The individual should be counselled about the risks and appropriate blood and HIV tests carried out. As the risk of seroconversion for HIV is estimated from six weeks onwards (Cockcroft and Williams, 1993), a commonly used schedule is to test at six weeks, then three, six and twelve months. Documentation should clearly record the extent of the exposure and the appropriate steps taken following the incident.

Rest

1. *Equipment required*
Cervical collar (various sizes); triangular bandage/collar and cuff; specialized splints (wrist, knee and ankle supports of various sizes, left and right); elbow/axillary crutches; stretcher; wheelchair.

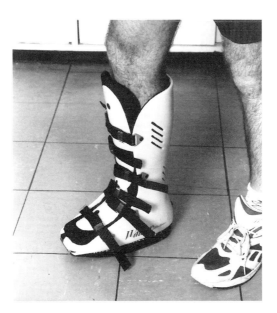

Figure 4.10 Immobilizing ankle brace to restrict unwanted movement.

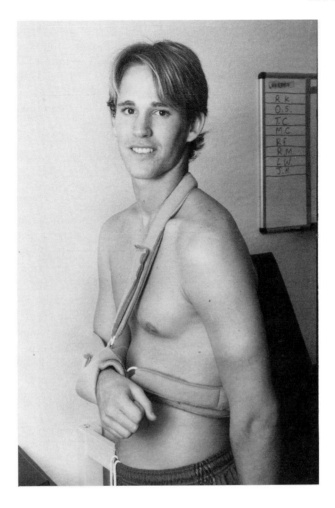

Figure 4.11 Immobilization of shoulder in a Polysling. Note the waist strap to prevent lateral rotation.

2. *Why?*

In order to allow the healing inflammatory process to take place in the ideal initial environment of stasis. Inflammation should not be thought of as a detrimental occurrence but as a necessary first stage in the healing process. It is the base upon which all the other phases of rehabilitation have to work. There is no precise definition of the period involved, with three to six days being the suggested upper time limit (Christie, 1991; Garrett and Lohnes, 1990; Enwemeka, 1989; Andriacchi *et al.*, 1988) for the following stages to take place:

- Damage to blood vessels and release of substances into the area to begin the healing process (Christie, 1991; Carlstedt and Nordin, 1989; Andriacchi *et al.*, 1988).
- Immediate vasoconstriction followed by vasodilatation of the blood vessels.
- Permeability of the blood vessels increases allowing blood, plasma and tissue fluid to flood the area.

- Platelets attach themselves to any available collagen and release phospholipids to initiate the clotting mechanism.
- Fibrin and fibronectin, along with the tissue collagen, develop a lattice which is a temporary plug to the leaking vessels (Martinez-Hernandez and Amenta, 1990).
- Leucocytes and macrophages begin the clean up operation of any tissue that has invaded the area.
- The dual role of certain substances – plasma, platelets, leucocytes and mast cells – is that they also release other substances into the area. Plasma releases bradykinin, which helps increase vasodilitation; platelets, leucocytes and mast cells release histamine, which is also a vasodilator and increases vascular permeability.
- Prostaglandins increase vascular permeability and attract leucocytes, as well as initiating the next stages of repair.

The typical signs and symptoms of this inflammatory process are:

Pain
Temperature
Redness
Swelling

with a resultant

Loss of function.

Pain occurs due to an increase in pressure on the soft tissues, and the stimulation of pain receptors. Temperature, swelling and redness occur due to exudate release into the extracellular spaces, brought about by the localized vasodilatation and increased vascular permeability. Loss of function is the result of the pain which inhibits normal neurological reflexes necessary for movement, the mechanical restrictions of the oedema present and the reduction in muscle strength, also caused by the oedema and tissue damage (Kibler, 1990).

| Case study | *Figure 4.12 demonstrates the classic signs of inflammation – pain, swelling, redness, temperature and loss of function. Here is a picture of a player who suffered a series of insect bites to his backside, a very painful injury! Visually it demonstrates the inflammatory process well, but why the loss of function? This player was meant to be a substitute in his next game, but was unable to take his seat on the bench due to the pain produced by the bites!* |

The whole inflammatory process then proceeds to further stages of repair, around which a structured rehabilitation programme can be planned. The following stages have been given loose time scales which are very much dependent on the severity of the injury, individual characteristics and the ability of the player to understand the meaning of rest in the early repair stages!

Stages of healing
- Day 7 – increase in the tensile strength of the injured area due to an increase in the amount of collagen (Garret and Lohnes, 1990; Hunt and Van Winkle, 1980).

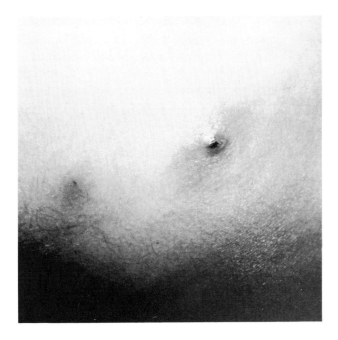

Figure 4.12 Infected insect bite to the gluteus maximus.

- Day 12 – replacement of initial collagen (Type 3) by a more mature, stronger collagen (Type 1).
- Day 21 – proliferation phase, with scarring becoming more dense, a maturing of the collagen fibres and dispersion of excess fluid.
- Day 21 – 365+ – the maturation phase is completed during this time, with the scar tissue changing due to an increase in the density of the collagen. This in turn will increase the overall strength, with better organization of the fibres which in turn produces a more complete scar (Christie, 1991; Andriacchi *et al.*, 1988).

Danger

Following surgical intervention or where injury involves laceration to the skin, the type of scar tissue that forms is determined by the degree of motion permitted. If the wound is immobilized completely and for too long, dense, contracted scar tissue will form which can have a detrimental effect on a full functional recovery. Early mobilization encourages the formation of loose or areolar connective tissue which allows movement through set ranges. This type of connective tissue contains cavities that can fill with liquid or air and allows the site to function like a collapsible sponge (Bloom and Fawcett, 1968).

This remodelling phase usually lasts at least six months. The scar will contract with subsequent maturation of the site with collagen and the tensile strength of the scar will slowly increase. This shrinkage and strengthening phase is of benefit in the long term healing process, particularly if recurrent problems are to be avoided.

3. *How?*

In the acute phases of the injury process it must be remembered that rest is only necessary at the injury site and not for the whole body (except in spinal injuries).

Most players will have no problems in performing this activity! Time off from work may be necessary depending on the severity of the injury and occupation of the player.

Danger

The ratio of rest to activity is important, as too little rest prevents formation of the granulation tissue matrix necessary for good, solid wound recovery. Too much rest can produce different complications, such as:

- Muscle atrophy or strength loss, which can be between 2–6% per day for the first eight days of immobilization (Muller, 1970).
- Reduction in muscle electrical activity (Rosemeyer and Sturz, 1977).
- Susceptibility of different fibre types. It has been shown that with immobilization, a shift in fibre population occurs with a wastage of slow (Type 1 or red) twitch muscle fibres (Desplanches *et al.*, 1987; Booth and Kelso, 1973) and an increase in activity of fast (Type 2 or white) twitch fibre types (Crockett and Edgerton, 1975; Fischbach and Robbins, 1969). These two fibre types are responsible for the muscle time response to stimulation. Most muscle groups per person contain a set ratio for the fibre types, the exception to the rule being the antigravity or postural muscles. This particular group can be further subdivided into single and multijoint antigravity muscles. The rate of atrophy varies and is dependent on the proportion of fast and slow twitch fibres. Single joint antigravity muscles which have a relatively high proportion of slow twitch fibres, e.g. vastus medialis, soleus, are the first to atrophy with immobilization. This is then followed by the multijoint antigravity muscles, e.g. erector spinae, rectus femoris, gastrocnemius (Lieber *et al.*, 1988). It has also been reported that extensor muscle groups tend to atrophy quicker than flexors (Roy *et al.*, 1987; Eccles, 1944).
- Changes occur in the chemical properties of muscle. There is a decrease in the levels of creatine and creatine phosphate (MacDougall *et al.*, 1977), succinate dehydrogenase and citrate synthase – aerobic enzymes, which again reflect the susceptibility of the contractile proteins (Jaspers and Tischler, 1982) and slow twitch muscle fibres to atrophy (Desplanches *et al.*, 1987; Edstrom, 1970).
- With immobilization, the oxygen supply to the soft tissue changes:
  There is a decrease in the maximum oxygen uptake (Saltin and Rowell, 1980; Sargeant *et al.*, 1977)
  There is an increase in total blood flow (Ferguson *et al.*, 1957), but with an impairment of blood flow distribution (LeBlanc *et al.*, 1985), so affecting oxygen supply to the necessary areas.
  The number of mitochondria is reduced early in the inflammatory process (Luthi *et al.*, 1989).
- There is an increase in the amount of intramuscular connective tissue which encourages atrophy and reduces the strength of the injured muscle tissue (Williams and Goldspink, 1984).

The player's first question following injury is usually, 'When will I be back playing?'. This depends on the severity of the injury and the gradual progression of the rehabilitation programme. Muscle tissue often does not make a full recovery (Grimby *et al.*, 1980; Houston *et al.*, 1979) even with the correct rehabilitation schedule, and often requires a retraining period two to three times as long as the period of immobilization.

1. *Equipment required*

Ice

Ice cubes for ice massage; crushed ice for towels and plastic bags; cryogel packs; towels (to make ice towels); cryocuff flasks and attachments; plastic bags; Velcro straps; water (for ice immersion).

2. *Why?*

Ice is used in the acute stages of soft tissue injury, and in the eyes of the player the most important benefit is to reduce the level of pain (Weston *et al.*, 1994; Belitsky *et al.*, 1987). This is because it reduces the conductivity of the nerve fibres, so much so that when the temperature is less than 10°C, total anaesthesia is present (Ellis, 1961; Travell, 1952). This in turn releases the reflex arc and reduces skeletal muscle spasm by decreasing the sensitivity of the muscle spindle (Mense, 1978).

More important to the medical team is the physiological effect of reducing tissue metabolizm after the application of ice (Jozsa and Reffy, 1978; Clarke *et al.*, 1958). When an injury occurs, producing damage to the various soft tissue structures, the cells within these tissues die off as there is an insufficient supply of 'food' and oxygen for them to exist. This is due to the detrimental effect of the injury on the localized blood supply. Each cell within the tissue has its own

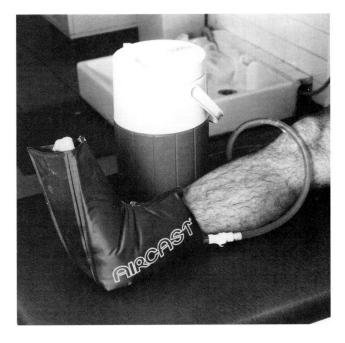

Figure 4.13 Cryocuff flask and ankle attachment providing ice therapy and compression.

metabolic rate and if this level is not maintained, secondary ischaemic cellular damage occurs to add to the primary cellular and vascular damage caused by the initial trauma. As more cells die off, more free protein becomes present which in turn enhances the osmotic pressure of the extracellular space, with a resultant increase in oedema. When ice is applied, it creates a hypometabolic state within the cellular structures producing less secondary cell destruction. This reduction in the degree of inflammatory death produces a smaller injury site to treat, a primary advantage to both the player and the medical personnel concerned.

It is often stated that ice is beneficial in the acute stages of injury because of its effect on the vascular stuctures. There have been many confusing and contradictory studies published in regard to cryotherapy and its effect on the circulation of the body. Vasoconstriction would appear to occur in the earlier stages of the cooling period after the application of ice (Thorsson *et al.*, 1985) due to an initial reflex sympathetic response, the reduced activity of noradrenaline-based metabolizing enzymes and an increase in blood viscosity (Taber *et al.*, 1992). Lewis (1930) suggested that following the initial reduction in blood flow there is a compensatory increase due to dilatation of the blood vessels of the muscle, caused by interruption of the sympathetic nervous system. This produces constantly changing increases and decreases in the blood flow in a cylindrical manner, labelled 'the Hunting response'; Knight *et al.*, (1980) showed that this only occurs in fingers which have been cooled to 20°C prior to ice water immersion. This is further supported by Shepard *et al.* (1983), who suggested that this reaction appeared to be most pronounced in anatomical areas prone to frostbite. Knight (1989) has more recently suggested that there is an obvious hyperaemia of the skin, with little change to the deeper vascular structures.

3. How?

McMaster *et al.* (1978) produced the following league table of the temperature effects different ice applications have on cellular tissue.

COLDEST
Ethyl chloride spray
Ice towels/bags
Ice packs
Ice massage
Immersion
COLD

Depth of treatment is certainly not an area that is considered by many physiotherapists, but logically it should be considered in the treatment equation. It has been shown on many occasions that after the application of ice, the temperature changes are not uniform throughout the different tissues (Martsen *et al.*, 1975; Benson and Copp, 1974; Bierman, 1955; Bierman and Frielander, 1940). Temperature changes in the thigh muscle after the application of ice are faster than in the ankle or forearm, but slower than in the fingers (Palmer and Knight, 1996). The body part that is to be treated with any form of cryotherapy must therefore determine the length of ice pack application. Other factors to be

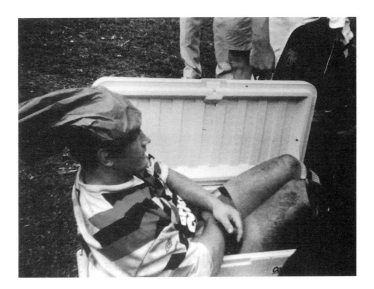

Figure 4.14 Total ice immersion!

considered include the mode of application and the degree of subcutaneous fat (Waylouis, 1967). The average recommended time is 20–30 minutes on and 90 minutes off (Knight, 1982).

From a safety aspect, it is important to remember that ice can burn. Pre-assessment of the skin type of the player and the anatomical site of injury is therefore imperative. There have been several cases of players suffering peripheral nerve injury following ice application (Covington and Barrett, 1993). Such instances have tended to occur in areas of the body where there is very little subcutaneous fat, with nerve pathways close to the surface of the skin. Common sites to be wary of include the anterior aspect of the pelvic bone, the superior aspect of the clavicle and the lateral aspect of the knee and elbow. It has been suggested that this type of nerve palsy has been caused by the compression factor onto nerve tissue rather than the direct application of ice (Green et al., 1989; Collins et al., 1986). To reduce the possibility of such a complication, it is recommended that extra insulation such as a wet towel be placed between the skin and the ice pack, with the compression bandage wrapped lightly over the area.

Compression

1. *Equipment required*
Cotton wool; adhesive wool felt; bubble packing; crepe bandages (various sizes); elastic cohesive bandages; elasticated tubular support bandage (Tubigrip).

2. *Why?*
Pressure is applied to the area of injury in order to reduce the physiological and functional effects of any effusion that may develop. Swelling is the natural response of the body to injury, yet it often complicates the injury situation by producing pain and encouraging muscle atrophy and joint stiffness (Wilkerson, 1985a). External compression over the injury site increases the internal tissue pressure in response to the reduction in pressure which occurs at the site of

trauma due to the leakage of fluid from the damaged blood vessels (Wilkerson, 1985b). As the inflammatory state continues and cells die off, the presence of protein encourages further fluid attraction to the area, so some degree of compression is needed in the first 72 hours after injury.

3. How?

Initially, non intermittent compression using various types of bandaging is applied. Before applying any external compression, all bony contours need to be padded out in order to produce a uniform surface and avoid pressure gradients over the area. This is possible using adhesive wool felt or various density adhesive foam padding, cut to the appropriate size and shape. It is important to remember that the site of injury may continue to swell over the first 72 hours, so the choice of dressing applied to the area is very important. The ideal material should have some give, yet be easily removed in order to reapply various treatment modalities. Elastic adhesive bandages and zinc oxide tape should therefore be avoided in the acute stages of injury. After 72 hours, single cell and sequential compression devices are often applied to the injury site and surrounding tissue structures. Some research exists, with limited support in terms of the positive effects of either treatment device (Rucinski et al., 1991).

Case study

Players must be made aware that compression is not meant to strangulate the circulatory system and so produce a tourniquet. A footballer who attended the casualty department after fracturing his tibia and fibula was put into plaster to immobilize the fracture site. Having suffered severe pain prior to this, he felt much better with the immediate relief the support of the plaster gave to him after application. It did not occur to him that the loss of sensation in his foot was of any relevance, so when he attended the Outpatient clinic the next day for a plaster check, he could not believe it when he was told he would have to be admitted to the ward. Overnight, two of his toes had become gangrenous and needed to be amputated.

It is imperative that any physiotherapist working in sports medicine explains the effects of any adverse symptoms which may develop after applying any form of compression. Never assume the knowledge of the individual or it may be too late.

Elevation

1. Equipment required

Slings (for upper limb injuries); foot stool (for lower limb injuries)

2. Why?

In order to use gravity to help assist in the removal of any oedema, as well as preventing 'pooling' of fluid. Gravity can be a help or a hindrance in the injury situation. Elevation can also assist venous drainage of blood and other fluids from the injury site into the main circulatory and lymphatics.

3. How?

Elevation in both upper and lower limb injuries must be above the level of the heart, particularly when sleeping.

Swelling or **effusion** at a site of injury is a common objective symptom which indicates the presence of an inflammatory reaction. This occurs due to an increase in blood pressure caused by a rise in blood volume following injury. Also, the tissue fluid now contains a greater percentage of protein materials than normal, which alters the pressure gradient between the blood vessel and interstitial space. This normally favours the blood vessel, but the rise in osmotic pressure in the tissue fluid causes swelling to develop. In mild cases of inflammation this movement of protein molecules only occurs from the venous system, probably due to the effects of histamine (Evans, 1990). It should also be remembered that swelling is a postoperative complication following surgery and needs to be addressed accordingly.

Effusion into a joint space can have an effect on normal function. Normally intra-articular pressure is 5–10 mm Hg lower than atmospheric pressure, which causes the soft tissue structures to cling closely to the periphery of the articular surfaces of the joint (Wyke, 1972). Should swelling and subsequent distension of the capsule occur following an injury, then the increase in pressure created produces a measurement greater than the normal level of atmospheric pressure. This has been shown to increase the level of neural inhibition and so affect function (Spencer *et al.*, 1984). This in turn produces a detrimental effect on torque values (De Andrade, 1965) and an elongation in reaction times (Wilkerson and Nitz, 1994) of muscle tissue. Both these factors play an important role in stabilizing the joint structures.

Static exercise

1. *Equipment required*
An active nerve supply to the desired muscle group.

2. *Why?*
To help maintain muscle strength as far as possible and to aid in the removal of oedema.

3. *How?*
Certain muscle groups, such as the quadriceps via the action of articularis genu on the suprapatellar pouch and gastrocnemius, with isometric contractions may reduce oedema far more quickly by utilizing this exercise modality than joint elevation and compression alone.

General

Other factors should also be considered in the acute injury situation. It is suggested that the intake of excess alcohol can produce a vasodilatory effect on the blood vessels and thus increase the severity of the injury. Anti-inflammatories may be prescribed by the team or player's own doctor, which in the acute stages can be very beneficial. Topical creams such as Lasonil or Movelat may give a localized anti-inflammatory effect, but depth of penetration is often questioned.

Using the injury assessment plan, certain diagnostic statements should be possible. A more detailed treatment programme can now be drawn up, with constant reassessment made to ensure provision of the appropriate treatment depending on the stage of healing and recovery.

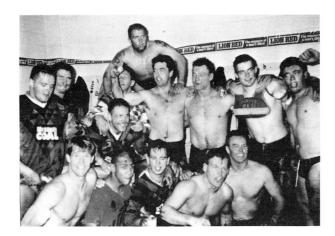

Figure 4.15 Same team – different psychological profiles.

Psychological factors

At the same time as the physical assessment, the psychological profile of the player is a key factor in the recovery process. This can and will change throughout the period of injury, depending on the physical nature and stage of repair of the injury.

Different profiles exist, though several common types predominate.

The regular visitor

Some players react dramatically to the slightest knock or twinge, but with the right amount of pampering after the game and in the treatment room, recovery is usually fairly quick.

The worrier

Other players can worry and brood over every injury no matter how serious or trivial the problem is. These individuals rarely miss a game and yet lay a seed of doubt about their fitness level before a game, often as a defence mechanism in case of a poor performance. Reassurance is constantly needed and can only be given after a thorough examination of each problem. The first time any state of injury is trivialized could be the first time there is a serious injury.

The unlucky player

Certain players seem destined to go from one injury crisis to another. This is often due to the somatotype and biomechanics of the player, which do not lend themselves to the training and playing regimes demanded by the coach or sport itself. A serious injury early in the career often produces a shift in the centre of gravity of the body and places a greater stress on the non injured side. This extra strain may be excessive, and another injury state develops. A reverse shift, back to the side of the original injury now occurs, and a new problem or aggravation of the original injury arises. This whole pattern becomes one vicious circle as the body tries to adapt to the latest problem, until the player drops to a lower level of competition or retires.

The artful dodger

These are the players who fit their training and playing schedules around their social calendars, using an injury to manipulate the situation as they desire. Careful clinical judgement is required here, as a direct confrontation may create a bigger problem. On the other hand, to neglect the situation is unfair to the majority of genuine players. These players are often the most skilful in the team, those the team cannot do without. The key is to treat them as every other player. Preferential treatment for one will prejudice the physiotherapist's relationship with the other players. Rehabilitation is required, not just for the site of injury, but for all the other body parts, so make up for missing training with extra work for these areas. This will often stimulate a reaction to get out of the treatment room as quickly as possible, which may temporarily solve the problem. Star players should get identical care to that of the youngest apprentice; the same injury requires the same aftercare, regardless of the personality of the player.

The invincible player

This uncomplaining and apparently 'never injured' player can create problems in the opposite direction. This individual feels that to set foot in the medical room demonstrates a sign of physical and mental weakness, and will try to train through every injury, only reporting in when it has reached a chronic state. It is therefore very important for the medical personnel to regularly monitor and question these players on their present states of health, in the hope that any developing problems can be sorted out in the acute stages.

The older player

Older, experienced players often need to be handled differently, even though their treatment programme will be similar to that of the other players. There may be a 20–25 year lifespan difference between the youngest and oldest player at the club. Senior players who have never experienced serious injury before have to adapt to this alien physical state, and often find it very difficult to do so. They can change personality, literally overnight, even though the injury will heal in time. It is also often hard for these players to recognize that their rate of recovery will be slower than that of a player half their age with an identical injury. Serious injuries in older players may end their careers; the young players have time on their side. Education, reassurance and a thorough rehabilitation programme are important. The players' confidence in the team physiotherapist is vital, and any doubts may encourage them to look for answers to their injury problems elsewhere. This scenario must be avoided. Tackle the problem as early as possible, before it develops too rapidly.

Often players will exhibit a mixture of these categories and it is important for the physiotherapist to react accordingly in the early stages. Know your players, and the job becomes much easier.

Treatment notes

Injury can occur without pain and pain can occur without injury. The degree of pain experienced by an injured player is a phenomenon that is not purely related to physical features. It is also determined by previous experiences, and the ability to understand the causes and the subsequent consequences of the sensation. There are many variables that influence the ability to cope with pain. These include:

Cultural values (Kozambi, 1967)
Earlier experiences (Melzack and Scott, 1957)
Understanding of pain (Beecher, 1959)
Attention, anxiety and distraction (Melzack *et al.*, 1963)
Individual differences (Kroeber, 1948).

All these factors must be considered when dealing with the many different personal characteristics exhibited by individual players.

References

Andriacchi, T., Sabiston, P., DeHaven, K. *et al.* (1988). Ligament: injury and repair. In: *Injury and Repair of the Musculoskeletal Soft Tissues.* pp. 103–128. Park Ridge, IL: A.A.O.S.

Beecher, H. K. (1959). *Measurement of Subjective Responses.* Oxford: Oxford University Press.

Belitsky, R., Odam, S. and Hubley-Kozey, C. (1987). Evaluation of the effectiveness of wet ice, dry ice and cryogen packs in reducing skin temperature. *Phys. Ther.,* **67,** 1080–1084.

Benson, T. B. and Copp, W. P. (1974). The effects of therapeutic forms of heat and ice on the pain threshold of the normal shoulder. *Pharmacol. Rehab.,* **13,** 101.

Bierman, W. and Frielander, M. (1940). Penetrative effects of cold. *Arch. Phys. Med. Rehab.,* **21,** 585–592.

Bierman, W. (1955). Therapeutic use of cold. *J.A.M.A.,* **157,** 1189–1192.

Bloom, W. and Fawcett, D. W. (1968). *A Textbook of Histology,* 9th ed. Philadelphia: WB Saunders.

Booth, F. W. and Kelso, J. R. (1973). Effect of hindlimb immobilization on contractile and histochemical properties of skeletal muscle. *Pfluegers Arch.,* **342,** 231–238.

Butler, D. S. (1991). *Mobilization of the Nervous System,* 1st ed. Edinburgh: Churchill Livingstone.

Carlstedt, C. A. and Nordin. M. (1989). Biomechanics of tendon and ligaments. In *Basic Biomechanics of the Musculoskeletal System,* 2nd ed. pp. 59–71. Philadelphia: Lea and Febiger.

Christie, A. L. (1991). The tissue injury cycle and new advances toward its tissue management in open wounds. *Ath. Train.,* **26,** 274–277.

Clarke, R., Hellon, R. S. and Lind, R. (1958). The duration of sustained contractions of the human forearm at different muscle temperatures. *J. Physiol.,* **143,** 454.

Cloward, R. B. (1959). Cervical discography. A contribution to the aetiology and mechanics of neck, shoulder and arm pain. *Annals Surg.,* **150,** 1052–1064.

Cockcroft, A. and Williams, A. (1993). Occupational transmission of HIV and management of accidental blood exposures. *Med. Int.,* **21(1),** 38–40.

Collins, K., Storey, M. and Peterson, K. (1986). Peroneal nerve palsy after cryotherapy. *Phys. Sportsmed.,* **14,** 105–108.

Covington, D. B. and Bassett, F. H. (1993). When cryotherapy injures. *Phys. Sportsmed.,* **21,** 78–93.

Cowan, F. M. and Johnson, A. M. (1993). HIV: controlling the epidemic. *Med. Int.,* **21(1),** 34–37.

Crockett, J. L. and Edgerton, V. R. (1975). Exercise and restricted activity effects on reinnervated and cross-innervated skeletal muscles. *J. Neurol. Sci.,* **25,** 1–9.

Cyriax, J. H. (1978). *Textbook of Orthopaedic Medicine – Diagnosis of soft tissue lesions,* Vol 1. London: Balliere Tindall.

Cyriax, J. H. (1982). *Textbook of Orthopaedic Medicine,* Vol 1, 8th ed. London: Balliere Tindall.

Davies, G. J. (1992). *A Compendium of Isokinetics in Clinical Usage,* 4th ed. S&S Publishers.

De Andrade, J. R. (1965). Joint distension and reflex muscle inhibition in the knee. *J. Bone Joint Surg.*, **47A**, 313–318.

Delorme, T. and Watkins, A. (1948). Techniques of progressive resistance exercise. *Arch. Phys. Med. Rehab.*, **29**, 263–273.

Desplanches, D. Mayet, M. H., Sempore, B. *et al.* (1987). Structural and functional responses to prolonged hindlimb suspension in rat muscle. *J. Appl. Physiol.*, **63**, 558–563.

Dusheiko, G. (1994). Acute viral hepatitis. *Med. Int.*, **22(11)**, 447–454.

Eccles, J. C. (1944). Investigations of muscle atrophies arising from disuse and tenotomy. *J. Physiol. (London)*, **103**, 253–266.

Edstrom, L. (1970). Selective atrophy of red muscle fibres in the quadriceps in long standing knee dysfunction injuries to the anterior cruciate ligament. *J. Neurol. Sci.*, **11**, 551–558.

Ellis, M. (1961). The relief of pain by cooling of the skin. *Br. Med. J.*, **1**, 250–252.

Enwemeka, C. S. (1989). Inflammation, cellularity and fibrillogenesis in regenerating tendon: implications for tendon rehabilitation. *Phys. Ther.*, **69**, 816–825.

Evans, D. M. D. (1990). Inflammation and healing. In *Cash's Textbook of General Medicine and Surgical Conditions for Physiotherapists* (ed. P. A. Downie), 2nd edn, pp. 12–29. London: Faber and Faber.

Feinstein, B., Langton, J. M. K., Jameson, R. M. *et al.* (1954). Sciatica in the intervertebral disc. An experimental study. *J. Bone Joint Surg.*, **40A**, 1401.

Ferguson, A. B., Vaughn, L. and Ward, L. (1957). A study of disease atrophy of skeletal muscle in the rabbit. *J. Bone Joint Surg.*, **39A**, 583–596.

Fischbach, G. D. and Robbins, N. (1969). Changes in contractile properties of disused skeletal muscles. *J. Physiol. (London)*, **201**, 305–320.

Friden, T., Zatterstorm, R., Lindstand, A. *et al.* (1990). Disability in ACL insufficency: An analysis of 19 untreated patients. *Acta Orthop. Scand.*, **61**, 131–135.

Garrett, W. B. Jr. and Lohnes, J. (1990). Cellular and matrix response to mechanical injury at the myotendinous junction. In *Sports Induced Inflammation.* pp. 215–224. Park Ridge: A.A.O.S.

Green, G. A., Zachzewski, J. E. and Jordan, S. E. (1989). Peroneal nerve palsy induced by cryotherapy. *Phys. Sportsmed.*, **17**, 63–70.

Grimby, G., Gustafsson, E., Peterson, L. *et al.* (1980). Quadriceps function and training after knee ligament surgery. *Med. Sci. Sport. Exc.*, **12**, 70–75.

Houston, M. E., Bentzen, H. and Larsen, H. (1979). Interrelationships between skeletal muscle adaptions and performance as studied by detraining and retraining. *Acta. Physiol. Scand.*, **105**, 163–170.

Hughtson, J. C., Andrews, J. R., Cross, M. J. *et al.* (1976a). Classification of knee ligament instabilities. Part 1. The medial compartment and cruciate ligament. *J. Bone Joint Surg.*, **58A**, 159–172.

Hughtson, J. C., Andrews, J. R., Cross, M. J. *et al.* (1976b). Classification of knee ligament instabilities. Part 2. The lateral compartment. *J. Bone Joint Surg.*, **58-A**, 173–179.

Hunt, T. K. and Van Winkle, W. Jr. (1980). Wound healing. In *Fracture Treatment and Healing.* pp. 1–34. Philadelphia: W.B. Saunders.

Irrgang, J. and Lephart, S. (1992). Reliability of measuring postural sway in normal individuals using the Chattecx Dynamic Balance System. *Phys. Ther.*, **72**, 566.

Jaspers, S. F. and Tischler, M. E. (1992). Correlation of quantity and the metabolism of protein in hindlimb muscles of hypokinetic rats. *Abstract. Fed. Proceed.*, **41**, 867.

Jozsa, L. and Reffy, A. (1978). Fine structural study of human skeletal muscle injuries due to blunt trauma. *Z. Rechtsmed.*, **82**, 145–152.

Kibler, W. B. (1990). Concepts in exercise rehabilitation of athletic injury. In *Sports Induced Inflammation*. pp. 759–769. Park Ridge: A.A.O.S.

Knight, K. L. (1982). Ice for immediate care of injuries. *Phys. Sportsmed.*, **10**, 137.

Knight, K. L. (1989). Cryotherapy in sports injury management. *Int. Perspec. Phys. Ther.*, **4**, 163–185.

Knight, K. L., Aquino, J., Johannes, S. M. *et al.* (1980). A re-examination of Lewis' cold induced vasodilitation of the finger and the ankle. *Ath. Train.*, **15**, 24–27.

Kozambi, D. D. (1967). Living prehistory in India. *Sci. Am.*, **216**, 105.

Kroeber, A. L. (1948). *Anthropology*. Harcourt.

LeBlanc, J. (1975). *Man in the Cold*. Springfield Charles Thomas (Publishers).

LeBlanc, A., Marsh, C., Evans, H. *et al.* (1985). Bone and muscle atrophy with suspension of the rat. *J. Appl. Physiol.*, **58**, 1669–1675.

Lewis, T. S. (1930). Observations upon the reactions of the vessels of the human skin to cold. *Heart*, **15**, 177–208.

Lieber, R. L., Friden, J. O., Hagens, A. R. *et al.* (1988). Differential response of the dog quadriceps muscle to external skeletal fixation of the knee. *Muscle and Nerve*, **11**, 193–201.

Luthi, J. M., Gerber, C., Classen. H. *et al.* (1989). Die verletzte und die immobilisierte muskelzelle: Ultrastrukturelle Betrachtungen. *Sportverletzung Sportschaden*, **3**, 58–61.

MacDougall, J. D., Ward, G. R., Sale, D. G. *et al.* (1977). Biochemical adaptions of human skeletal muscle to heavy resistance training and immobilisation. *J. Appl. Physiol.*, **43**, 700–703.

Maitland, G. D. (1991). *Peripheral Manipulation*. 3rd ed. Oxford: Butterworth-Heinemann.

Martinez-Hernandez, A. and Amenta, P. S. (1990). Basic concepts in wound healing. In: *Sports Induced Inflammation*. pp. 55–101. Park Ridge: A.A.O.S.

Martsen, F. A., Questad, K. and Martsen, A. L. (1975). The effect of cooling on post fracture swelling: a controlled study. *Clin. Orthop.*, **109**, 201.

McMaster, W. C., Little, S. and Waugh, T. R. (1978). Laboratory evaluations of various cold therapy modalities. *Am. J. Sports Med.*, **6**, 291–294.

Melzack, R. and Scott, T. H. (1957). The effects of early experience on the response to pain. *J. Comp. Physiol. Psychol.*, **59**, 155.

Melzack, R., Wall, P. D. and Weisz, A. Z. (1963). Masking and metacontrast phenomena in the skin sensory system. *Exp. Neurol.*, **8**, 35–46.

Melzack, R. (1973). *The Puzzle of Pain*. Harmondsworth: Penguin.

Melzack, R. (1986) Neurophysiological foundations of pain. In: *The Psychology of Pain* (ed. R. A. Sternbach), 2nd edn, pp. 1–24. New York: Raven Press.

Mense, S. (1978). Effects of temperature on the discharge of muscle spindles and tendon organs. *Pflugers Arch.*, **374**, 159–166.

Muller, E. A. (1970). Influence of training and of inactivity on muscle strength. *Arch. Phys. Med. Rehab.*, **51**, 449–462.

Nicholas, J. A. (1978). Report of the Committee on Research and Education. *Am. J. Sports Med.*, **6**, 295–304.

Palmer, J. E. and Knight, K. L. (1996). Ankle and thigh skin surface temperature changes with repeated ice pack application. *J. Ath. Train.*, **31(4)**, 319–323.

Renstrom, P. A. F. H. and Konradsen, L. (1997). Ankle ligament injuries. *Br. J. Sports Med.*, **31**, 11–20.

Rettig, A. C., Shelbourne, D. K., McCarroll, J. R. *et al.* (1988). The natural history and treatment of delayed union stress fractures of the anterior cortex of the tibia. *Am. J. Sports Med.*, **16**, 250.

Rosemeyer, B. and Sturz, H. (1977). Musculus quadriceps femoris bei immobilisation und remobilisation. *Zeitschrift fur Orthopeadie*, **115**, 182–188.

Roy, R. R., Bello, M. A., Bouisson, P. *et al.* (1987). Size and metabolic properties of fibres in rat fast twitch muscles after hindlimb suspension. *J. Appl. Physiol.*, **62**, 2348–2357.

Rucinski, T. J., Hooker, D. N., Prentice, W. E. Jr, *et al.* (1991). The effects of intermittent compression on oedema in postacute ankle sprains. *J. Orthop. Sports Phys. Ther.*, **14**, 65–69.

Saltin, B. and Rowell, L. B. (1980). Functional adaptions to physical activity and inactivity. *Fed. Proceed.*, **39**, 1509–1513.

Sargeant, A. J., Davies, C. T. M., Edwards, R. H. T. *et al.* (1977). Functional and structural changes after disuse of human muscles. *Clin. Sci. Mol. Med.*, **52**, 337–342.

Sheen, D. and Green, A. (1997). Are you positive? Aids, attitudes and physiotherapy. *Physiotherapy*, **83(4)**, 190–194.

Shepard, J., Rusch, N. and Vanhoutte, P. (1983). Effect of cold on the blood vessel wall. *Gen. Pharmacol.*, **14**, 61–64.

Smyth, M. J. and Wright, V. (1958). Experiments on pain referred from deep somatic tissue. *J. Bone Joint Surg.*, **36A**, 981.

Spencer, J. D., Hayes, K. C. and Alexander, I. J. (1984). Knee joint effusion and quadriceps reflex inhibition in man. *Arch. Phys. Med. Rehab.*, **65**, 171–177.

Taber, C., Countryman, K., Fahrenbruch, J. *et al.* (1992). Measurement of reactive vasodilatation during cold gel pack application to non-traumatized ankles. *Phys. Ther.*, **72**, 294–299.

Tegner, Y., Lysholm, J., Lysholm, M. *et al.* (1986). A performance test to monitor rehabilitation and evaluate ACL injuries. *Am. J. Sports Med.*, **14**, 156–159.

Thorsson, O., Lilja, B., Ahgren, L. *et al.* (1985). The effect of local cold application on intramuscular blood flow at rest and after running. *Med. Sci. Sports Exerc.*, **17**, 710–713.

Travell, J. (1952). Ethyl chloride spray for painful muscle spasm. *Arch. Phys. Med. Rehab.*, **33**, 291-298.

Tropp, H., Ekstrand, J., Gillquist, J. (1984). Stabilometry in functional instability of the ankle and its value in predicting injury. *Med. Sci. Sports Med.*, **16**, 64–66.

Waylouis, G. W. (1967). The physiological effects of ice massage. *Arch. Phys. Med. Rehab.*, **48**, 37–42.

Weston, M., Taber, C., Casagranda, L. *et al.* (1994). Changes in local blood volume during cold gel pack application to traumatized ankles. *J. Orth. Sports Ther.*, **19**, 197–199.

Williams, P. E. and Goldspink, G. (1984). Connective tissue changes in immobilised muscle. *J. Anat.*, **138**, 343–350.

Wilkerson, G. B. (1985). Treatment of ankle sprains with external compression and early mobilisation. *Phys. Sports Med.*, **13**, 83–90.

Wilkerson, G. B. (1985). External compression for controlling traumatic oedema. *Phys. Sports Med.*, **13**, 97–106.

Wilkerson, G. B. and Nitz, A. J. (1994). Dynamic ankle stability: Mechanical and neuromuscular interrelationships. *J. Sports Rehab.*, **3**, 43–57.

Wyke, B. (1972). Articualar neurology – a review. *Physiotherapy*, **58**, 94–99.

5

Care of the chronic injury

Only physiotherapists who work directly with teams and who are involved with providing medical facilities on a match day are likely to be treating a sports injury in an acute state. In most instances, the physiotherapist who works in a sports injury clinic or who is responsible for the injured player in a later stage of recovery is going to see the injury when it reaches the chronic stage. It is at this point that the clinically proficient physiotherapist will apply assessment, manual and electrotherapy skills to assist in a full and speedy recovery. Ability and confidence in these various techniques and in one's own judgement is essential in the sporting environment, where the physiotherapist may be the sole medical and clinical practitioner caring for the injured player.

Definition

A classification of sports injuries has been established which is based upon the international classification of diseases (ICD-CM-10) by the World Health Organization. This simplification was first suggested by Thorndike (1959) and has been presented by the American Medical Association (1966), Williams (1971) and Lysens and Ostyn (1984). This classification gives the following categories of medical diagnosis:

Sprain (of joint capsule and ligaments)
Strain (of muscle and tendon)
Contusion (bruising)
Dislocation or subluxation (of joint)
Fracture (of bone)
Abrasion (graze)
Laceration (open wound)
Infection
Inflammation.

Treatment modalities

Various manual and electrotherapy modalities are available to the physiotherapist which can be incorporated into the care of the injured sportsperson. Manual treatment techniques are vital if the practising physiotherapist is to survive in the medical world of sport, as financial limitations and inadequate allocation of necessary medical resources exist in the majority of sporting environments. At the same time, this should be acknowledged as a beneficial state to ensure maximum clinical knowledge and skills are gained, without having to rely on a power source and instruction manual.

Manual therapy

Spinal or peripheral manual therapy techniques are often labelled as manipulation or mobilization procedures. The descriptive terms 'active' and 'passive' should be included as they give a far better impression and a wider appreciation of the varying techniques available to the physiotherapist. Mobilization involves a low velocity, large amplitude passive movement, performed with patient control and within the normal limits of articular amplitude (Spitzer *et al.*, 1987). Manipulation is an abrupt, high velocity, short amplitude passive movement of a joint beyond its physiological range, but within the normal limits of articular amplitude (Spitzer *et al.*, 1987). Some techniques combine an active component, which is supplied by the player, with the passive movement, produced by the physiotherapist. In the sporting environment, such clinical skills are a vital tool to have available as a treatment choice and are essential for the many varying problems that will enter the medical room throughout the season. Many different techniques which involve mobilizations and manipulation with active and passive components are available, and the physiotherapist with sufficient experience and knowledge will integrate the different movements, positions and grades of treatment of these various procedures. Very few 'pure' physiotherapists who base all their treatment on one methodology exist nowadays, which demonstrates the profession's ability to encourage continued development whilst working as clinicians.

Some of the different and most common techniques available include the following:

Maitland (1986)

The Maitland concept is based upon a detailed and specific subjective and objective examination of the patient. From these findings, a choice of treatment is made to suit that particular individual. This type of assessment is used throughout the treatment programme, showing the possible value of a particular treatment technique. Further procedures may be introduced, if necessary, depending on the clinical picture demonstrated on reassessment.

The techniques of treatment involve the use of several variables and the physiotherapist must know how to relate these factors to the examination findings. These include:

Grades
Rhythm of movement
Amplitude
Position in range.

Basic treatment techniques exist to which many modifications can be introduced by the open minded physiotherapist. The choice of treatment is made with regard to the clinical findings and not to a diagnostic label given to the individual. Maitland (1986) suggests that two separate but interdependent compartments of thought are necessary. One contains the theoretical information, the other the clinical picture demonstrated by the patient. Interaction of the two should provide a diagnosis on which to base a treatment regime.

This concept of treatment is based upon the role of the physiotherapist complementing the work of the orthopaedic surgeon, particularly in the management of musculoskeletal conditions. The examination process involves a simple yet logical approach, assessing each joint component in turn to provide a diagnosis on the basis of applied anatomy.

Cyriax (1982)

From this, the injury can be classified into one of two categories:

1. Capsular pattern – Arthritis or nonmechanical lesion
2. Noncapsular pattern – Mechanical or extra-articular lesion.

The treatment process may then include any of the following modalities:

Massage
Traction
Mobilization
Manipulation
Deep transverse frictions
Corticosteroid injection.

This treatment concept is largely based on patient-generated forces in relation to treating spinal postural, dysfunction and derangement conditions. Mechanical pain arises due to one of these three causative factors, and treatment is largely based on patient self-care in terms of postural care and corrective exercise procedures. In order to appreciate the treatment ideals, three classifications need to be examined in more detail.

McKenzie (1981)

1. Postural
This occurs when the soft tissues surrounding the relevant vertebrae are placed under prolonged postural stress. Players who work in sedentary occupations which involve prolonged sitting are most at risk, and symptoms will therefore be more noticeable in the working environment than when playing or training. This is because the stresses are constantly changing when competing, unlike the static postures necessary in their everyday occupation. Spinal posture in sitting and standing needs to be examined and static, prolonged positions monitored for pain onset. Active spinal movements will be full and pain free.

Treatment techniques involve a complete assessment of daily spinal posture, with necessary adjustments to seats at home, work or in the car. Postural stance and sitting positions at work or at home can be adjusted where necessary. Postural retraining exercises are the priority in terms of prescribed active work.

2. Dysfunction
The player will often describe symptoms from a specific moment of trauma, yet the present symptoms are related more to the resultant loss of mobility and function. When dysfunction is due to poor posture or arthritic changes, the player will be unaware of the onset. Morning stiffness eases as the day progresses, though in chronic cases this relief will diminish. Functional tasks will become more difficult and compensatory movements in other joints may be necessary to

fulfil such tasks. Activity which avoids stress at the end of range will make the player feel much easier. The pain is intermittent, occuring only when the periarticular structures are placed on full stretch.

Poor posture with a reduced lordosis are classical visual signs. Flexibility is limited into extension; flexion may be full, but is only possible due to deviation. Treatment of a player with dysfunction problems must initially involve instruction on postural awareness. Symptoms can be controlled or aggravated by the postural stresses created by the individual. Exercises are used to improve the degree of flexion or extension, yet must be performed to avoid micro trauma. Elongation of the soft tissues can only take place without repeated trauma due to overstretching. Bouts of ten modified press ups or flexion in lying exercises, often repeated up to ten times per day, produce a stretching effect on the soft tissues. This regularity of exercise and understanding of the need to avoid traumatic pain on exercising are the key points when treating such an individual. Gravitational stress is eliminated in this initial exercise prescription, but is introduced as progression is required. Flexion may also involve deviation of the spine, and this may be due to adaptive shortening of soft tissue structures within the intervertebral segment or an adherent nerve root. Diagnosis is therefore very important before determining the appropriate mobilization schedule. Relevant associated lateral shifts of the spine also require self-correction by the player and can be treated with specific exercises that realign the spinal posture.

Mobilization techniques are required when little or no progress is made. Manipulation techniques can also be introduced if necessary.

3. *Derangement*

The onset of symptoms may arise from a single traumatic incident or from a sustained flexion strain. This can create pressure on the disc nucleus, and posterior movement of nuclear fluid produces disc derangement. The degree of derangement determines the severity of the symptoms and can be divided into a number of categories.

Treatment is based on the type of derangement present. The initial aim is to reduce the derangement and then maintain this reduction. The player progresses from static prone lying to full modified press ups, depending on the continuing symptoms. These must be performed at regular intervals throughout the day to have an effect on the disc tissue. Postural care and advice is important to prevent recurrence of the symptoms in everyday life. Flexion exercises are introduced once the derangement has been reduced in order to ensure a full functional recovery.

With the more severe derangements, other factors must be considered. Any related lateral shift must be corrected with the appropriate exercises before commencing on the extension-based protocol of the mild derangement. Referred pain from an entrapped or adherent nerve root may require the introduction of stretching techniques. These should only be introduced when flexion in lying exercises do not aggravate the disc tissue. Symptoms at this stage are due to an adherent nerve root and not the disc prolapse, and stretching can be included in the treatment regime.

A great emphasis is therefore placed on player's self-treatment and on prophylaxis; mobilizations and manipulation can be applied when self-treatment is insufficient.

These treatment techniques combine mobilizations with movement and have been effective in treating spinal and peripheral joint problems. A large emphasis is placed on restoring the glide component of joint motion in order to produce pain-free joint movement.

*Nags and snags
(Mulligan, 1992/93)*

For the cervical and upper thoracic spine, the player is treated in a weightbearing position and the direction of the mobilization is along the facet joint plane. A midrange oscillatory movement called a nag (natural apophyseal glide) is then performed.

Another spinal technique used follows the same principle, but involves a sustained rather than oscillatory component. This technique is called a snag (sustained natural apophyseal glide). Any active movement this time comes from the player, who is encouraged to actively perform the painful physiological movement whilst the physiotherapist applies sustained pressure.

Peripheral joint conditions are also treated by mobilization with movement techniques. The sustained mobilization is performed at right angles or parallel to the limited, painful movement, with the player providing the active component.

This technique appreciates that not all joint articulating surfaces are congruent with one another. Physiological movement is therefore a combination of rotation and glide, and treatment techniques place a large emphasis on the glide component to facilitate a full pain-free range of movement.

Kaltenborn (1989)

Adverse mechanical tension (AMT) is based upon 'tension tests', which were used as diagnostic standard tests. These have now been fully integrated into passive mobilizing treatment techniques (Butler, 1987; Maitland, 1986). Consideration is given to the fact that nerve tissue must be capable of adapting to body movements, and acts not just purely as an impulse conducting mechanism. This is particularly so in sport where the body produces endless combinations of movement patterns over different ranges and at different speeds. Not only is tension produced in the nerve, but movement of the surrounding mechanical interface tissues (Butler, 1987) takes place, affecting both extraneural and intraneural components. It should be remembered that tension tests may bring normal neural tissue into contact with other structures and provoke a pain response. Altering distal or proximal components of the test and knowledge of the correct subjective or objective response is essential in such situations.

*Adverse mechanical
tension (Butler, 1987)*

The base tests used include:

1. *Straight leg raise*
Classically, this test has been used to examine movement of the lumbosacral nerve roots in relation to the intervertebral foramen (Breig, 1978), with little consideration for the remaining sciatic tract in the lower limb. Movement of the tibial nerve has been shown to occur in both a cranial and caudal direction,

depending whether distal or proximal to the knee (Smith, 1956). Distal or proximal components which can alter and localize tension and movement include:

Ankle dorsiflexion
Ankle plantar flexion with inversion
Passive neck flexion
Hip medial rotation
Hip adduction
Spinal posture.

2. *Prone knee bend*
This test is used in relation to the second, third and fourth lumbar segments and the femoral nerve (Estridge *et al.*, 1982). This simple test involves the player flexing the knee from a prone starting position, with stabilization of the hip and thigh. Interpretation is predominantly based upon the subjective response. Additional modifications include:

Cervical flexion
Slump in side lying
Hip abduction, adduction, medial and lateral rotation.

3. *Slump test*
This standard test must be performed with the correct technique in order to validate interpretation of the player response. The standard test consists of:

Thoracic and lumbar flexion
Cervical flexion
Knee extension
Ankle dorsiflexion.

The terminal joints at opposite ends of the body, the head, knee and ankle, provide sensitization of the nerve. The test is positive if the player's symptoms are reproduced and/or there is a restriction in the asymmetrical range of movement.

4. *Passive neck flexion*
This provides tension in the opposite direction to the straight leg raise test. Passive neck extension and lateral flexion can also be introduced into this procedure.

5. *Upper limb tension tests*
This is equivalent to the straight leg raise in the lower limb (Kenneally *et al.*, 1988) and comprises of:

Abduction, extension and lateral rotation of the glenohumeral joint
Elbow extension
Forearm supination
Wrist extension
Finger extension.

From this starting position, proximal, distal and lower limb components can be introduced to focus on the injury site.

A work posture related technique for the upper limb is also possible (Butler, 1987), which puts more emphasis on the shoulder girdle position.

Following this testing procedure, passive mobilizing treatment techniques may be applied based on these standard positions. Mobilization of the nerve tissue is graded according to the range of movement required and subsequent pain response.

Danger

It is also very important to obtain a full medical history of the player, as many contraindications exist with regard to spinal manipulation and other allied treatments. In the sporting environment, it can be very easy for the physiotherapist to forget these important yet basic clinical rules in the hope that manipulation of a joint problem will provide an instant cure. Players and managers may try to apply pressure on the physiotherapist to use these 'instant cures', ignorant of complications which may occur due to inappropriate treatment. Any treatment technique which involves the production of movement or applied stress to joints and soft tissue structures, or which increases pressure in vessels or vascular sinuses, is contraindicated in the absence of a thorough clinical examination. This must include radiological investigations if organic disease is suspected.

Absolute contraindications

1. *Mobilization and manipulation techniques*
These include all oscillatory, combined movement, sustained vertebral pressures and neural tension techniques.
   (a) Malignancy which involves the vertebral column.
   (b) Disturbance of normal bladder or bowel functions due to a lesion of the cauda equina.
   (c) Active, inflammatory and infective arthritis.
   (d) Bone disease of the spine, e.g. osteoporosis, necrosis, osteomyelitis, etc.
   (e) Spinal cord injury.
   (f) More than one spinal nerve root on one side, or two adjacent roots in one lower limb only (Grieve, 1989).

2. *Manipulation only*
   (a) Spinal deformity due to old pathology, such as adolescent osteochondrosis.
   (b) Cervical and thoracic joint conditions which produce neurological symptoms in one or both limbs.
   (c) Congenital generalized hypermobility.
   (d) Advanced degenerative changes.
   (e) Severe root pain.
   (f) Undiagnosed pain.
   (g) Anticoagulant medication.

(h) Gout.
(i) Advanced diabetes.
(j) Vascular abnormalities, e.g. vertebral artery involvement, visceral arterial disease.
(k) Clinical factors such as acquired hypermobility or instability, protective spasm, joint irritability, poor patient compliance.

Care is necessary in the following situations:

Pregnancy
Spondylolisthesis
The presence of neurological signs
Dizziness.

Soft tissue mobilization

Manual therapy for soft tissue pathology has had very little literature coverage when compared to that of joint structures, in relation to injury. Following soft tissue injury, the tensile strength of damaged tissue will decrease due to a reduction in internal and external dynamic forces normally exerted on fully functional tissue (Amiel *et al.*, 1982). In certain research studies, a 50% drop in tensile strength has been recorded by day one (Garrett, 1990) or day two (Garrett and Lohnes, 1990) post-injury. It is restoration of this 'normal' tensile strength which is an important factor in the recovery of full fitness to the site of injury, and ultimately to the injured player. Several techniques exist which will assist in full recovery of the injury site, and prevent complications such as adhesion formation or less mobile scar tissue (Evans, 1980). The physiotherapist must therefore understand and recognize the correct stage of healing at which to introduce the appropriate manual techniques.

These include the following.

Massage

Massage is a basic component of many standard assessment and treatment techniques used by chartered physiotherapists, and is useful in many instances of sports physiotherapy. Classical massage techniques (Hollis, 1987) include:

1. *Effleurage*
This type of massage technique can be used to provide either a physical or a sensory effect, depending on the technique utilized by the physiotherapist. Skin contact is maintained throughout, with a gliding movement over the skin from the distal to proximal aspect. Variable factors in application include:

Depth
Speed.

2. *Petrissage*
Kneading, picking up and wringing techniques are all forms of petrissage mobilization. These involve maintaining hand contact with the skin and compressing, rolling or picking up the soft tissue structures.

3. *Tapotement*
This uses percussive movements to produce a stimulatory effect. Clapping, hacking and beating are various techniques which can be utilized to provide the necessary effect.

Within the sporting world, many claims have been made for the use of massage with very few controlled studies available. Most research papers are based on limited case studies and practical experiences, rather than scientific principles. However, many therapists use massage for several reasons:

(a) To alleviate muscle cramps and remove lactic acid (Kopysov, 1979).
(b) To increase pain threshold, flexibility and coordination (Hungerford and Bernstein, 1985).
(c) To stimulate circulation and improve the energy supply to muscle tissue (Balke *et al.*, 1989; Kuprian, 1981).
(d) To speed up healing and restoration of joint mobility (Hungerford and Bernstein, 1985).

The effects of positive physiological responses during submaximal exercise following massage have certainly been questioned (Shoemaker *et al.*, 1997; Callaghan, 1993; Boone *et al.*, 1991). It is suggested that any recuperative benefits may be more psychological than physiological.

Frictions

The physiotherapist applies mobilization through their fingers or thumbs to the affected soft tissue structures with a deep yet soft application of force. The locked digits must not move or glide over the skin surface, as the only movement should come from the underlying tissues to which the force is being applied. For small areas, the first and second fingers are used to apply and reinforce the desired pressure: larger areas will require the use of all the fingertips on one hand, reinforced by the other. Two methods of application exist:

1. *Circular*
This technique involves several circular movements with a gradual increase in pressure depending on the pain response of the player. This type of mobilization is used to loosen thickened oedema, particularly in the soft tissue structures around a joint.

2. *Transverse*
Transverse frictions are applied transversely to the line of collagen fibres, but not in the same plane. The aim is to produce localized hyperaemia, encourage correct collagen fibre orientation, prevent or loosen the formation of adhesions or scar tissue and to provide an analgesic effect.

This technique is an important component of treatment techniques used by Cyriax (1984). Certain authors (Chamberlain, 1982) recommend immediate use after ligament sprain to maintain passive mobility of the tissue, even though collagen tissue will not be present in the scar until the fourth to sixth day (Peacock, 1984; Nordin and Frankel, 1980). The physiotherapist must remain aware of the healing state of an injury before immediately proceeding with such recommendations. It must be remembered that this or any other time scale in the healing process is not set in stone, and other factors such as typeset, degree of tissue demagogue and sex of the player will affect the average time measurements.

The effects of friction mobilization are based on theory and individual case studies, with little or no scientific background to support its use.

Passive physiological joint movements

Passive physiological joint movements (PPJM) involve applying a longitudinal stretch to the soft tissue structures (Maitland and Corrigan, 1994) and can be used as an objective test procedure or as a mode of treatment. The physiotherapist must consider the frontal, sagittal and transverse components of the relevant tissues and apply these factors accordingly. In the tension testing phase, subjective player response, objective tissue resistance, quality and range of movement should be noted. As a treatment modality, following a sufficient warm-up, PPJM can be utilized from the fourth to sixth day depending on the clinical findings on reassessment. Careful tensioning of the wound has been shown to promote correct realignment of the new collagen fibres in relation to those of the surrounding undamaged tissue (Loitz *et al.*, 1989). These movements should be practised at home by the player, three times per day in the initial stages and up to two hourly in more chronic situations.

Specific soft tissue mobilization

This technique of specific soft tissue mobilization (SSTM) is suggested by Hunter (1994) and is based upon clinical results. SSTM involves applying a manual force in the same plane as the muscle fibres, stretching the tissues longitudinally. The degree of force applied is based on the stage of healing and the subjective/objective response of the player. From day five, when fibroblasts begin to lay down collagen fibres in the regeneration phase of recovery, to day 14, when a sound base of collagen will be present (Garrett and Lohnes, 1990; Peacock, 1984), an oscillatory force is applied respective to the pain of the player. Application begins with a treatment protocol of 3×30 seconds initially to 3×60 seconds by day 14. After day 14, SSTM can be combined with PPJM and the force applied based upon the resistance felt by the physiotherapist. This is performed until a change in quality of movement is experienced, and resistance will gradually decrease as mobility improves. In the chronic injury situation these resistance-dominant techniques may be the initial choice of treatment.

Proprioceptive neuromuscular facilitation

Proprioceptive neuromuscular facilitation (PNF) is used in many rehabilitation programmes and is based on the principles of functional human anatomy and neurophysiology. Proprioceptive, cutaneous and auditory factors are utilized to produce a functional effect in motor output. The principles of PNF are based on the neurophysiological mechanisms involved in the stretch reflex and their association with stimulation of certain stretch receptors, the muscle spindle and Golgi tendon organs. The respective stimulatory and inhibitory effects these two receptors produce with regard to tension within the muscle tissue can then be utilized in various treatment applications.

The physiotherapist must utilize the specific techniques which will assist that particular individual. These can either strengthen and facilitate a particular agonist muscle group, or stretch and inhibit the antagonistic group.

1. *Strengthen*

Various techniques can help in developing muscular strength, endurance and coordination. Repeated contraction is useful when a player has weakness at a specific point or throughout the full range of movement. This involves repeated isotonic work of the weakened muscle group until fatigue occurs. A stretch is then applied to facilitate the weak component and produce a more coordinated movement when repeated.

Slow reversal techniques are used to improve the range of movement in an agonistic muscle group and produce correct timing in normal agonist/antagonist muscle patterns. Isotonic contraction of the antagonist is immediately followed by isotonic contraction of the agonist, to assist the agonistic contraction.

Co-contraction of agonist/antagonist muscle groups is assisted by using rhythmic stabilization techniques. These involve sequential isometric contraction of the agonist/antagonist muscle groups, working the two relevant muscle groups in turn.

2. *Stretch*

When the player complains of muscle tightness and exhibits associated limited range of movement, a contract-relax technique can be used. The player is instructed to contract the antagonistic muscle group against the manual resistance of the physiotherapist. On relaxation, the limb is moved through a full range, passively, until resistance is felt. The hold-relax technique involves isometric contraction of the antagonist followed by concentric contraction of the agonist. This will produce similar effects and prevents the inexperienced physiotherapist from applying too much overpressure.

Variations on these basic techniques can be introduced by altering the type of muscle work involved. These variations include:

Passive
Active-assisted
Active
Isometric
Isotonic.

In anterior cruciate instabilities of the knee, it is well documented that facilitation of the hamstring muscle group is an important factor in the rehabilitation programme. The action of biceps femoris as an opposing external rotatory force to anterolateral subluxation of the tibial condyles (Muller, 1983), and semimembranosis/pes anserinus in opposition to anteromedial displacement, are important muscle functions which can be activated by modifying classical PNF techniques (Engle and Canner, 1989). Initially, emphasis should be placed on stimulating the neuromuscular components of both the hamstring and other lower limb synergists to produce a functional pattern of muscular activity. Hold-relax, contract-relax and rhythmic stabilization techniques can be utilized, with variations of joint angles and type of muscle work introduced at the appropriate stage. Emphasis should be placed on the changeover phases from concentric to eccentric activity which occur during the normal movement cycle in the quadriceps and hamstring muscle groups. Isometric muscular activity is also an

Treatment notes

important component of functional recovery, and can be incorporated using the various PNF techniques described. These considerations should also be given to other types of injuries, such as quadriceps and hamstring soft tissue lesions, which can benefit from similar functional movement patterns.

Traction

Manual or mechanical traction is often used in the treatment of cervical, thoracic and lumbar spine conditions as well as in certain peripheral joint injuries. In terms of the effects and uses of traction, opinion varies considerably, with clinical experience and individual case studies being the major influences on treatment choice for the physiotherapist. Randomized clinical trials (Pocock, 1991; Bloch, 1987) contain many flaws in the methodology used, and any positive or negative results have been open to question. Rationale for using lumbar traction is based upon mechanical and neuroreflectory mechanisms (Geiringer *et al.*, 1988; Saunders, 1983), rather than any possible effects on an existing annular tear or prolapsed disc nucleus. In applying a traction force, counterforces are produced by the friction of the body on the traction table. This resistive force depends on numerous variables such as the angle of pull, the position of treatment, muscular tension and skin stretch (Saunders, 1983).

The traction force can be applied in three forms, continuous, intermittent or manual:

1. *Continuous traction*

This can be applied either as an inpatient on a hospital ward or as an outpatient in a physiotherapy department. If traction is applied with associated bed rest, the poundage exerted on the spine is relatively low in relation to the patient's body weight. The main purpose is to keep the player on near permanent bed rest; if the injury is disc-related, such small poundage will have little benefit to the injured individual (Cyriax and Cyriax, 1983).

Traction on an outpatient basis is a more practical, rational and clinically correct method of treatment. Traction couches can be used for both cervical and lumbar applications, and in a small treatment room can be utilized for any other treatment procedures or physical assessments.

The factors which can vary the effects of traction include:

(a) Position
The use of a traction stool or a number of pillows can have a marked effect on the degree of lordosis and angle of pull on the cervical and lumbar spine. The use of such items can neutralize or eliminate the spinal lordosis and localize the pull along the axis of the vertebra.

Many variations of the appropriate starting position, particularly for the lumbar spine, have been suggested. Various symmetrical and asymmetrical lying postures, involving supine, prone or a side lying posture have been used (Sherriff, 1988). Objectively, the choice is dependant on the antalgic position of the player, the position of most comfort, or the one in which the selected form of traction can most easily be applied.

Active exercise incorporated into a period of cervical traction has clinically been shown to be beneficial in certain individual cases, where

the patient is suffering from a history of degenerative and facet joint problems (Gilworth, 1991).
(b) Amount and duration of treatment
Traction of the cervical spine with a weight greater than 9 kg (20 lb) produces vertebral separation of 1–1.5 mm, with the normal cervical lordosis eradicated at pulls of about 9–11 kg (20–25 lb) (Grieve, 1982). In the lumbar spine, the degree of initial poundage applied is calculated from the body weight of the patient. A traction force of greater than 25% body weight is likely to produce spinal elongation (Colachis and Strohm, 1969); any positive effects using a weight less than 25% body weight are thought to be produced by muscle relaxation (Onel et al., 1989; Gillstrom et al., 1985).

Treatment time varies between 20–40 minutes, with an average of 30 minutes being the suggested minimum (Cyriax and Cyriax, 1983) for the lumbar spine.

Subsequent treatment poundages and times are based on reassessment following the initial treatment. If the player fails to make any improvement after the initial treatment session, only the poundage should be increased. Once a subjective or objective improvement occurs in the symptoms of the player, then the effective poundage is continued with an increase in the length of treatment time.
(c) Frequency of treatment
Daily treatment is recommended by most authors (Cyriax and Cyriax, 1983). The beneficial results of isolated traction treatment, however, appear to be short term in effect (Van der Heijden et al., 1995).

2. *Intermittent*
Rhythmical longitudinal movements produced by intermittent traction produce different effects to those associated with a frank distractive force. These may include:

(a) A simple passive mobilization of stiff joint segments.
(b) An inhibitory effect on the afferent neural system, producing pain relief.
(c) Reduction of muscle spasm.
(d) Stretching effect on soft tissue structures.
(e) A physiological benefit to the arterial, venous and lymphatic systems of the patient.

A relatively small poundage, enough to equal or overcome the apposition forces produced by the joint and the surrounding soft tissue structures, is often sufficient to produce such effects. In the highly irritable condition, the traction period can be held for up to one minute in duration, with a lesser degree of pull maintained during the intermittent rest periods. If the aim of intermittent traction is to increase mobility, as with an oscillatory mobilization technique, the held traction position should be maintained for a much shorter period of time in order to allow as many repeated movements as possible within the allocated total treatment time.

3. Manual

Isolated manual traction or traction in combination with other mobilization or manipulation procedures may be the only or preferential mode of applying a traction force as a treatment procedure. Techniques which involve manual traction and cervical rotation should not be utilized before a 30 second sustained rotation vertebral artery test has been performed in either direction, and produced a negative result. Quantifiable measurement of the force applied is not possible, but many combinations of application exist for the enterprising and skilled physiotherapist which mechanical traction units cannot provide.

Intermittent pneumatic compression

Intermittent pneumatic compression (IPC) units are used to help in the removal of excess oedema following soft tissue injury. Various sized anatomical attachments can be connected to a central compression power unit, most consisting of multi-individual airtight compartments to provide sequential segmental compression.

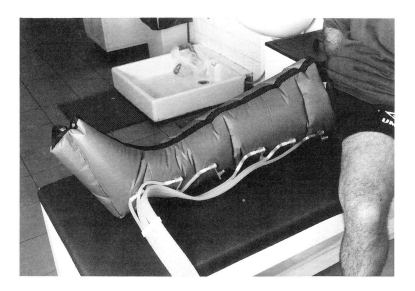

Figure 5.1 Sequential segmental compression.

Physiologically, the principal effects of IPC are as follows.

1. To remove oedema

The external pressure applied to the injured limb will assist in preventing oedema and help to remove excess tissue fluid from the interstitial spaces into the venous and lymphatic network (Pflug, 1975).

2. Circulatory

IPC has been shown to produce variable effects on the circulatory volume. The physical effect of increasing or decreasing circulation is dependent on:

Site of application
Blood vessel structure
Treatment variables.

1. Treatment variables which must be recorded include:

   Pressure measurement
   Total treatment time
   Ratio of compression/relaxation time.

2. Several randomized studies have shown that the use of intermittent pneumatic compression devices can independently reduce the amount of swelling present following injury (Airaksinen, 1989; Airaksinen *et al.*, 1988).
3. Combination treatments using ice or electrical muscle stimulation are often used in the clinical setting.
4. It is suggested that slow inflation/deflation rates of IPC produce a reduction in blood flow, with an increase when faster cycles are used (Sayegh, 1987).

Electrotherapy

Electrotherapy is widely used in physiotherapy practice, yet there is very little agreement both nationally or internationally about treatment dosages or which type of wave form will give the optimum results in specific injury conditions. In recognizing this shortfall, the Chartered Society of Physiotherapy and the Department of Health in the United Kingdom have conducted several surveys on this subject. From these, certain critical reviews on the various forms of electrotherapy have been produced and published, with regular updates to demonstrate the information available. Each chartered physiotherapist, therefore, whilst acknowledging the importance of individual clinical experience, must also recognize the need to apply a critical approach to standard electrotherapy practices. Regular reviews of the literature available are therefore necessary to find out what evidence exists to substantiate the claims of efficiency and underlying physiological effects of each treatment modality.

Treatment notes

Most treatment rooms in the sporting environment contain a range of standard equipment that would be found in any everyday outpatient physiotherapy department. How well equipment is utilized depends on the clinical skills of the physiotherapist and not on the number of extra gadgets the manufacturing companies keep adding to make the units more marketable. The main factor in how well equipped this area is depends on the amount of money available to the medical team. In most instances financial support will be limited, which will have an effect on the choice of equipment available to the physiotherapist. Fortunately a lot of electrotherapy units are available in portable form, with the facility to operate from a battery unit if required. Some manufacturers are able to offer portable units which are capable of several different types of modality within one individual shell.

   Safety for both player and physiotherapist is an important factor when buying a piece of electrical apparatus. Basic health and safety standards should never be forgotten, even in the sporting environment. Most treatment areas are small, as space is of a premium for many clubs. Often the player who enters the room will still be sweating, or has recently had a shower. The skin surface needs to be dried before any form of electrotherapy treatment is used, to prevent the possibility of a burn occuring. Power sources should be positioned close to the unit to avoid any trailing wires which individuals may trip over. Ice packs and damp towels should be kept well clear of any electrical source. Machinery should be serviced at the recommended intervals suggested by the manufacturer. Health and safety rules do not only apply to the hospital environment.

Case study	*The very first treatment room I worked in was situated in the old tearoom of the club. When I first entered the room, there were two fixed height plinths, a safe for all the medical supplies and two electrotherapy units. These facilities surprised me, as financially the club was struggling. One of the units looked like an old shortwave diathermy unit, yet was positioned well away from any power source. When I went to move the machine, I realized that it was now functioning as a bucket to catch the rain from a leak in the roof and was full of water! The other unit, an ultrasound, looked like the first prototype ever designed in the history of electrotherapy. I immediately arranged for this to be serviced and was told by the engineer that it probably had not emitted any degree of ultrasonic waves for the last five years. I wonder how many injured players had jumped off the bed in that time saying 'That feels much better now, after that treatment'. So much for the placebo effect! For the next six years, though, and in this very basic environment, I learnt so much about working in sport, the injuries that occur and how to manage a medical department on a shoestring budget. The practical learning process during that time, I am sure, has been invaluable to me as my career has progressed.*

Infrared

Infrared (IR) is a treatment modality which heats the superficial body tissues by radiation. Within the electromagnetic spectrum, IR lies between microwave and visible light with a wavelength of $0.78–1000\,\mu m$. Clinical wavelengths are mainly between 0.7 and $1.5\,\mu m$, with maximum depth of penetration into the skin occurring with wavelengths of $1.2\,\mu m$. Depth of penetration is also affected by the following variables:

Treatment source of IR used
The angle at which the ray hits the skin surface
Absorption properties of the skin surface being treated
The degree of wavelength scattering produced by the skin microstructure.

Long wavelengths only penetrate to 0.1 mm, while shorter wavelengths may penetrate up to a depth of 3 mm (Kitchen and Partridge, 1991).

The biological effects produced by IR are the result of tissue heating and are listed below.

1. *Metabolic*
An increase in superficial skin temperature produces a subsequent increase in relative metabolic activity (Low and Reed, 1994).

2. *Circulatory*
Direct heating of the skin tissue produces an increase in circulation due to vasodilatation of the superficial vessels. This occurs either due to the direct

heating and increased metabolic effect produced, or indirectly via the vasometer nerve supply. This has been shown to be limited to the cutaneous circulatory system, with little change in the underlying muscular tissue (Lehmann *et al.*, 1974).

3. Neurological

Pain relief brought about the rise in tissue temperature is often regarded by the patient to be an effective method of treatment. This subjective evaluation suggests benefits must exist. The difficulty arises in establishing the mechanism by which this occurs.

The pain gate mechanism (Melzack and Wall, 1965) has often been associated with the effects of heat giving pain relief. It is suggested that heating soft tissue structures generates impulses which have an inhibitory effect and close the pain gate. Heating is also thought to increase the speed of motor and sensory conduction velocities (Currier and Kramer, 1982). An increase in speed of motor conduction can increase the speed of a reflex response, and possibly the speed of muscle contraction. In sensory terms, an increase in endorphin release brought about by an increase in sensory conduction could affect the pain gate mechanism. New information and limited supporting evidence suggests these mechanisms are open to question.

Superficial heating mechanisms such as IR, may reduce muscle spasm through inhibitory effects on the muscle spindle and Golgi tendon organs (Lehmann and de Lateur, 1982). Other supporting literature suggesting a definite physiological link is sparse.

4. Cellular

Certain cellular components such as amino acids and ground substance may be affected by IR radiation (Westerhof *et al.*, 1987; Kligman, 1982).

5. Collagen Extensibility

Heat has been shown to alter the extensibility of collagen tissue in *in vitro* studies (Ciullo and Zavins, 1983; Warren *et al.*, 1971). The physiotherapist has put this to use, heating collagen tissue prior to applying a passive stretch or when using active exercises to facilitate the lengthening of scars or contractures. At the same time it should be remembered that in the *in vivo* situation, the force applied in active and passive movement will be much less than that used in the *in vitro* situation, so identical benefits may not necessarily occur.

Hot packs, wax baths, hot water bottles and hot baths produce a heating effect by conduction rather than by radiation. Similar effects are produced to those listed for IR radiation, though it has been documented that blood flow and pulse volume only increase during treatment time (Baker and Bell, 1991). This increase has been measured at two to three times the resting state (Downey *et al.*, 1968), with this response limited to the superficial structures only (Lehmann *et al*, 1974).

Conduction heating

Continuous shortwave diathermy (SWD) operates from within the radio frequency band of 10–100 MHz, the most common treatment frequency being 27.12 MHz (Low and Reed, 1994). There is no direct stimulatory effect on nerve

Shortwave diathermy

tissue, due to this high frequency level. The intensity of the current however is great enough to produce a direct heating effect on the tissues.

SWD can be applied in two forms:

1. *Condenser field*

Electrodes are placed on either side of the injured body part and act as capacitor plates. The tissues of the body and any insulating material form a dielectric. When the current is applied, rapidly alternating charges are set up on the electrodes and give rise to a rapid, even, alternating electrical field across them. In the human body, the tissue fluids act as electrolytes, substances which contain ions. The application of an alternating electrical field causes displacement of these ions and the resultant drifting and collision of the particles will produce a heating effect. Electrolytes also contain dipoles, molecules which consist of two oppositely-charged ions, with one end bearing a negative charge and the other a positive. The particle as a whole is electrically neutral, but once an electrical field is applied the electrical dipole created rotates so that each end lies as far as possible away from the nearest electrode bearing the same charge. This polarization of atoms and molecules to create dipoles, and subsequent rearrangement of their position produces friction with a resulting heating effect (Delpizzo and Joyner, 1987).

2. *Inductive*

An insulated cable is either wrapped around the injured body part or wrapped into a flat spiral and then placed adjacent to the body tissues, which act as an electromagnetic conductor. With this method of treatment, a magnetic field exists on top of the electrostatic field which occurs in the condenser field mechanism. This magnetic field is situated around the centre of the cable and produces heat within the superficial tissues due to the production of eddy currents, circular currents which occur at right angles to the magnetic lines of force. The effects of these two fields vary depending on the level of impedance of the tissue type being treated.

The physiological effects of continuous SWD therefore occur due to various thermal mechanisms, which include:

1. *Rise in tissue temperature*

This is dependent on the physical properties of the tissue site, such as vascularity and tissue type, being treated (Guy, 1982). It should also be noted that different commercially available units have been shown to give varying patterns of heat emission (Lehmann *et al.*, 1983).

2. *Increase in circulation*

Increases in blood flow have been shown to occur following the application of SWD, with a temperature of 45°C producing a maximal effect (Lehmann and de Lateur, 1982; Lehmann, 1971). The effect of SWD on different anatomical sites has been shown to produce variable circulatory changes, depending on the vascularity of the tissue (Millard, 1961).

3. *Reduction of pain*
SWD is claimed to produce a rise in pain threshold levels and have an effect on the speed of nerve conduction (Low and Reed, 1994; Benson *et al.*, 1974).

1. Treatment parameters should be fully recorded in order to be able to progress the treatment schedule on reassessment of the injured player. These should include:

   Frequency
   Average power
   Treatment time
   Method of application.

2. Treatment time would appear to affect any resultant tissue temperatures. Short duration application of five minutes (Hansen and Kristensen, 1973) has been shown to produce higher tissue temperatures than treatment times of 20–30 minutes (Verrier *et al.*, 1977; Abramson *et al.*, 1960). Rather than having a derogatory effect, a lower tissue temperature would suggest a greater increase in circulation, removing the excess heat.

3. The physiotherapist should be aware of the impedance values of different tissue types in order to fully understand and utilize the appropriate heating mechanism. Blood and muscle tissues are classified as having low impedance, whilst ligamentous, tendon and fatty tissues have high impedance values. In the cable method of treatment, low impedance tissues will utilize the properties of the magnetic field created, particularly if superficial heating is required. With higher impedance tissues, the effects of the electrostatic field should predominate.

4. Treatment application using the inductothermy method has been shown to produce greater tissue temperatures than the condenser field approach (Verrier *et al.*, 1977).

5. Changes in blood flow have been shown to be less after applying shortwave diathermy than those following gentle to moderate exercise (Wyper and McNiven, 1976; Millard, 1961).

6. Most research into the effects of continuous shortwave diathermy on soft tissue lesions has been carried out on animals. The physiotherapist should therefore remember that the healing of animal tissue varies from that of human tissue by being mainly skin contraction over the wound (Basford, 1989).

Treatment notes

Pulsed shortwave diathermy (PSWD), often referred to as pulsed electromagnetic energy (PEME), pulsed electromagnetic field (PEMF) or pulsed electromagnetic energy treatment (PEMET), operates at 27.12 MHz just like continuous SWD, but has an output which is pulsed. The pulsing parameters available, such as pulse length and frequency, can be altered to affect the number of rest phases between each pulse. A high peak power can then be applied at each pulse, keeping the average power and any subsequent heating effect low.

Pulsed shortwave diathermy

Physiologically, the treatment effects of PSWD include:

1. *Rise in tissue temperature*
As with continuous SWD, thermal heating has been well documented as occurring with PSWD (Lehmann and de Lateur, 1982; Erdman, 1960) albeit at a lower intensity and often below the detection level of the player being treated. This effect is dependent on the total average power, the peak power and frequency level.

2. *Accelerated healing of acute inflammatory symptoms*
The following effects are demonstrated:

Removal of oedema
Repolarity of the injured cell membrane
Increased rate of phagocytosis
Increase in enzyme activity
Aid in transport across the cell membrane
Increased rate of fibrin and collagen deposition and organization
Increased nerve growth and repair.

Various physiological mechanisms have been put forward to explain these effects. One theory suggests that the increase in energy provided by PSWD 'stirs up' the various components and activities within the injured cell, accelerating the healing process (Low and Reed, 1994). Another suggests that PSWD helps to repolarize the damage to the cell membrane which occurs following injury (Collier, 1984; Hayne 1984). The presence of 'frequency windows' is another concept suggested in certain literature which suggests that when PSWD is applied at specific frequencies or amplitudes, cellular tissue will absorb this energy. This then stimulates or enhances some components of cellular activity (Charman, 1990; Tsong, 1989).

Treatment notes

1. As with continuous SWD, certain treatment parameters should be recorded to ensure treatment outputs can be related to healing of the injury. These include:

   Peak power
   Average power
   Pulse length
   Pulse frequency
   Treatment time.

2. Not all PSWD units exhibit the same characteristics, so dosage levels which appear to be similar may be quite different if comparing two different treatment units.
3. PSWD is most beneficial on acute soft tissue injuries, helping to accelerate the tissue healing processes. Objective markers such as oedema, range of movement and functional disability have all been shown to improve

following the application of PSWD (McGill, 1988; Barclay *et al.*, 1983; Wilson, 1972).
4. Beneficial effects of treatment would appear to require 60 minutes or more of treatment per 24 hours (Low, 1995).
5. Differences in treatment parameters and protocols may account for the diverse results that have arisen in various clinical trials (Kitchen and Partridge, 1992). Relevant research must provide this information to validate any treatment claims.

Ultrasound

Ultrasound is a mechanical wave similar to audible sound, with a frequency which is much greater than that detectable by the human ear. It can be used for diagnostic purposes (frequency, 10 MHz) as well as for the therapeutic uses (frequency 0.75–3 MHz) when applied by physiotherapists.

The ultrasonic beam is generated by applying an alternating current across a piezo-electric crystal. This causes distortion of the crystal with a series of changes in shape, the frequency of which depend on the way the crystal has been cut. The resulting oscillatory movement sets the particles of the tissue substance in motion and so produces the ultrasonic wave. As the ultrasound beam passes through the various tissue types, energy is lost with increasing depth due to absorption, reflection, refraction and scattering of the wave.

The physiological effects produced by therapeutic ultrasound include:

1. Rise in temperature
Heating has been shown to occur in the soft tissue structures during the application of ultrasonic therapy (Borrell *et al.*, 1980; Lehmann *et al.*, 1978). It has been demonstrated that it requires $1 W/cm^2$ at $1 MHz$ to raise the temperature 0.86°C (Williams, 1987), suggesting any thermal effects are dependent on the intensity level applied.

The heating effect produced is also dependent on several other individual factors:

Tissue type
Blood flow to the region
Frequency of ultrasound applied.

Instant heating will occur in both continuous and pulsed modes, although total heating over a set time period will be much less when using a pulsed beam, especially with long rest periods.

2. Circulatory changes
In early research it has been demonstrated that arterial blood flow increases on application of ultrasound (Dyson, 1987; Abramson *et al.*, 1960). Clinically, this is supported in literature comparing other treatment modalities to ultrasound and the direct effects on blood flow in muscular tissue (Baker and Bell, 1991).

On the other hand, ultrasound has also been shown to produce vasoconstriction of the small arterioles with a subsequent decrease in blood flow (Rubin *et al.*, 1990). This would obviously be detrimental if sufficient to produce a localized ischaemic or hypoxic reaction. If a standing wave is allowed to develop due to nonmovement of the transducer head on application, detrimental effects have also been reported on endothelial tissue, so affecting the efficiency of the circulatory system (Leighton *et al.*, 1988; Dyson, 1987).

3. *Cellular changes in the acute inflammatory stage of injury*
Various cellular changes which are important in the inflammatory phase of healing have been reported (Mortimer and Dyson, 1988; Dyson, 1987; Bjork *et al.*, 1983; Hogan *et al*, 1982). These include:

Increased histamine release
Mast cell degranulation with subsequent increase in activity
Increase in calcium ion transport
Stimulation of fibroblast activity
Increase in platelet activating factor
Increase in vascular permeability
Increase in angiogenesis to restore adequate blood flow to the injury site.

4. *Changes in the regeneration and remodelling phases of recovery*
In the early stages of healing, up to the maturation phase which begins at approximately two weeks, ultrasound has been shown to have various positive effects (Murrell *et al.*, 1990; Dyson, 1989) on recovery. These include:

Increased protein synthesis
Increased fibroblast activity
Increased collagen deposition.

However, *in vitro* studies which involved exposure of healing tissue to ultrasound showed no improvement, or even a derogatory effect in some cases (Stevenson *et al.*, 1986).

5. *Pain relief*
This may occur directly, due to the thermal effects produced by high intensity, low frequency, continuous ultrasound (Kramer, 1987) or indirectly, due to the reduction in oedema and inflammation (Wells *et al.*, 1988).

6. *Bone healing*
Unstable fractures may experience delayed bony union due to the proliferation of cartilage following the application of ultrasound (Dyson, 1989). Various animal studies, however, suggest that bone repair may be stimulated by the use of such a treatment modality (Pilla *et al.*, 1990; Dyson and Brookes, 1983).

1. Treatment parameters which should be recorded include:

   Frequency
   Pulse ratio
   Time of irradiation
   Intensity
   Size of transducer
   Size of area to be treated.

2.

Depth of penetration (Ward, 1986)		
Frequency/tissue type	1 MHz	3 MHz
Muscle	4 cm	1.1 cm
Bone	0.058 cm	0.006 cm

Table 5.1 *Depth of treatment using ultrasonic therapy*

3. The use of ultrasound in any treatment programme should be related to the stage of healing and the level of dosage applied (Maxwell, 1992).
4. The use of an appropriate coupling medium is also very important. Treatment using an ultrasonic transducer without application of a coupling medium produced a degree of reflection at the air/skin interphase of 99.9% (Williams, 1987). The medium used must be able to prevent any air pockets from developing between the transducer and the player, yet retain a viscosity which allows easy application.
5. The use of an anti-inflammatory gel or cream as a coupling medium is often considered to enhance the effectiveness of ultrasound in the acute stages of injury, a process known as phonophoresis. Many commercially available topical creams, however, have not been formulated to act as efficient ultrasound couplants, and may prevent or reduce transmission. A league table of efficient and non-efficient mediums has been produced (Benson and McElnay, 1988).
6. Continuous and pulsed beam regimes are possible using ultrasonic therapy. If heating is the predominant effect required, temperature rise will be greatest where the frequency is highest and an intensity of $0.5–3\,W/cm^2$ is applied when in the continuous mode. To emphasize the nonthermal stimulatory effects during treatment, pulsing the beam with an intensity of $0.1–0.2\,W/cm^2$, produces a lower time average intensity and ensures any excessive heating, cavitational or standing wave effects are avoided during the 'off' phase (Dyson, 1990).
7. A cylindrical beam of ultrasound approximately the diameter of the transducer is emitted by the various transducers available (Hoogland, 1989).

Longwave ultrasound units have also been produced with claims that they are more effective on deeper tissues, provide a more even pattern of energy absorption and have a lower risk factor than conventional ultrasound. As the beam produced from a 45 KHz unit has a much greater beam divergence than treatment from a MHz unit, with an associated greater proportion of reflected energy (Ward, 1986), the suggested depth of treatment of these units must be questionable. Any physical benefits would appear to be short-term, in the form of pain relief due to a greater superficial thermal effect when compared to conventional ultrasound (Robertson and Ward, 1997). A comparison with more conventional methods of superficial heating would be more relevant.

Interferential therapy

Interferential therapy involves the application of two medium frequency currents, within the frequency range of 4000–5000 Hz. This range is utilized in order to keep skin impedance to a minimum. The first of these currents has a fixed frequency of 4000 Hz, the second a variable frequency of 4000–4250 Hz. The electrodes used are placed so that the two waves produced cross at the site of the lesion being treated. As the two currents oscillate, the rise and fall of the two wave patterns can occur either at the same time (in phase) or can oppose each other (out of phase). When in phase, the amplitude produced by the two currents is greater than that produced by each individual wave form. When out of phase, the differing wave patterns cancel the effects of each other out. The result is that a third low frequency current is produced, known as the 'beat frequency', which ranges from 0–250 Hz. The beat frequency can be either constant or rhythmical, a factor that determines the physiological effects desired by the physiotherapist. These include the following:

1. *Pain relief*

It is suggested there are a number of different mechanisms which may be implicated in the relief of pain using interferential therapy (De Domenico, 1982). These include:

Activation of pain-gate mechanism
Stimulation of descending pain suppression system
A physiological block of nocioceptive input
Removal of active chemicals on the pain nerve endings at the injury site
A placebo effect.

Different treatment frequencies have been suggested dependent on the relative mechanism for pain relief. To selectively stimulate the large diameter afferent fibres and the 'pain gate' mechanism, a 100 Hz frequency is recommended (Low and Reed, 1994; De Domenico, 1982). To activate the descending pain suppression system by increasing activity in fibres descending from the ralphe nucleus, a frequency of 15 Hz is suggested (De Domenico, 1982). Release of endorphin and enkephalin, the natural pain killers of the human body, may be stimulated with frequencies of 10–25 Hz (Low and Reed, 1994).

2. *Muscle contraction*

Interferential therapy produces an asynchronous muscle contraction as the large fibre motor nerves are only stimulated as the peak amplitude of the beat frequency is reached. Various frequency recommendations have been suggested for muscle function; Savage (1984) suggests using a sweep of 5–50 Hz, whilst Goats (1990) prefers a 40–80 Hz sweep.

3. *Increase in circulation*
It is claimed that interferential frequencies in excess of 80 Hz have an inhibiting effect on A delta and C nerve fibre activity. Since the muscular walls of the small arterioles of the body are innervated by sympathetic fibres, a depressive effect on this system is calculated to produce a vasodilatory effect on the circulatory supply. This increased blood flow may assist in removal of the pain producing substances from the area (De Domenico, 1982).

In contrast to this it is also stated that different types of excitable tissue propagate impulses at widely differing speeds. When this is combined with the differing stimulus duration requirements of each tissue type, there is an optimum frequency at which stimulation, instead of inhibition, occurs (Deller, 1984). The following treatment frequencies are claimed, therefore, to provide a stimulatory effect on the named tissue type.

Frequency	Tissue type
0–5 Hz	Sympathetic nerves
10–150 Hz	Parasympathetic nerves
10–50 Hz	Motor nerves
90–110 Hz	Sensory nerves
130 Hz	Nociceptive
0–10 Hz	Unstriped muscle

Table 5.2 *Recommended treatment frequencies using interferential therapy*

4. *Accelerated bony repair*
Several studies have demonstrated accelerated callus formation following the application of interferential therapy (Ganne et al., 1979). This suggests that other damaged soft tissue structures may also benefit from similar treatment, though more research into this area is required.

1. Treatment variables to be recorded include:

   Pad position
   Size of electrode
   Swing pattern
   Number of electrodes used
   Treatment frequency
   Treatment time
   Suction/malleable/labile application.

2. It must be appreciated by the physiotherapist that low frequency interferential therapy may well not only stimulate the target tissues, but also other tissue types through which they pass.

Treatment notes

Case study

In my first year as a qualified chartered physiotherapist, I attended a week-long course on interferential therapy. At that time, interferential therapy was a new treatment concept in this country and the outpatient department was keen to purchase a unit, providing one of the staff had been trained in the subject. This being my first course, and keen to impress myself on other members of staff, I came back full of enthusiasm pronouncing this as a treatment modality which could be effective in the majority of conditions seen in any outpatient department. For the next six months most of my treatment regimes involved the use of interferential therapy, as I felt confident in the effects it could produce. In hindsight, I realize that it made me very blinkered in my approach to each patient's needs and I am thankful that it occurred so early in my career. It is very easy to create an unbalanced approach to your methods of treatment unless you can appreciate and be critical of any treatment modality used. Experience as to when to use the many treatment variables we have available as chartered physiotherapists is essential if we are to avoid becoming trained technicians.

Muscle stimulation

Muscle stimulation using faradic or trophic methods of treatment is often used in the clinical environment of a hospital physiotherapy outpatient department. In sports medicine, only isolated severe injury conditions may benefit from such treatment and this equipment is therefore very rarely the first piece of apparatus a chartered physiotherapist would purchase. With the majority of injuries that

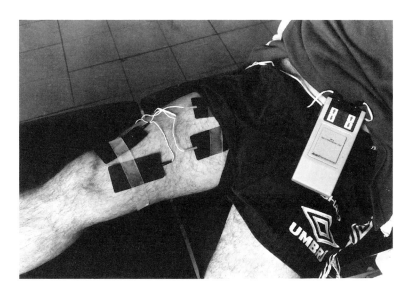

Figure 5.2 Trophic stimulation.

occur, voluntary active muscle work in the simplest of forms is possible, and is a far more effective mode of contraction for an active sportsperson. Neither method is a satisfactory substitute for voluntary exercise (Lloyd *et al.*, 1986).

Laser

The term 'laser' is an acronym of light amplification by stimulated emission of radiation and in physiotherapy practice involves the use of low-level laser therapy (LILT). The light beam produced is part of the electromagnetic spectrum, utilizing a wavelength of 630–1300 nm. This includes both visible light and the near part of the infrared spectrum.

To produce laser light, an electrical power source is applied to an appropriate lasing medium, as different solids, liquids and gases have been found to produce lasers of different yet defined wavelengths. This medium is situated in a chamber between two mirrors, one of which is semipermeable. On applying the power source, negative electrons situated around the nucleus of each atom absorb the applied energy. This will cause the electron to jump to a higher energy shell and the atom becomes 'excited'. This only lasts momentarily, and as the electron falls back to its lower energy state and level it emits energy in the form of a photon. This then produces a chain reaction with other surrounding atoms to produce an identical photon. As the level of energy builds up within the chamber, photons will eventually pass through the semipermeable mirror towards the tissue surface. This beam may then be reflected, transmitted, scattered and absorbed (Goldman et al., 1989).

The physiological effects of LILT are dependent on the type of tissue which is exposed to radiation and the dosage and type of laser used. Several studies have shown no favourable therapeutic response to LILT (Lundeberg et al., 1987; Siebert et al., 1987) to counter the following statements. Most supportive relevant literature, however, covers two particular areas:

1. *Tissue healing*
The effect of LILT on soft tissue injuries is very similar to that of ultrasound. Relevant studies (Hickman and Dyson, 1988; Abergel et al., 1987; Mester et al., 1985) have demonstrated:

Increases in fibroblastic activity
Increases in collagen production
Increase in angiogenesis
Increases in associated tensile strength.

2. *Nerve conduction*
Any effects of LILT associated with pain relief may occur directly due to nerve tissue repair (Rockhind et al., 1988), or indirectly due to a reduction in the level of inflammation associated with soft tissue repair.

1. To standardize treatment regimes, numerous treatment variables must be recorded. These include:

Type of unit
Wavelength of unit
Average power
Peak power
Continuous or pulsed frequency
Treatment time
Beam surface area
Distance from the applicator to the skin.

Treatment notes

2. Depths of penetration have been reported to be between 1–4 mm (King, 1989), as wavelength of the laser and light penetration through tissue are relevant variable factors. Using laser sources with a wavelength of between 300–1000 nm, 99% of the radiation penetrating the skin is absorbed in the first 3.6 mm of tissue (Goldman *et al.*, 1989).

3. It is suggested that there may be an indirect effect on deeper tissue (Saliba and Foreman, 1990).

4. Few positive clinical studies exist in relation to damaged human tissue (Kitchen and Partridge, 1991).

EMG

EMG (electromyographic) activity generated by active muscle tissue can be monitored by using either surface or fine wire EMG units. The majority of physiotherapy work involves the use of the former technique, though there are several disadvantages to be aware of when interpreting the data. Most of the commercial units available are only able to take a sample measurement of 20–50 Hz of the EMG activity of the muscle, which is approximately only one-twentieth of the information provided by the EMG signal regarded as being scientifically acceptable (Ng *et al.*, 1996). Furthermore, due to the fairly large detection area of the surface electrodes this raw signal may contain overflow from other background muscle activity which will distort the information produced. This means it cannot be selective to small muscles in close proximity to larger muscles, and can only be used on superficial tissue. Limits also apply when interpreting the data. If muscle A produces a larger amplitude than muscle B, it must not be interpreted that muscle A is producing more force than muscle B. This only demonstrates a greater amount of myoelectrical activity in muscle A, a factor which is itself complicated by many other factors such as size of the muscle fibres and nature of the interface between skin and electrodes (LSUMC, 1995). Data related to states of muscle imbalance must also be clearly interpreted as the effect of two muscles working as a force couple can very easily be misinterpreted. It must be understood that the work values of each muscle can only be expressed as a proportion of the normal activity levels of that muscle, and not as equal values. The most reliable method of recording this information is to use a maximal isometric voluntary contraction (MIVC) (Knutson *et al.*, 1994). In an imaginary situation, two muscle groups, A and B, might be shown to have a disproportionate effect on MIVC testing. If muscle A has the greatest percentage level of activity in stabilizing a joint, fatigue will soon develop in this muscle group with recruitment of inappropriate synergists (White and Sahrmann, 1994). If an increase in force was to be applied to the couple, muscle B is more likely to be the dominant factor in resisting this situation, which creates an imbalance in the force couple, a factor not represented when using EMG as a biofeedback unit.

In support of the use of EMG units as an adjunct to treatment and rehabilitation routines, the signal produced does demonstrate the point of muscle activation in movement and functional patterns. Much information in terms of muscle activity during functional movement has been gleaned using EMG units. It has been shown that prior to upper limb movement, activity of transversus abdominis provides a stabilizing affect on the torso (Hodges, 1995; Richardson, 1995), a factor which should be addressed in all early stages of upper limb rehabilitation. In the exercise stage of rehabilitation, EMG signals have demonstrated muscle activity timing in open and closed kinetic chain exercises (Cook *et al.*, 1992), important information in lower limb injuries (Gryzlo *et al.*, 1994). It has also been used in conjunction with isokinetic rehabilitation to further enhance biofeedback on muscle activity (Osternig *et al.*, 1984).

In treatment terms, EMG units are most commonly used in rehabilitation of the shoulder joint (Beall *et al.*, 1987) and in patellofemoral pain in the knee (Selfe, 1995; Wise *et al.*, 1984) and provide motivational biofeedback along with postural re-education. Initially this can be used to establish ideal muscle ratios during early scapular stability work, providing the aforementioned MIVC ratio has been calculated, with a more functional role in the later stages of sports-specific rehabilitation.

Treatment notes

Danger
The thermal effects of several electrotherapy modalities/units can, if used or looked after carelessly, cause damage to either the player or the physiotherapist themselves. In this age of 'compensationitis', strict clinical practice must therefore be maintained even in the sporting environment. Burns and scalds can occur due to overdoses, or during normal levels of radiation. Subcutaneous fat has been shown to heat up much more quickly than muscle tissue (Guy *et al.*, 1974), and alternative forms of treatment must be considered when treating the obese player. Scalds can easily occur and care should be taken to remove any synthetic materials or dressings from the treatment area. If moisture is present on the skin surface, treatment should be stopped and the area dried before proceeding with any form of heating, such as shortwave diathermy.

A good subjective history should inform the physiotherapist if the player has had previous surgery to the area. Loss of superficial sensation or the presence of metallic fixation devices are contraindicated with some treatment modalities (Delpizzo and Joyner, 1987). Individuals with pacemakers should avoid the treatment room when any form of electromagnetic therapy is being used, as reports of adverse effects have been reported in the literature available (DHW, 1980).

Female players and physiotherapists must take care if there is a possibility of pregnancy, or if they use intrauterine contraceptive devices such as the coil, when using treatment modalities that produce an electromagnetic field. Research suggests it is wise rather than proven to avoid exposure in such situations (Taskinen *et al.*, 1990; Nielson *et al.*, 1979).

With low level laser therapy, the main hazards associated with the treatment modality are damage to the retina and anterior aspect of the eye, and the skin (CSP, 1991). This is due to focusing the high power density beam over a very small surface area. Goggles should be worn by both the physiotherapist and patient to prevent this situation arising.

In sport, it is vitally important that chartered physiotherapists liaise with other members of the medical team in order to gain a full perspective of the correct approach for every injury that enters the medical room. In the remainder of this chapter, the aim is to make the physiotherapist aware of the role the club doctor and specialist can play in the many chronic injury situations that may arise. An understanding of their position and function in the overall medical approach is essential, especially when explaining the treatment plan to the injured player and in designing the necessary rehabilitation programme.

Doctor

The club doctor has an important role to play in the treatment of both the acute and chronic injury. Liaison between the different members of the medical team is essential in order to produce a broad spectrum of appropriate care for the injured player once an injury has occurred. There are many treatment modalities that a doctor with a good base of general medicine and sports injury experience can bring into the medical department of a club, which will benefit players and other personnel.

Medication

In certain medical situations which arise in sports medicine, the club doctor will often need to prescribe prescription drugs to assist in the natural recovery of the problem. Numerous different scenarios arise in the sporting environment, but the most common medicaments required include

1. Anti-inflammatory – Voltarol retard, tablets and injection.
2. Antibiotic – penecillin, augmentin, flucloxicillin, klaracid, cicatrine powder.
3. Pain relief – paracetemol, diamorphine (naloxane, in case of respiratory distress).
4. Antifungal – zovirax, dactacort, canesten.
5. Antihistamine – clarityn.
6. Antidiarrhoeal – imodium.
7. Antiemetic – notilium (tablets, suppositries, injection).
8. Nasal decongestants – afrazine.
9. Indigestion – antacid tablets and liquid.
10. Asthmatic – bricanyl, serevent, ventolin.
11. Player specific drugs.

Danger

Acute infections of the hand usually occur due to the invasion of the nailbed area by pyrogenic organisms. This is often referred to as a 'whitlow' and has all the typical signs of acute inflammation. Early diagnosis and treatment with antibiotic drugs usually prevents a spread of the infection into the more proximal parts of the hand. If the condition deteriorates, then the player should be admitted to hospital for surgical debridement of the area in order to prevent damage to the tendons or run the risk of a more serious incidence of osteomyelitis.

In the foot, superficial fungal infections are most common inbetween the toes or in the nailbed itself. These tend to remain localized and can be treated with topical antifungal agents. Recurrence of such problems is not uncommon amongst players with a poor standard of foot hygiene.

Following surgery, bacterial infection may occur superficially in the wound. Immediate referral to the player's general practitioner is necessary in order to commence antibiotic therapy as quickly as possible. Active exercise should be reduced to allow the infection time to settle. If an injury has required internal fixation following a fracture, rejection of the foreign matter inserted can produce a far deeper and more serious site of infection. Immediate referral to the consultant involved and administration of the appropriate antibiotics can prevent the possibility of more drastic measures being necessary.

Swelling into a joint space following injury can appear over different time periods. The decision of the club doctor to perform the aspiration should be based on clinical grounds. If the player is to be admitted to hospital, the aspiration is best performed in such an environment, either as an isolated or as part of a surgical procedure.

Joint aspiration

An instant effusion indicates a haemarthrosis; a more delayed reaction is usually due to the buildup of synovial fluid. In some cases, infection may be the root cause of the chronic problem. Aspiration of the joint is a useful diagnostic and treatment procedure in both inflammatory and non-inflammatory joint disease. Appropriate conditions would include:

Septic arthritis
Haemarthrosis
Crystal synovitis
Acute large effusion
Effusion interfering with function.

Aspiration to aid recovery is sometimes necessary to remove blood, pus or large effusions. Blood is an irritant and leads to synovitis, which will severely impair function. Infection will produce a marked inflammatory reaction and the degree of pus will hamper the effect of antibiotics.

An aseptic technique ensures the risk of iatrogenic infection is kept to a minimum. To minimize discomfort during aspiration, a 1–2% solution of lignocaine without adrenalin may be injected through the skin and underlying tissues into the pain-sensitive joint capsule. Specialist creams can also be applied to the area to numb the skin, although this can take up to 15–20 minutes to be effective. Palpation of anatomical landmarks is essential to increase the possibility of first time success, and to ensure the player does not become uptight about the situation.

If there is the possibility of infection, the synovial fluid should be sent for Gram stain, total and differential white blood count and bacterial culture so the appropriate medication can be prescribed. If a crystal synovitis is present, polarized light microscopy is necessary.

In a chronic injury situation, the use of an appropriate steroid injection can have beneficial effects. The best effects appear to be in cases of chronic scarring, though any success depends on an accurate diagnosis and injection application. Such an injection should not be used if any source of infection is present.

Steroid injection

Long-acting steroids, such as corticosteroid and methylprednisolone, are used in various dosages depending on the size of the joint to be injected. Shorter acting steroids like hydrocortisone are used for injection into soft tissues, as the longer acting steroids may lead to fat atrophy (Nichols, 1989) if used in such instances. Following the injection, the player should be warned that the injection site may be painful for the first 24 hours, and that there should be complete rest for the first couple of days. Any benefits may not be apparent for at least a week.

Much controversy exists as to the benefit of such injections. Inhibition of collagen synthesis, reduction in the speed of tendon repair, lower elastic limits and atrophy of fatty tissue (Nichols, 1989) are all states of repair not beneficial to a player in the long-term healing process of an injury, yet have been shown to occur following steroid injection. Many research papers suggest that following steroid injection, the Achilles tendon is more susceptible to complete rupture (Kleinman and Gross, 1983; Chechick *et al.*, 1982; Halpern *et al.*, 1977), but these are based purely on anecdotal cases. Only one paper (DaCruz *et al.*, 1988) avoids using individual case studies, and shows no incidence of rupture following steroid injection. Cyriax (1982) states that Achilles tendon rupture associated with steroid injections is due to incorrect technique and not due to the effects of the treatment.

Local anaesthetic

The decision to use this procedure in a player who is about to play must be made on ethical grounds and discussed by the medical team and the player. Anatomical factors and an accurate clinical diagnosis are determining medical features in this decision, and should not be pushed to one side by other considerations, such as managerial and player pressure. Isolated, important matches may also encourage the use of such a procedure. Even though this is not medically defensible, it is realistically a factor that many club doctors have to consider. The player involved must be made fully aware of the risks involved, and a signed acknowledgement from the player should be obtained to cover the use of this procedure. Ethical guidelines covering this topic have been produced by the World Medical Association and International Olympic Committee (1981).

Consultant

Certain acute conditions such as fractures or dislocations require immediate surgical intervention to stabilize the injury site and allow the healing process to commence.

Danger
Non-union at a fracture site occurs when all repair processes have ceased and bony continuity has not been fully restored. This may occur for several reasons:

Inadequate blood supply
Infection
Inadequate period of immobilization
Poor reduction of fracture site
Inadequate internal fixation
Delayed diagnosis
Patient noncompliance with medical state.

The bone ends become either atrophic or hypertrophic. Occasionally a synovial cavity will form between the two bone ends to form a false union, a pseudarthrosis. The only treatment option at this stage is removal of the synovium and internal fixation of the fracture site. Bone grafting may be necessary to gain union.

Once a player is allowed to return to full contact sport, there is always the possibility of refracturing the initial injury site. This is particularly so after the removal of a brace, a cast or any type of internal fixation. Players who return to play with a fracture site still internally fixed also run the risk of fracturing around the fixating nails or screws due to the difference in tensile strength between the bone and metallic components. This is particularly so with rugby players who have suffered a fracture to the forearm or wrist, and in the femur or tibia in the adolescent.

The majority of other soft tissue injuries will in the initial phase be treated conservatively using the various techniques available to the club doctor and chartered physiotherapist. Once the acute inflammatory symptoms have resolved, reassessment may demonstrate a more sinister clinical picture which requires the services of the orthopaedic or general surgeon. The ability to recognize and refer such players is an important clinical requirement of the medical team so that any corrective surgery which is required can be carried out as quickly as possible.

After a thorough examination and any necessary investigative procedures, the surgeon may feel there is a need to consider a surgical approach to the problem. This will depend on many factors such as the nature and severity of the injury, effectiveness of conservative procedures, degree of healing time, level of player participation and patient compliance. Further notes on surgical procedures are included in Chapters 6 and 7.

References

Abergel, R. P., Lyons, R. F. and Castel, J. C. (1987). Biostimulation of wound healing by lasers: experimental approaches in animal models and fibroblast cultures. *J. Dermat. Surg. Oncol.*, **13**, 127–133.

Abramson, D. L., Bell, Y., Rejal, H. *et al.* (1960). Changes in blood flow, oxygen uptake and tissue temperatures produced by therapeutic physical agents. *Am. J. Phys. Med.*, **39**, 87–95.

Airaksinen, O., Kolari, P. J., Herve, R. *et al.* (1988). Treatment of post-traumatic oedema in lower legs using intermittent pneumatic compression. *Scand. J. Rehab. Med.*, **20**, 25–28.

Airaksinen, O. (1989). Changes in post-traumatic ankle joint mobility, pain and oedema following intermittent pneumatic compression therapy. *Arch. Phys. Med. Rehab.*, **70**, 341–344.

Amiel, D., Woo, S. L. Y., Harwood, F. L. *et al.* (1982). The effect of immobilisation on collagen turnover in connective tissue: a biochemical-biomechanical correlation. *Acta Orthop. Scand.*, **53**, 325–332.

Baker, R. J. and Bell, G. W. (1991). The effect of therapeutic modalities on blood flow in the human calf. *J. Orthop. Sports Phys. Ther.*, **13(1)**, 23–27.

Balke, B., Anthony, J. and Wyatt, F. (1989). The effects of massage treatment on exercise fatigue. *Clin. Sports Med.*, **1**, 189–196.

Barclay, V., Collier, R. J. and Jones, A. (1983). Treatment of various hand injuries by pulsed electromagnetic energy. *Physiotherapy*, **69(6)**, 186–188.

Basford, J. R. (1989). Low energy laser therapy: Controversies and new research findings. *Lasers Surg. Med.*, **9**, 1–5.

Beall, M. S., Diefenbach, G. and Allen, A. (1987). Electromyographic biofeedback in the treatment of voluntary posterior instability of the shoulder. *Am. J. Sports Med.*, **15**, 175–178.

Benson, H. A. E. and McElnay, J. C. (1988). Transmission of ultrasound energy through topical pharmaceutical products. *Physiotherapy*, **74(11)**, 587–588.

Bjork, J., Lindbom, L., Gerdin, B. *et al.* (1983). Paf-acether (platelet activating factor) increases microvascular permeability and affects endothelium-granulocyte interaction in microvascular beds. *Acta Physio. Scand.*, **119**, 305–308.

Bloch, R. (1987). Methodology in clinical back pain trials. *Spine*, **12**, 430–432.

Boone, T., Cooper, R. and Thompson, W. R. (1991). A physiologic evaluation of the sports massage. *Ath. Train.*, **26**, 51–54.

Borrell, R. M., Parker, R. and Henley, E. J. (1980). Comparison of *in vitro* temperatures produced by hydrotherapy, paraffin wax treatment and fluidotherapy. *Physical Therapy*, **60**, 1273–1276.

Breig, A. (1978). *Adverse Mechanical Tension in the Central Nervous System*. Stockholm: Almqvist and Wiksell.

Butler, D. S. (1987). Adverse mechanical tensions in the nervous system: Applications to repetition strain injury. *Proceedings of the Manipulative Therapists Association of Australia*, Fifth Biennial Conference, Melbourne.

Callaghan, M. J. (1993) The role of massage in the management of the athlete: a review *Br. J. Sports Med.*, **27**, 28–33.

Chamberlain, G. (1982). Cyriax's friction massage: A review. *J. Orthop. Sports Phys. Ther.*, **4(1)**, 16-22.

Chartered Society of Physiotherapy (1991). Guide lines for the safe use of lasers in physiotherapy. *Physiotherapy*, **77(3)**, 169–171.

Charman, R. A. (1990). Exogenous currents and fields – experimental and clinical application. (Part 5 of Bioelectricity and electrotherapy – towards a new paradigm?) *Physiotherapy*, **76(12)**, 743–750.

Chechick, A., Amit, Y., Israli, A. *et al.* (1982). Recurrent rupture of the achilles tendon induced by corticosteroid injection. *Br. J. Sports Med.*, **16**, 89–90.

Ciullo, J. V. and Zarins, B. (1983). Biomechanics of the musculotendinous unit: relation to athletic performance and injury. *Clin. Sports Med.*, **2(1)**, 71–86.

Colachis, S. C. and Strohm, B. R. (1969). Effects of intermittent seperation of lumbar vertebrae. *Arch. Phys. Med. Rehab.*, **50**, 251–258.

Collier, R. (1984) Physics and physiological effects of pulsed electromagnetic fields (as far as known). Lecture, Stoke Mandeville.

Cook, T. M., Zimmerman, C. L., Lux, K. M. *et al.* (1992). EMG comparison of lateral step-up and stepping machine exercise. *J. Sports Phys. Ther.*, **16(3)**, 108–113.

Currier, D. P. and Kramer, J. F. (1982). Sensory nerve conduction: heating effects of ultrasound and infrared. *Physiotherapy Canada*, **34**, 241–246.

Cyriax, J. H. (1982). *Textbook of Orthopaedic Medicine*. London: Butterworths.

Cyriax, J. H. (1984). *Textbook of Orthopaedic Medicine*, Vol. 2. London: Bailliere Tindall.

Cyriax, J. H. and Cyriax, P. J. (1983). *Illustrated Manual of Orthopaedic Medicine*, 2nd ed. Oxford: Butterworth-Heinemann.

DaCruz, D. J., Geeson, M., Allen, M. J. *et al.* (1988). Achilles paratendinitis: an evaluation of steroid injection. *Br. J. Sports Med.*, **22**, 64–65.

De Domenico, G. D. (1982). Pain relief with interferential therapy. *Aust. J. Physio.*, **28(3)**, 14–18.

Deller, A. G. McC. (1984). Physical principles of interferential therapy. In *Interferential Therapy*. London: Faber and Faber.

Delpizzo, V. and Joyner, K. H. (1987). On the safe use of microwave and shortwave diathermy units. *Aust. J. Physio.*, **33(3)**, 152–162.

Department of Health and Welfare (Canada) (1980). Canada wide survey of non-ionizing radiation-emitting medical devices. 80-EHD-52.

Downey, J. A., Darling, R. C. and Miller, J. M. (1968). The effects of heat, cold and exercise on the peripheral circulation. *Arch. Phys. Med. Rehab.*, **49**, 309–313.

Dyson, M. (1987). Mechanisms involved in therapeutic ultrasound. *Physiotherapy*, **73**, 116–120.

Dyson, M. (1989). The use of ultrasound in sports physiotherapy. In *Sports Injuries (International Perspectives in Physiotherapy 4)*, (Grisogono, ed.). Edinburgh: Churchill Livingstone.

Dyson, M. (1990). Oral communication; The 4th international biotherapy laser association seminar on laser biomodulation, Guys Hospital, London.

Dyson, M. and Brookes, M. (1983). Stimulation of bone repair by ultrasound. In *Proceedings of the Third Meeting of the World Federation of Ultrasound in Medicine and Biology*, (R. A. Lerski and P. Morley, eds), pp. 61–66. Oxford: Pergamon.

Engle, R. P. and Canner, G. C. (1989). Proprioceptive neuromuscular facilitation (PNF) and modified procedures for anterior cruciate ligament (ACL) instability. *J. Orthop. Sports Phys. Ther.*, **11(6)**, 230–236.

Erdman, W. J. (1960). Peripheral blood flow measurements during application of pulsed high frequency currents. *Am. J. Orthop.*, **2**, 196–197.

Estridge, M. N., Stanley, M. D., Rouhe, A. *et al.* (1982). The femoral stretching test. *J. Neurosurg.*, **57**, 813–817.

Evans, P. (1980). The healing process at cellular level: A review. *Physiotherapy*, **66(8)**, 256–259.

Friedman, M. J., Berasi, C. C., Fox, J. M. *et al.* (1984). Preliminary results with abrasion arthroplasty in the osteoarthritic knee. *Clin. Orthop.*, **182**, 200.

Ganne, J. M., Speculand, B. and Mayne, L. H. (1979). Interferential therapy to promote union of mandibular fractures. *Aust. New Zealand J. Surg.*, **49**, 81.

Garrett, W. E. Jr. (1990). Muscle strain injuries: Clinical and basic aspects. *Med. Sci. Sports Exerc.*, **22**, 436–443.

Garrett, W. E, Jr. and Lohnes, J. (1990). Cellular and matrix response to mechanical injury at the myotendinous junction. In *Sports-induced Inflammation* (W. B. Leadbetter, J. A. Buckwalter and S. L. Gordon, eds.), pp. 215–224. Park Ridge: A.A.O.S.

Geiringer, S. R., Kincaid, C. B. and Rechtien, J. J. (1988). Traction, manipulation and massage. *Rehabilitation Medicine. Principles and Practice*, (J. A. DeLisa, ed.). Philadelphia: Lippincott.

Gillstrom, P., Ericson, K. and Hindmarsh, T. (1985). Autotraction in lumbar disc herniation. A myelographic study before and after treatment. *Arch. Orthop. Trauma. Surg.*, **104**, 207–210.

Gilworth, G. (1991). Cervical traction with active rotation. *Physiotherapy*, **77(11)**, 782–784.

Goats, G. C. (1990). Interferential current therapy. *Br. J. Sports Med.*, **24(2)**, 87–92.

Goldman, L., Michaelson, S. M., Rockwell, R. J. *et al.* (1989). Optical radiation, with particular reference to lasers. In *Nonionizing Radiation Protection* (M. Suess and D. Benwell-Morison, eds.). 2nd edn. WHO Regional Publication, European Series, 25.

Grieve, G. P. (1982). Neck Traction. *Physiotherapy*, **68(8)**, 260–265.

Grieve, G. P. (1989). Contra-indications to spinal manipulation and allied treatments. *Physiotherapy*, **75(8)**, 445–453.

Gryzlo, S. M., Patek, R. M., Pink, M. *et al.* (1994). Electromyographic analysis of knee rehabilitation exercises. *J. Orthop. Sports Phys. Ther.*, **20(1)**, 36–43.

Guy, A. W. (1982). Biophysics of high frequency currents and electromagnetic radiation. In *Therapeutic Heat and Cold* (J. F. Lehmann, ed.). 3rd edn. Baltimore: Williams and Wilkins.

Guy, A. W., Lehmann, J. F. and Stonebridge, J. B. (1974). Therapeutic applications of electromagnetic power. *Proc. Int. Elec. Electron. Eng.*, **62**, 55–75.

Halpern, A., Horowitz, B. and Nagel, D. (1977). Tendon ruptures associated with corticosteroid therapy. *West J. Med.*, **127**, 378–382.

Hansen, T. I. and Kristensen, J. H. (1973). Effect of massage, shortwave diathermy and ultrasound upon ^{133}Xe disappearence rate from muscle and subcutaneous tissue in the human calf. *Scand. J. Rehab. Med.*, **5**, 179–182.

Hayne, C. R. (1984). Pulsed high frequency energy – its place in physiotherapy. *Physiotherapy*, **70(12)**, 459–466.

Hickman, R. A. and Dyson, M. (1988). The effect of laser therapy on angiogenesis during dermal repair. *Am. Soc. Laser Med. Surg. Abst. Lasers Surg. Med.*, **8**, 186.

Hodges, P. (1995). Dysfunction of transversus abdominis associated with chronic low back pain. *Proceedings of the Ninth Biennial Conference of the Manipulative Physiotherapists Association of Australia.*

Hogan, R. D., Burke, K. M. and Franklin, T. D. (1982). The effect of ultrasound on haemodynamics in skeletal muscle: Effects on arterioles. *Ultrasound Med. Bio.*, **8**, 45–55.

Hollis, M. (1987) *Massage for Therapists.* Oxford: Blackwell Scientific.

Hoogland, R. (1989). *Ultrasound Therapy*, 2nd edn., BV Enraf-Nonius Delft, Rotgenweg 1, PO Box 483, 2600 A L Delft, The Netherlands.

Hungerford, M. H. and Bornstein, R. (1985). Sports Massage. *Sports Med. Guide*, **4**, 4–6.

Hunter, G. (1994). Specific soft tissue mobilisation in the treatment of soft tissue lesions. *Physiotherapy*, **80(1)**, 15–21.

International Olympic Committee (1981). Principles and ethical guidelines of health care for sports medicine. *World Med. J.*, **28**, 83.

Keneally, M., Rubenach, H. and Elvey, R. (1988) The upper limb tension test;

the SLR test of the arm in: 'Physical therapy of the cervical and thoracic spine' *Clinics in Physical Therapy* (ed. R. Grant). Edinburgh: Churchill Livingstone.

Kitchen, S. S. and Partridge, C. J. (1991). Review of low level laser therapy. *Physiotherapy*, **77(3)**161–168.

Kitchen, S. and Partridge, C. (1992). Review of shortwave diathermy continuous and pulsed patterns. *Physiotherapy*, **78(4)**, 243–252.

King, P. R. (1989). Low level laser therapy – a review. *Lasers Med. Sci.*, **4**, 141–150.

Kleinman, M. and Gross, A. E. (1983). Achilles tendon rupture following steroid injection: report of three cases. *J. Bone Jt. Surg.*, **65A**, 1345–1346.

Kligman, L. H. (1982). Intensification of ultraviolet induced dermal damage by infra-red radiation. *Arch. Dermat. Rsrch.*, **272**, 229–238.

Knutson, L., Soderberg, G., Ballantyne, B. *et al.* (1994). A study of various normalisation procedures for within-day electromyographic data. *J. EMG Kineisiol.*, **4(1)**, 47–59.

Kopysov, V. S. (1979). Use of vibrational massage in regulating the per-competition condition of weight lifters. *Soviet Sports Rev.*, **14**, 82–84.

Kramer, J. F. (1987). Sensory and motor nerve conduction velocities following therapeutic ultrasound. *Aust. J. Physio.*, **33(4)**, 235–243.

Kuprian, W. (1981). Massage. In *Physical Therapy for Sports*, pp. 7–51. Philadelphia: W. B. Saunders.

Lehmann. J. F. (1971). Diathermy. In *Handbook of Physical Medicine and Rehabilitation*, (F. H. Krusen, F. J. Kottke and J. Elwood, eds.). Philadelphia: WB Saunders.

Lehmann, J. F., Warren, C. G. and Scham, S. M. (1974) Therapeutic heat and cold *Clin. Orthop.*, **99**, 207–237.

Lehmann, J. F. and deLateur, B. J. (1982). Therapeutic Heat. In *Therapeutic Heat and Gold*, (J. F. Lehmann, ed.). pp. 404–562.

Lehmann, J. F., Warren, C. G. and Scham, S. M. (1974). Therapeutic heat and cold. *Clin. Orthop.*, **99**, 207-237.

Lehmann, J. F., Stonebridge, J. B., de Lateur, B. J. *et al.* (1978). Temperatures in human thighs after hot pack treatment followed by ultrasound. *Arch. Phys. Med. Rehab.*, **59**, 472–475.

Lehmann, J. F., McDougall, J. A., Guy, A. W. *et al.* (1983). Heating patterns produced by shortwave diathermy applicators in tissue substitute models. *Arch. Phys. Med. Rehab.*, **64**, 575–577.

Leighton, T. G., Pickwick, M. J. W., Walton, A. J. and Dendy, P. P. (1988) Studies of the cavitational effects of clinical ultrasound by sonoluminescence: 1. Correlation of sonoluminescence with the standing wave pattern in an acoustic field produced by a therapeutic unit *Phys. Med. Bio.*, **33**, 1249–1260.

Lloyd, T., De Domenico, G. and Strauss, G. R. (1986). A review of the use of electro-motor stimulation in human muscle. *Aust. J. Physio.*, **32**, 18–30.

Loitz, B. J., Zernicke, R. F., Vailas, A. C. *et al.* (1989). Effects of short term immobilisation versus contiuous passive motion on the biomechanical and biochemical properties of the rabbit tendon. *Clin. Orthop. Rel. Res.*, **224(7)**, 265–271.

Louisiana State University Medical Center (1995). *A Practical Guide to Electromyography*, LSUMC.

Low. J. (1995). Dosage of some pulsed shortwave clinical trials. *Physiotherapy*, **81(10)**, 611–616.

Low. J. and Reed, A. (1994). *Electrotherapy Explained: Principles and Practice*, Oxford: Butterworth-Heinemann.

Lundeberg, T., Haker, E. and Thomas, M. (1987). Effects of laser versus placebo in tennis elbow. *Scand. J. Rehab. Med.*, **19**, 135–138.

Lysens, R. J. J. and Ostyn, M. S. (1984). Prolegomena bij de preventie van sportetsels. *Hermes*, **17**, 85–94.

Maitland, G. D. (1986). *Vertebral Manipulation*. 5th edn. Oxford: Butterworth-Heinemann.

Maitland, G. D. and Corrigan, B. (1994) *Musculoskeletal and Sports Injuries*. Oxford: Butterworth-Heinemann.

Maxwell, L. (1992) Therapeutic ultrasound. *Physio.*, **78(6)**, 421–426.

McGill, S. N. (1988). The effect of pulsed shortwave therapy on lateral ligament sprain of the ankle. *New Zealand J. Physio.*, **10**, 21–24.

McKenzie, R. A. (1981). *The Lumbar Spine: Mechanical Diagnosis and Therapy*. New Zealand: Spinal Publications.

Melzack, R. and Wall, P. D. (1965). Pain mechanisms: a new theory. *Science*, **150**, 971–979.

Mester, E., Mester, A. F. and Mester, A. (1985). The biomedical effects of laser application. *Lasers Surg. Med.*, **5**, 31–39.

Millard, J. B. (1961). Effect of high frequency currents and infra red rays on the circulation of the lower limb in man. *Annals Phys. Med.*, **6(2)**, 45–65.

Mortimer, A. J. and Dyson, M. (1988). The effect of therapeutic ultrasound on calcium uptake in fibroblasts. *Ultrasound Med. Bio.*, **14**, 499–506.

Muller, W. (1983). *The Knee: Form, Function and Ligament Reconstruction*. pp. 2–115. New York: Springer-Verlag.

Murrell, G. A., Francis, M. J. O. and Bromley, L. (1990) Modulation of fibroblast proliferation by oxygen free radicals *Biochem. J.*, **265**, 659–665.

Ng, J., Richardson, C., Kippers, V., Parnianpour, M. *et al.* (1996). Clinical applications of power spectral analysis of electromyographic investigations in muscle function. *Man. Ther.*, **2**, 99–103.

Nichols, A. W. (1989). Achilles tendinitis in running athletes. *J. Am. Brd. Fam. Pract.*, **2(3)**, 196–203.

Nielson, N. C., Hansen, R. and Larsen, T. (1979). Heat induction in copper bearing IUDs during shortwave diathermy. *Acta Obstet. Gyn. Scand.*, **58**, 495.

Nordin, M. and Frankel, V. H. (1980). Biomechanics of collagenous tissues. In *Basic Biomechanics of the Skeletal System* (V. H. Frankel and N. Nordin, eds). pp. 87–109. Philadelphia: Lea and Febiger

Onel, D., Tuzlaci, M., Sari, H. *et al.* (1989). Computed tomographic investigation of the effect of traction on lumbar disc herniations. *Spine*, **14**, 82–90.

Osternig, L. R., Hamill, J., Corcos, D. M. *et al.* (1984). Electromyographic patterns accompanying isokinetic exercise under varying speed and sequencing conditions. *Am. J. Phys. Med.*, **63(6)**, 289–297.

Peacock, E. E. (1984). *Wound Repair*, 3rd edn. London: WB Saunders.

Pflug, J. J. (1975). Intermittent compression in the management of swollen legs in general practise. *Practitioner*, **215**, 69–76.

Pilla, A. A., Figueiredo, M., Nasser, P., *et al.* (1990). Noninvasive low intensity pulsed ultrasound: a potent accelerator of bone repair. *Proceedings of the 36th Annual Meeting, Orthopaedic Research Society*, New Orleans.

Pocock, S. J. (1991). *Clinical Trials*. Chichester: John Wiley.

Richardson, C. A. (1995). Muscle control-Pain control. What exercises would you prescribe? *Manual Therapy*, **1**, 2–10.

Robertson, V. J. and Ward, A. R. (1997). Longwave ultrasound reviewed and reconsidered. *Physiotherapy*, **83(3)**, 123–130.

Rockhind, S., Barr-Nea, L., Bartal, A. *et al.* (1988). New methods of treatment of severely injured sciatic nerve and spinal cord. *Acta Neuro.*, **Supplement 43**, 91–93.

Rubin, M. J., Etchison, M. R., Condra, K. A. *et al.* (1990). Acute effects of ultrasound on skeletal muscle, oxygen tension, blood flow and capillary density. *Ultrasound Med. Bio.*, **16**, 271–277.

Saliba, E. N. and Foreman, S. H. (1990). Low power lasers. In *Therapeutic Modalities in Sports Medicine* (W. E. Prentice, ed.). St. Louis: Times Mirror/Mosby College Publishing.

Saunders, H. D. (1983). Use of spinal traction in the treatment of neck and back conditions. *Clin. Orthop. Rel. Res.*, **179**, 31–38.

Savage, B. (1984). *Interferential Therapy*, London: Faber and Faber.

Sayegh, A. (1987). Intermittent pneumatic compression, past, present and future. *Clin. Rehab.*, **1**, 59–64

Selfe, J. (1995). The use of biofeedback in the treatment of anterior knee pain. *J. Assoc. Ch. Physios. Orthop. Med.*, **Spring**, 6–13.

Sheriff, J. (1988). A flexible approach to traction. *International Federation of Orthopaedic Manipulative Therapists Papers and Poster Abstracts*, Cambridge.

Shoemaker, K. J., Tiidus, P. M. and Mader, R. (1997) Failure of manual massage to alter limb blood flow: measures by Doppler ultrasound *Med. Sci. Sports Excse.*, **29(5)**, 610–614.

Siebert, W., Seichert, N., Siebert, B. *et al.* (1987). What is the efficacy of 'soft' and 'mid' lasers in therapy of tendinopathy? *Arch. Orthop. Trauma. Surg.*, **106**, 358–363.

Smith, C. G. (1956). Changes in length and posture of the segments of the spinal cord with changes in posture in the monkey. *Radiology*, **66**, 259–265.

Spitzer, W. *et al.* (1987). Scientific approach to the assesment and approach of activity-related spinal disorders: A monograph for clinicians. *Spine*, **12**, 7S.

Standard Nomenclature of Athletic Injuries (1966). Chicago: Am. Med. Assoc.

Stevenson, J. H., Pang, C. Y., Lindsay, W. K. and Zuber, R. M. (1986) Functional, mechanical and biochemical assessment of ultrasound therapy on tendon healing in the chicken toe *Plas. Recon. Surg.*, **77**, 965–970.

Taskinen, H., Kyyronen, P. and Hemminki, K. (1990). The effects of ultrasound, shortwaves and physical exertion on pregnancy outcome in physiotherapists. *J. Epidem. Comm. Health*, **44**, 196–201.

Thorndike, A. (1959). Frequency and nature of sports injuries. *Am. J. Surg.*, **98**, 316–324.

Tsong, T. Y. (1989). Deciphering the language of cells. *Trends Bio. Sci.*, **14**, 92.

Van der Heijden, G. J. M. G., Beurskens, A. J. H. M., Dirx, M. J. M. *et al.* (1995). Efficacy of lumbar traction: A randomised clinical trial. *Physiotherapy*, **81(1)**, 29–35.

Verrier, M., Falconer, K. and Crawford, J. S. (1977). A comparison of tissue temperature following two shortwave diathermy techniques. *Phys. Canada*, **29(1)**, 21–25.

Ward, A. R. (1986). *Electricity Fields and Waves in Therapy*. Merrickville: Science Press.

Warren, C. G., Lehmann, J. F. and Koblanski, J. N. (1971). Elongation of rat tail tendons: effect of load and temperature. *Arch. Phys. Med. Rehab.*, **51**, 465–474.

Wells, P. E., Frampton, V. and Bowsher, D. (1988). *Pain Management and Control in Physiotherapy*. London: Heinemann

Westerhof, W., Siddiqui, A. H., Corman, R. H. *et al.* (1987). Infra-red hyperthermia and psoriasis. *Arch. Dermat. Res.*, **279**, 209–210.

White, S. and Sahrmann, S. (1994). A movement system balance approach to management of musculoskeletal pain. In *Physical Therapy of the Cervical and Thoracic Spine*. (R. Grant, ed.), 2nd edn. Edinburgh: Churchill Livingstone.

Williams, J. G. P. (1971). Aetiological classification of injuries in sportsmen. *Br. J. Sports Med.*, **5**, 228-232.

Williams, R. (1987). Production and transmission of ultrasound. *Physiotherapy*, **73(3)**, 113–116.

Wilson, D. H. (1972). Treatment of soft tissue injuries by pulsed electrical energy. *BMJ*, **2**, 269–270.

Wise, H., Fiebert, I. and Kates, J. (1984). EMG biofeedback as treatment of patellofemoral pain syndrome. *J. Orthop. Sp. Phys. Ther.*, **6(2)**, 95–103.

Wyper, D. J. and McNiven, D. R. (1976). Effects of some physiotherapeutic agents on skeletal muscle blood flow. *Physiotherapy*, **63(3)**, 83–85.

6

Related issues and lower limb injuries in soccer

Soccer, or Association football as it is known throughout the world, has a well-documented history. From Chinese history dating back to 206 BC, references are made to a game which involved 'tse chu' meaning to 'kick with foot, ball made of leather and stuffed'. The Japanese also had a game which was a derivative of kemari, a game played by eight men kicking a ball within a pitch approximately 14 metres square. Other nationalities such as the Ancient Greeks, Italians and British also had their derivatives of the game, and in 1863 the Football Association was formed in England to provide one set of rules for the eleven member clubs, which were mainly in the London area. Soon after, though, the supporters of the different variations went their separate ways and two separate games were formed – soccer and rugby. As the Football Association grew, internationals started to take place between countries and the introduction of professionals into the game brought about the formation of the Football League. Other countries followed the organization of the British, and in 1904 the Federation Internationale de Football Association (FIFA) was born. The game today has now spread to all corners of the globe, and numerous domestic and international competitions exist throughout the world.

Research

Outdoor soccer is currently one of the most popular sports in the world played by both sexes covering different age groups. It is a team sport involving 10 outfield players and one goalkeeper per team, with a standard game consisting of two halves lasting 45 minutes each with a 15 minute break inbetween. A player has to be able to perform numerous functional activities with and without the ball, at a high intensity, in intermittent bursts (Table 6.1).

Various physiological characteristics have been demonstrated in recent studies, information that is essential for any physiotherapist involved in the rehabilitation of soccer players. These include:

1. The average player will cover approximately 9–12 kilometres per game in total, and may be required to head the ball about 100 times per game (Tysvaer and Storli, 1981).
2. Player analysis has shown that during a game, the ratio of aerobic to anaerobic work is approximately 9:1 (Mayhew and Wenger, 1985) and at the end of the game most players will have empty glycogen stores, be dehydrated and have a raised body temperature (Ekblom, 1986).

Table 6.1 *Functional characteristics of a soccer player*

With the ball	*Without the ball*
Tackling	Walking
Passing	Jogging
Heading	Cruising
Dribbling	Sprinting
Shooting	Cutting
Controlling the ball	Angular runs
Catching the ball (goalkeeper)	Collision
Crossing	Acceleration/deceleration
Driving	Turning
	Jumping

3. Less than 2% of the distance covered by a player in a game is with the ball.
4. Premier League players change activity every five to six seconds and have short rest periods of three seconds every two minutes (Reilly and Thomas, 1976).
5. Sprints average about 15 metres and occur every 90 seconds.
6. The distance covered by an outfield player consists of 37% jogging, 25% walking, 20% cruising, 11% sprinting and 7% moving backwards (Reilly and Thomas, 1976).

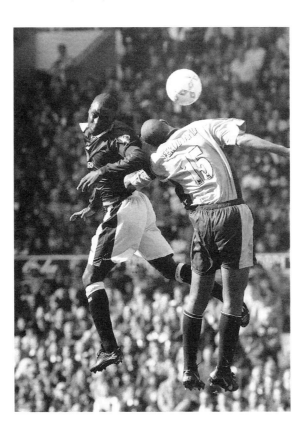

Figure 6.1 Heading.

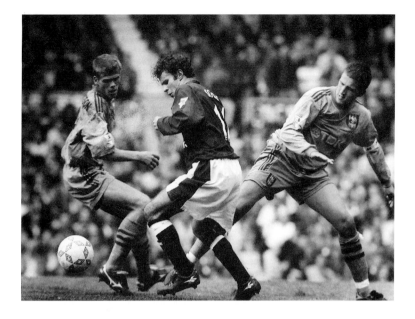

Figure 6.2 Dribbling.

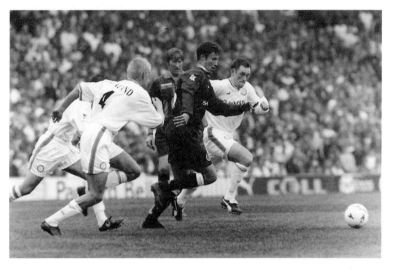

Figure 6.3 Intermittent short sprints are an important cardiovascular characteristic of the soccer player.

Incidence

In analysing the research on injury incidence in soccer very little relative comparison is possible, as many variables exist which have no standard definition. Injury definition, standard of rehabilitation and medical facilities available and anatomical injury/tissue diagnosis are all variables that have many different definitions throughout the research papers available.

Despite these discrepancies, it would seem that the risk of injury is influenced by three factors:

1. *Age*

The incidence of injury would appear to increase with the age of the male player (Schmidt-Olsen *et al.*, 1985 and 1991). This may be explained by better flexibility or less weight in the younger player, resulting in reduced speed in any collisions (Keller *et al.*, 1987).

In female soccer there is no clear indication of age and the effect on the incidence of injury.

2. Gender

Female soccer players have a higher incidence of injury than their male counterparts at youth (Maelhum *et al.*, 1986) and elite level (Engstrom *et al.*, 1991). These studies suggested that this was due to a lower level of skill, technique and degree of physical fitness in the female players involved.

3. Level of competition

It is suggested that injury incidence is highest in the match situation for elite players and in training for those at a lower level of competition (Ekstrand and Tropp, 1990; Nielson, 1989). These results occurred due to the differences in speed and intensity in the game situation allied to the physical conditioning and training conditions in the practice situation. Another explanation is the influence of foul play that may occur in the match situation as compared to training. Hoy *et al.* (1992) found 19% of injuries were due to violation of the rules; this correlates with observations by Ekstrand *et al.* (1983), who found that 12% of all injuries were the result of foul play.

Positional differences

Differences exist between the injury patterns of the goalkeeper and the outfield player. The most common anatomical sites for injuries in a goalkeeper are the head (concussion 9%, dental damage 5.1%) and hand (dislocated fingers 16%, soft tissue 4.7%) (Berbig and Biener, 1983). The outfield player is more prone to injury in the knee and ankle (Schmidt-Olsen *et al.*, 1991; Nielson, 1989), although the most common chronic overuse injuries occur in the adductor and Achilles tendon (Ekstrand and Gillquist, 1983a and b).

In the female soccer player the same injury pattern appears to exist, with the most common injury sites being the knee and ankle (Engstrom *et al.*, 1991), although the most chronic overuse problems occur in the iliotibial tract and compartment syndromes in the shin (Brynhildsen *et al.*, 1990). This can be explained by the variation in biomechanical characteristics of the lower extremities between males and females.

Anatomical site

In a game such as soccer the majority of injuries occur in the lower limb, with figures of 61–90% of the total number of injuries being recorded (Inklaar, 1994). There is a general agreement that the most common sites of injury are the joints, with figures varying between 39.4% (Lewin, 1989) and 49% (Hoy *et al.*, 1992) as opposed to 26.8% in muscle and tendon. The majority of studies suggest that the ankle is the most frequently injured joint, accounting for 15–20% of all injuries (Sadat-Ali and Sankaran-Kutty, 1987; Keller *et al.*, 1987).

Permanent injury

Chronic or serious injury can cause permanent physical damage and may force a player to continue playing at a lower standard of football or give the game up completely (Engstrom *et al.*, 1990; Nielson, 1989).

Long-term mechanical instability of the knee and ankle has been noted in numerous reports for both male (Windsor Sports Insurance Brokers, 1997; Tropp *et al.*, 1985) and female (Brynhildsen *et al.*, 1990) soccer players.

Aetiology

Knowledge of soccer injuries and their aetiology is limited, inconsistent and far from complete. Numerous studies exist, but are limited due to the many variables such as level of competition, gender and age, or involve isolated case studies which have no value in identifying the risk factors involved (Walter *et al.*, 1985). Intrinsic or personal risk factors such as flexibility, muscle strength and foul play have been discussed in Chapter 2. Others exist, and need to be mentioned at this stage:

1. Injury recurrence
A relatively high percentage of re-injuries occur in soccer (Nielson, 1989; Lysens, 1987), which suggests there is inadequate rehabilitation in terms of restoring full functional stability, flexibility, muscle strength and maximal anaerobic and aerobic capacities before returning to play. It would also suggest that some players are returning to play before an injury has fully healed.

2. Physical maturity
Single studies involving either gender have suggested more risk factors for injury from soccer in certain player characteristics. Backous *et al.* (1988) showed that there was a higher incidence of injury amongst the tall and weak boys who played soccer than in the immature (short and weak) or mature (tall and strong). Lack of coordination and lower strength levels may have contributed to these results. In women soccer players it has been suggested that the premenstrual and menstrual period of the ovarian cycle is the most susceptible time for injuries to occur (Moller-Neilson and Hammar, 1989). The same study also found a lower rate of injury amongst oral contraceptive users, with a different ovarian cycle to non users. Other studies are needed to support these isolated findings.

The extrinsic (environmental) risk factors such as protective equipment, footwear and playing surfaces have also been mentioned in Chapter 2, yet other elements exist in the risk of injury in soccer:

1. Training load
A higher incidence of injury has been noted in games compared to practice matches (Ekstrand and Tropp, 1990; Neilson, 1989), and in preseason training compared to training in season (Mackay and Hillis, 1996; Engstrom *et al.*, 1991; Neilson, 1989).

2. Direct collisions
In soccer it has been recorded that 63–73% of injuries are caused by collision with a second person, 84% of which involve an opposing player (Minarovjech, 1980; Napravnik, 1980).

Different prophylactic programmes may be necessary for the different age, sex and skill groups which participate in soccer the world over. To produce these, however, more adequate methods of research and standard definitions of all variables are required.

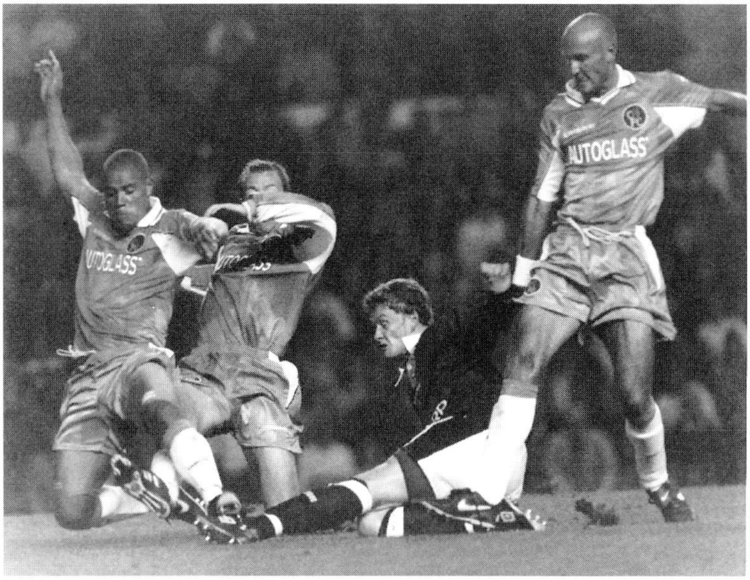

Figure 6.4 Collision with opposing players produces the majority of injuries in the soccer player.

Children

Before discussing specific injuries which occur in soccer, it is important to recognize the aetiology of injury amongst children and adolescents who participate in collision sports, and the types of injuries which are peculiar to this age group as compared to adults.

It is important that coaching and medical staff should recognize that children are not adults and therefore cannot be expected to train, perform and respond to injury as an adult would. This appears in several dimensions:

1. Children exercise at a level closer to their maximum capacity and may not be as aware of fatigue as it develops.
2. Their level of aerobic fitness is different to that of an adult. Figures of $47-51\,ml/kg^{-1}\,min^{-1}$ in boys and $37-50\,ml/kg^{-1}\,min^{-1}$ in girls have been recorded, an aerobic capacity generally higher than a non-athletic adult.

   Anaerobic exercise is not as easily assessed in children, but performance tends to be reduced when compared to adults due to the smaller muscle mass and lower enzyme concentrations present.

   At young ages, children show a higher correlation between aerobic capacity and anaerobic power than during adolescence. Many children excel at both speed and endurance sports and then specialize in the sports which utilize their dominant energy system as they reach adolescence.
3. The body profiles of children change as they develop and gaining weight to compete in collision sports is an area of great debate. Adolescents have to consider their dietary intake, and body composition can be monitored by the use of skin calipers. Excess fat is just extra baggage to carry when performing. Many adult players use weight training as a method of gaining strength with subsequent changes of their body profile. In the child and adolescent, strength gains can be made using a weights programme, but many dangers are

present in the form of acute and chronic injuries. In the pre adolescent, gym work should be confined to circuit training and skills related work. In 1985 the American Orthopaedic Society for Sports Medicine (AOSSM) hosted a workshop for the relevant medical and coaching departments involved with sport for children. They concluded that the benefits outweighed the risks involved, and recommended the following guidelines for adolscent weight training:

(a) Supervision by appropriately qualified coaching staff.
(b) The weights programme should be included in an overall planned training programme.
(c) Use only apparatus that will accommodate the size and degree of maturity of the adolescent.
(d) The apparatus used should be safe, free of defects and be serviced regularly.
(e) A physical examination is mandatory before participation is allowed.
(f) The individual must be mature enough to accept coaching advice and instruction.
(g) Emphasis should be on concentric work only, with no attempts to perform a maximum lift. A full range of motion is essential on every lift.
(h) All training should be preceded by a warm-up and warm-down.
(i) Intensity of work should be two to three times per week, and of 20–30 minutes duration. Resistance should only be used when the adolescent can demonstrate the correct technique. Sets should consist of 6–15 repetitions with 1–3 sets per exercise. The weight should be increased by one to three pounds only after 15 good, complete repetitions can be managed.

Seeing these factors, very few adolescents will be able to appreciate the need for such restrictions, particularly when they have no pain to inform them that an injury is developing.

4. They are more prone to head injuries because of their higher proportion of skin surface area to body volume when compared with adults.
5. They are subject to injuries that are unique to children, due to the softer nature of the bone structure and the growth plates (epiphyses) which are present in each bone.

The growth pattern of the child is the result of a complex interaction of genetics, nutrition, psychology and the possible presence of specific diseases that may hinder the developmental process.

Initially, any developmental irregularities in the child should be referred to the qualified medical professional, whether it be club surgeon, doctor or chartered physiotherapist. This could be anything from an abnormal curvature of the spine, a marked leg length discrepancy, or poor knee, shin and foot posture. All these factors will affect the gait pattern and will gradually produce a chronic problem. Always be alert for the child who complains of a pain which has developed over the last few months, rather than the last couple of days. The sprains and pulls are easy to treat, but the injuries that have had an insidious onset should be thoroughly examined.

In order to help in the initial stages, a reduction in the amount of exercise, training and competition is necessary. Most children who are promising footballers also tend to be good allround athletes, and various school, town, county and national teams in different sports may require their skills. There are many top professional players in sport today who have had to decide at an early age which sport to take up as a career, even though they have played at an international level in two or more different sports.

| Case study | *The following schedule is one I was given by an injured 16 year old footballer still at school, supposedly studying for his GCSE exams five months later. It is one typical of many injured children often seen by the medical team.* |

Table 6.2 *A weekly training diary of an injured schoolboy footballer*

	Morning	Afternoon	Evening
Monday		Basketball practice	Soccer training (town team)
Tuesday	Physical ed. (school)		Soccer training (amateur team)
Wednesday			Basketball match (school)
Thursday		Physical ed. (school)	Soccer training (amateur team)
Friday		Basketball practice	
Saturday	Soccer match (school)	Soccer match (town team)	
Sunday	Soccer match (amateur)		

Eleven activity sessions per week out of a maximum of 21. (Note: A full time professional footballer would only be asked to take part in nine sessions per week.)

He developed a chronic adolescent knee injury and attended for his initial assessment four months after the original symptoms arose. The longest rest period he had taken was two days. In order to give the injury a chance to heal, his leg was immediately immobilized for six weeks to ensure he did not participate in any sport. Rehabilitation following this took a further four months, before he played again.

Similar stories exist in other sports. The following schedule is one I obtained from an injured 12 year old girl in the non-collision sport of swimming.

This young girl was put into the 14–16 years age group for training, as she was far too good for the other swimmers of her own age. She struggled to keep up, and subsequently developed pain under the acromial arch due to a fault that developed in her technique. Three months after the initial injury, and only because she was going

	Morning	Afternoon	Evening
Monday		Physical ed. (school)	Swimming training (club)
Tuesday	Swimming training (club)		Swimming training (club)
Wednesday	Swimming training (club)	Physical ed. (school)	School netball
Thursday			Swimming training (club)
Friday	Swimming training (club)		
Saturday		Gala or swimming training	
Sunday	Swimming training (club)		

Table 6.3 *A weekly training diary of an injured adolescent swimmer*

backwards in relation to her times and failure to win a national event, her parents decided to seek medical help. When the schedule was written down in front of them, they were surprised at the intensity of training expected of their daughter. What brought the matter home was when it was calculated that this girl was performing 24 000 rotational movements of her shoulders each week (12 000 per shoulder).

One of the most worrying statistics in relation to the injured adolescent is the increase in overuse injuries. To be sport-specific at an early age subjects the child to the identical physical stresses of the game each and every day. Quantity (in relation to the amount of training and playing time) technique, posture and equipment have all been found to be causative factors in injury.

In my first season at a football club, I decided to assess the types of injuries occuring in the 16–18 year old age group. Only those that caused a player to miss one game or more were included. I divided the injury types into four categories:

Case study

1. *Genetic injuries – non-football related injuries, e.g. tonsilitis, sinus washouts, chicken pox.*
2. *Trauma injuries – injuries collected due to trauma in the training or game situation.*
3. *Overuse injuries – e.g. stress fractures, osteochondritic conditions.*
4. *No injuries – players who received no serious injuries in that particular season.*

The results were as follows:

Table 6.4 *Injury Classification in Subject Group*

	Genetic	Trauma	Overuse	No injury
%	18	22	44	14

I then compared these results with those from the English Football Association Excellence Scheme Study, which evaluated injuries amongst the elite 16 year old footballers who attended the National School at Lilleshall. The main objective was to look at the degree of overuse injuries in 16–18 year old players who were just starting out in their chosen careers.

Table 6.5 *Comparative overuse injuries from the National School, Lilleshall (UK)*

	1992	1993
Overuse (%)	35	41.6

Virtually identical percentages were noted for overuse injuries, a worrying statistic considering the age range of the players analysed.

There are several factors which must be considered in this area of overuse:

- Research suggests that bone may grow faster than muscle and other soft tissues (Micheli, 1983), which produces a relative muscle tightness and subsequent decrease in flexibility. Other research has shown that flexibility decreases as adolescence is reached (Leighton, 1956 and 1964).
- The development of muscle tissue in young athletes is primarily under hormonal control. Mechanical factors such as muscular tension are necessary for proper growth in the musculotendinous units of each muscle (Williams and Goldspink, 1971). However, muscle tendon imbalances can easily occur due to an inadequacy in strength or flexibility.
- Adolescents can go through growth spurts, which it is suggested increase the possibility of muscle-tendon imbalance problems (Micheli, 1983).
- The growth plates in the bone tissue are at their weakest during puberty and at the end of growth. Acute and chronic injuries can develop in these particular sites and the mixture of growth and injury can dramatically affect the normal development of the bone cells.

  It must also be remembered that different bones ossify at different times, with full maturity between the ages of 18–21 years. Young players up to that age can still therefore develop adolescent-type injuries, a factor often forgotten when trying to diagnose a particular injury.

- Adolescents will change shape at different stages of their development. Alteration of this development by dietary intake and weight training needs constant monitoring.
- Other factors affecting development include posture, hormones, diet, training, exercise, medical disorders, alcohol and drugs.

In order to try and rectify this problem wherever possible, the English Football Association have issued advisory leaflets containing information for parents, coaches and players. Other recommendations include reducing the size of the ball, the playing pitches, the number of players per team and the duration of the match, whilst increasing the number of substitutes depending on the age group involved.

Childrens' injuries

In the child or adolescent, sport is a very important part of their developing years. Injuries to this particular age group can be very different to those of the adult and consideration must be given to the developmental and growing characteristics of such individuals.

Growth injuries can occur in the sporting child and arise in the two main centres responsible for such development:

1. *Epiphysis*
The epiphyses are situated at the ends of the bones and are responsible for longitudinal growth.

2. *Apophyses*
These areas are sited at the attachment of the musculotendinous tissue to the bone, and accommodate the longitudinal growth of the bone by allowing associated lengthening of the muscle and tendon.

These two centres can be affected by the strong pull of the developing muscles and the forces they produce when a child has a growth spurt. They can also be affected by the stresses exerted in playing competitive sport. Length of bone and the soft tissues may alter the leverage system of the surrounding joints, producing excessive loading at one end of the fulcrum point of movement. Other complications include unequal development of bone length, often seen by a leg length discrepancy in the lower limb, and angulation deformities, which produce a cosmetic or functional problem and may need correction in time.

Osteochondrosis is a disease of the growth or ossification centres of the bone. This is stimulated by trauma, with most conditions being present in the spine or lower limb due to the stresses produced by weightbearing, which obviously increase during sporting activity. Following necrosis to the injury site, repair and regeneration occur but leave an alteration in the physical structure of the bone tissue affected. This in turn can produce symptoms in other areas proximal or distal to the problem.

The most common sites in the upper limb (Julsrud, 1988) are:

Table 6.6 *Common sites of osteochondrosis in the upper limb*

Eponym	Anatomical site
Brailsford	Head of radius
Burns	Distal end of ulna
Friedrich	Clavicle
Froehlich	Humeral condyles
Hass	Humeral head
Kienboeck	Lunate
Legg	Epicondyle of the humerus
Panner	Humeral head
Preiser	Scaphoid
Schaefer	Proximal end of radius

In the spine and pelvis (Julsrud, 1988):

Table 6.7 *Common sites of osteochondrosis in the spine and pelvis*

Eponym	Anatomical Site
Buchman	Iliac crest
Calve	Vertebral body
Oldberg/Van Neck	Ischiopubic junction
Pierson	Symphysis pubis
Scheurmann	Lower thoracic/upper lumbar

In the lower limb (Julsrud, 1988):

Table 6.8 *Common sites of osteochondrosis in the lower limb*

Eponym	Location
Blount	Proximal end of the tibia
Diaz/Mouchet	Talus
Felix	Lesser trochanter of the femur
Freiberg	Second metatarsal head
Haglund	Navicular
Iselin	Fifth metatarsal head
Kohler	Patella
Lewin	Distal end of tibia
Mandi-Buchman	Greater trochanter of the femur
Osgood-Schlatter	Tibial tuberosity
Perthes	Head of the femur
Ritter	Head of the fibula
Sever	Calcaneus
Sinding-Larsen-Johansson	Patella, inferior pole
Valtancoli	Ischial tuberosity

Danger

Avascular necrosis is most common in very young children and primarily affects the weightbearing joints. It occurs in the epiphyseal area of the bone due to disease or repeated minor trauma to the main blood supply of the growth plate, the epiphyseal artery. The main sites of possible necrosis include:

1. Hip

Loss of the intracapsular blood vessels from the obturator artery may occur due to trauma or disease. Related disorders include:

Fractured neck of femur
Dislocated hip
Burns
Surgical damage to blood supply of the hip
Perthes disease
Slipped femoral epiphyses
Congenital dislocation of the hip
Sickle cell anaemia.

Other miscellaneous causes include steroids, alcoholism, liver disease, renal disease, radiation and systemic lupus erythematosus.

2. Knee

Associated avascular necrosis is the primary pathological change which occurs in osteochondritis dessicans. This is then followed by secondary changes in the overlying articular cartilage (Hopkinson *et al.*, 1985).

3. Pubic bone

Avascular necrosis of part of the pubic bone is often associated with osteitis pubis.

4. Elbow

Osteochondrosis of the capitulum is also referred to as Panner's disease (Panner, 1929), which occurs due to a vascular impairment. This will eventually lead to an avascular necrotic state.

5. Hand

The carpal bones of the hand are prone to avascular necrosis following trauma due to fracture or dislocation. The articulating surface of the lunate is so extensive that it lends itself to such chronic changes even if the injury is treated promptly and correctly. Spontaneous necrosis may also occur in the lunate, Kienbock's disease, which can be confirmed by a bone scan or, in chronic cases, radiological changes. When diagnosed early, the lunate must be immobilized in the hope that protection from any repetitive stress will allow revascularization. A prompt diagnosis may be difficult due to the lack of initial symptoms.

In the scaphoid, fractures to the waist and proximal pole of the bone may disrupt the vascular supply. Healing can then be slow, or in severe cases, non-union may occur.

Fractures that occur in a child are often referred to as **greenstick fractures**, as the site of injury often resembles that of a snapped twig, with an incomplete fracture line held together by some connecting bone tissue. This will produce angulation of the bone and the degree of displacement will determine the healing time required. Severe trauma may also produce an **avulsion fracture** at the apophyseal attachment of the musculotendinous tissue to the bone, and a period of immobilization will be necessary to prevent long-term problems.

Injuries

In order to prevent repetition of information, specific injury notes will be divided into two sections, in both Chapter 6 and Chapter 7.

1. Chapter 6. Soccer injuries – lower back, pelvis and lower limb.
2. Chapter 7. Rugby injuries – head, neck, trunk, upper limb and pelvis.

Much overlap exists with regard to specific injuries in these two sports and referral to the appropriate section of each chapter will provide the necessary information on a particular injury. A basic reference may be made to the appropriate physiotherapy modalities or rehabilitation schedules used for specific injuries. More detailed notes regarding physiotherapy and rehabilitation modalities are covered in Chapters 4, 5 and 8. Where appropriate surgical notes have been included in Chapters 6 and 7 to give the reader a wider appreciation of injury prognosis. Injuries in both children and adults will be covered in each section.

Lumbar spine

Stress fractures of the lumbar spine most commonly occur at L5 in the neural arch, between the upper and lower posterior apophyseal joints. The onset of the symptoms is identical to that of any other stress fracture in the human body, with an insidious onset of pain which comes on immediately and gradually gets worse. Players with an increased lumbar lordosis are most at risk, as such a posture increases the tendency to posterior element failure. Confirmation of such a diagnosis requires investigative scans, and following a sufficient rest period for the fracture to heal, a carefully structured rehabilitation programme is required to prevent recurrence of the symptoms.

Anterior movement of the vertebral body, a **spondylolisthesis**, is most common at L4 vertebra on L5, or L5 on S1. This is often in association with other spinal pathologies such as disc protrusion, with or without impingement on neural tissue. Symptoms vary from mild backache to severe radiating pain, depending on the grade of shift. Initial care involves a period of reduced activity or total rest in severe cases. Long-term relief from the symptoms depends on the chronic nature of the problem. Early diagnosis coupled with a lumbar stabilization and pelvic re-education exercise programme (Saal and Saal, 1989) can help to produce a more neutral spinal posture. In severe cases, surgery is necessary to stabilize the shift, using either a bone graft or screw fixation.

Disc lesions in soccer players commonly present with a pathology of degeneration followed by protrusion and then prolapse. Players with severe initial symptoms may need a period of bed rest for two to four days. Prolonged bed rest of more than four days may lead to debilitation, and is not

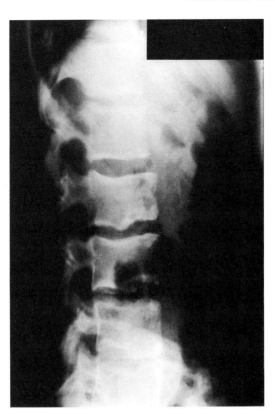

Figure 6.5 Gross degenerative changes of the lumbar spine . . . in a 16 year old soccer player.

recommended for treating acute low back problems in athletes (Bigos and Davis, 1996). Mobilizing, manipulative, exercise and the functional rehabilitation skills of the chartered physiotherapist will be tested to the maximum in order to ensure a full physical and psychological recovery from such an injury.

Degenerative changes in the lumbar spine, **spondylosis**, occur with the natural ageing process of any player. Reduced disc spaces, osteophytic lipping and generalized degenerative changes at numerous levels are commonly seen on the radiographs of both senior and junior professionals. A realistic long-term prognosis should be considered along with the short-term requirements of match fitness.

Referral to Chapter 7, 'Spine', is also suggested with regard to this anatomical site.

Surgical notes

Disc prolapse is no more common in collision sports players than it is in the general population. The vast majority of people with disc prolapses will see a great improvement in their symptoms within four to six weeks, and players can probably start training again as soon as their symptoms permit. However, in people whose symptoms are not resolving within that timespan and who have a definite pathology on MRI scanning, there is little doubt that they improve more rapidly if treated surgically. The key reference in this respect is Weber (1983), which is an old study but not bettered as yet. He randomized people with sciatica and treated half surgically, half conservatively. The surgically-treated group got back to normal activities much more quickly than the conservatively-treated group, although at five and ten years there was no difference.

Spondylolysis is more common in sportsmen and women, although spondylolytic defects occur in an unknown percentage of the general population. The pars defect is a well established source of pain. The treatment of choice in the young athlete without advanced disc degeneration secondary to segmental instability is local *in situ* repair – a fusion of the pars defect. There are a number of techniques for doing this, but all involve putting a compression device across the defect, excising the fibrous tissue from the defect and filling it with bone graft. The results of this procedure are excellent, with over 90% of players returning to sports at their previous level. The outlook is much less rosy in individuals with spondylolytic spondylolisthesis and secondary disc degeneration. If they get to the stage where they have radicular pain, then although surgical treatment in the form of decompression and fusion may return them to a normal sedentary life there is little chance of continuation in sporting activity.

Abdomen
Diagnosing the cause of groin and abdominal pain can be difficult as there may be more than one contributing factor (Ekberg *et al.*, 1988).

Abdominal trauma in many collision sports, such as soccer (Maehlum and Daljord, 1984) and American football (Murphy and Drez, 1987), result in the 10% of abdominal injuries produced in sports-related incidents (Diamond, 1989). These injuries and their management are described in greater detail in Chapter 3, but notice should be taken of any player who develops pain in the associated anatomical area of the **spleen, liver, kidney** and **pancreas**. Other common symptoms of abdominal injury include sweating, thirst, rapid pulse, low blood pressure and haematuria, and such positive signs require urgent medical evaluation. Bed rest, and in severe cases surgery, will be required.

The groin is the portion of the anterior abdominal wall below the level of the anterior superior iliac spines. The most common cause of groin pain is a **strain** of the adductor longus, rectus abdominis, iliopsoas or rectus femoris muscles (Renstrom and Peterson, 1980). These can be acute injuries with all the typical signs of inflammation, or chronic, where a more nagging ache is produced by the presence of scar tissue. In the acute injuries, anti-inflammatories, physiotherapy and a progressive rehabilitation programme will settle many of the immediate problems. The more chronic problems will need referral to the orthopaedic surgeon, who may use a corticosteroid injection (Mozes *et al.*, 1985) or have to resort to a soft tissue release in the more severe cases. Calcification can readily develop into the musculotendinous and tenoperiosteal junctions of such injuries and give chronic long-term symptoms.

No disease of the human body, belonging to the province of the surgeon, requires in its treatment a better combination of accurate, anatomical knowledge with surgical skill than Hernia in all its varieties.

Sir Astley Paston Cooper, 1804 (Nyhus, 1994).

Recognition of the **sportsman's hernia**, or **Gilmore's groin** (Leather, 1989) as it was originally labelled, only occurred from the early 1980s. More modern and anatomically correct names include **indirect hernia, abdominal/pelvic wall disruption** or **groin disruption syndrome**. This is a condition which can presently be repaired surgically, with a recovery period of four to six weeks postoperatively. It is most common in men due to the embryonic descent of the testes, and can cause many months of problems before a firm diagnosis has been made. On the contrary, some players who have such an injury have continued to play for many months following diagnosis, or without recognizing the problem, though this depends on the ability of the individual to cope with the sensation of pain. Functionally, however, it becomes more and more difficult for a player to maintain fitness levels and perform various activities in the game situation. It must also be recognized that such chronic groin pain may be due to an incompetent abdominal wall, with or without a detectable inguinal hernia (Malycha and Lovell, 1992). In terms of reaching a diagnosis, the majority of indications of the problem come in the subjective examination

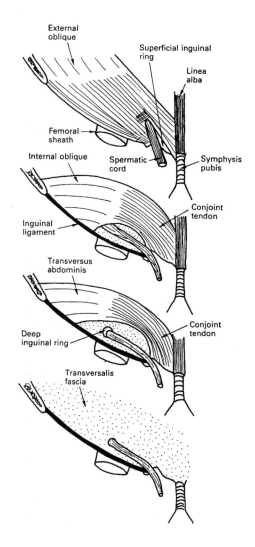

Reproduced with permission from Palastanga *et al.*, 1994

rather than the physical, objective assessment. The symptoms to be aware of include:

- Rarely a specific date of trauma, with gradual onset of the symptoms.
- Dull, intermittent 'toothache' type pain.
- The intensity of pain eases as the level of activity increases and then becomes more severe as fatigue sets in.
- Very rarely are there any associated adductor symptoms.
- 15% of players will complain of bilateral symptoms.
- The pain is aggravated by coughing, sneezing, kicking, sprinting and getting out of bed or the car, particularly the day after a game.
- Physical signs include a dilated superficial inguinal ring on palpation, a positive cough impulse, and tenderness on the affected side. The size of the inguinal ring is not a watertight physical sign, as a tight inguinal ring may suggest the absence of an indirect hernia. Exploratory surgery has often refuted the reliability of this test, with indications of early 'hernia' type changes in the external oblique and posterior wall.

Reference should also be made to Chapter 7, 'Abdomen' injuries for the acute trauma type injury to this area, as opposed to the degenerative condition described above.

Surgical notes

Surgically, the players are usually found to have torn the external oblique aponeurosis, the conjoined tendon, and have a dilated superficial inguinal ring. The two most common types of surgery involve open or laparoscopic techniques. If the muscular opening is too wide to draw together and suture, a patch of Prolene mesh may be used to repair the defect, which allows tissue fluid and fibrous tissue to pass and grow through the holes. Rehabilitation following surgery takes between four and eight weeks, and needs to be functional in relation to the particular sport of the player.

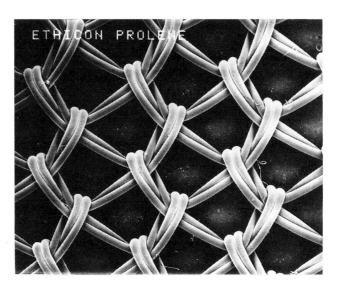

Figure 6.6 Ethicon Prolene mesh used in the repair of the abdominal wall.

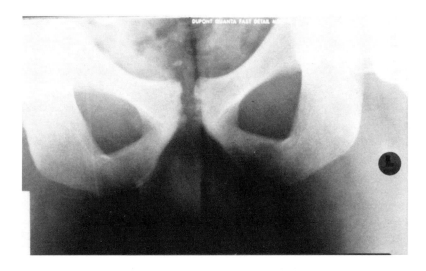

Figure 6.7 Degenerative changes in the symphysis pubis of a 17 year old footballer.

Reference should be made to Chapter 8, 'Abdomen', for a suggested rehabilitation protocol following surgical repair of the abdominal wall.

Treatment notes

Osteitis pubis (Beer, 1924) is an orthopaedic condition which is common in soccer players who are training and/or playing to excess, particularly on hard surfaces. It usually develops following chronic repetitive movement of the symphysis pubis, which produces shearing and tensile forces and subsequent laxity in the symphysis ligaments (Gamble *et al.*, 1986). The player tends to complain of vague low abdominal pain along the pubic bone or in the pubic symphysis. The diagnosis is confirmed by 'stork view' (standing on one leg) radiographs, with a fraying or roughening of the periosteum of the symphysis pubis. Ligamentous instability is present if a step in the joint line exists of 3 mm or more. Computerized tomography (CT) or bone scans might reveal an increase in radionuclide uptake in the region. Rest (which in severe cases may be for several months and up to a year), restructuring the training programme of the player, and the use of anti-inflammatory medication give the best relief.

Pelvis

In the younger soccer player, pain and limitation of movement in the hip joint should always be reguarded with caution. **Epiphyseal, apophyseal** and other stress-related injuries have already been mentioned and should be considered on initial assessment. A **slipped femoral epiphysis**, where a shearing force on the femoral head causes an acute slip of the upper femoral epiphysis, can occur due to trauma or be insidious in onset. Examination will give limitation of all hip movements, particularly medial rotation (Gross, 1984), and a Trendelenberg gait pattern may be noted. X-ray investigations will confirm such a condition. Acute symptoms will require bed rest and traction. A large displacement will require manipulative reduction under anaesthetic with the epiphysis internally fixated with pins.

In the older player, **degenerative changes** in the hip joint cannot be discounted when trying to diagnose chronic joint pain. Results of case studies of former soccer players suggest that a link exists between playing soccer and

Hip

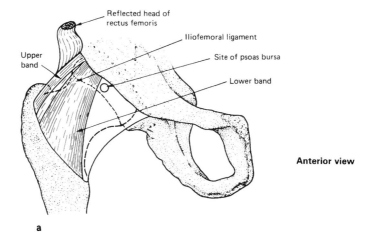

a

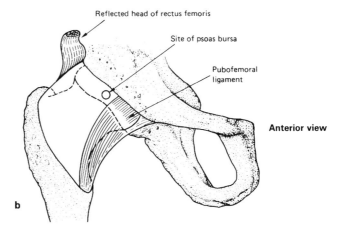

b

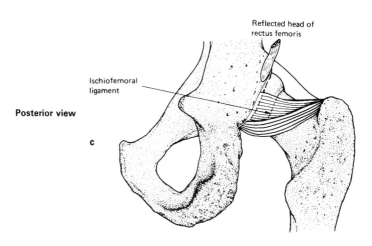

c

Reproduced with permission
from Palastanga *et al.*, 1994

osteoarthritis of the hip (Vingard *et al.*, 1993). The older player is not exempt from the natural ageing process and on top of this is subject to minor injuries, repeated overuse and an increase in bodyweight. Degeneration will begin in the non-weightbearing areas of the acetabulum, as a degree of compression is necessary for bone cell nutrition. Eventually the weight-bearing areas become affected and the protective articular cartilage is eroded, exposing the subchondral bone. The non-weightbearing areas then start to develop osteophytes, or areas of calcification, and the articular surface becomes a roughened, uneven contour. The inflammatory symptoms produced and the compensatory biomechanical changes will produce subjective, objective and functional symptoms. With regard to active and passive movement of the joint, capsular tightening produces limited movement, most noticeably in flexion and medial rotation. Anti-inflammatories, corticosteroid injections, counterirritants, graded mobilizations, passive stretching and adaptations in the training programme of the player can all provide temporary relief and extend playing careers. However, medical advice should be based on sensible counselling in the light of what the future holds, if common sense does not prevail.

Preseason training and fatigue towards the end of the season tend to produce their own special crop of injuries, and **trochanteric, ischial** or **psoas bursitis** is not uncommon. The bursae are present to reduce friction between prominent bony structures and overlying soft tissue. Irritation of the bursal tissue produces a localized inflammatory reaction, with a resulting sensation of 'toothache' type pain. Often there is a training or biomechanical cause to the problem, which needs to be attended to before using an appropriate anti-inflammatory treatment modality such as electrotherapy or prescribed medication. A period of rest from the aggravating activity is imperative to give the bursitis any chance of resolving.

Thigh
A **fracture** of the femur is not a common injury in soccer, but one which can occur in any collision sport. After examination and the appropriate radiological investigations, reduction and internal fixation may be necessary, particularly if early mobilization is sought. Rehabilitation commences once the fracture site is stable, and progresses according to the healing and functional progress of the player.

Case study

During a soccer match, a colleague of mine was treating one of the players in the team. The player had suffered a blow to the lower third of the femur, and as he limped to the touchline, he shouted to my colleague that he had got a 'dead leg' and would try and run the injury off. A minute later, the player realized he would be unable to continue and walked to the touchline. As it was a very cold day he was told to go and have a shower immediately, so he walked straight into the dressing room. Within minutes, this lad's father returned to the side of the pitch to say his son was in a lot of pain and the injury site had started to swell. He was immediately immobilized and transferred to the local hospital, where an X-ray showed he had suffered an undisplaced fracture to the lower one third of his femur. Fortunately for him, as he was only 17, the epiphyseal plate at the distal end of the femur was still present. The fracture line extended from the lateral aspect of the femur to the epiphysis, which then reflected the crack up the

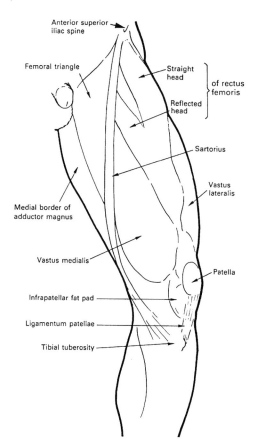

Anterior superior
iliac spine

Femoral triangle

Straight
head

of rectus
femoris

Reflected
head

Sartorius

Vastus
lateralis

Medial border of
adductor magnus

Vastus medialis

Patella

Infrapatellar fat pad

Ligamentum patellae

Tibial tuberosity

Reproduced with permission
from Palastanga *et al.*, 1994

shaft of the femur, so preventing invasion into the knee joint. An intercondylar fracture would obviously have been far more serious than the fracture he suffered, and after internal fixation he returned to play seven months later.

Muscular aches, sprains, strains and **ruptures** of the quadriceps and hamstring muscle groups are common injuries in the world of soccer and should not be taken lightly. These should be subdivided, assessed and treated accordingly.

1. Muscular ache
This is often referred to as delayed onset muscle soreness (DOMS) and develops 24–48 hours after unaccustomed or intense exercise. On investigation, the individual will have a raised creatine phosphokinase (CPK) level and show all the typical signs of an inflammatory reaction. This is due to the breakdown of muscle cells produced by the type or intensity of exercise, and can vary from a mild ache to a disabling pain. Treatment tends to vary from anti-inflammatories and rest to a light stretching or exercise programme, depending on the severity of the symptoms. See also Chapter 2, 'Flexibility'.

2. *Sprains* (mild/grade 1)

3. *Strains* (partial tears/moderate/grade 2)

4. *Ruptures* (complete tears/severe/grade 3)

The later three injury states all involve an acute phase with a sudden onset of immediate and often incapacitating pain. Often the player will say that they had a feeling of tightness prior to the acute symptoms.

Signs and symptoms are best shown in the following table:

Severity	Pain/ spasm	Swelling	Colour/ bruising	Loss of ROM	Loss of Function
Sprain	+	Slight, if any	None	Slight	Slight
Strain	++	Moderate	Possible	Moderate	Moderate
Rupture	+++ (initially)	Severe	Extensive	Severe	Severe*

Table 6.9 *Signs and symptoms of the varying degrees of muscle injury*

(Note that functional activities may be possible from overflow of other active muscle groups.)

Physiotherapy and appropriate active rehabilitation is essential in the acute, subacute, remodelling and functional stages of recovery, as well as in the early stages of full training and playing, in order to reduce the possibility of recurrence. An understanding and appreciation of the active, concentric and eccentric role of the hamstring muscle group is necessary to produce an effective rehabilitation schedule.

In the case of such injuries, certain relative factors have been associated with muscle injury:

(a) Hamstring strength imbalances (Heiser *et al.*, 1984; Burkett, 1970)
(b) Lack of hamstring flexibility (Worrell *et al.*, 1991)
(c) Muscle fatigue (Dorman, 1971)
(d) Insufficient warm-up (Safran *et al.*, 1988).

Rehabilitation following injury should include all the above factors, as evidence exists that all have an influence on the likelihood of hamstring strain (Worrell and Perrin, 1992)

Due to the nature of the game, the thigh is also an area which receives a large number of blows which often lead to **contusions (haematomas)** of different degrees. If the player is able to flex the hip/knee joint in the acute stages up to and beyond 90 degrees, then the injury should settle very quickly. Severe trauma or failure to constantly reassess this type of injury, however, may produce complications.

Danger

Myositis ossificans is a localized tissue reaction that progresses to the formation of non-neoplastic bone and cartilage (Connor, 1983; Gilmer and Anderson, 1959), and can develop if bleeding persists. It is particularly common in adolescents and young males competing in active sport (Ellis and Frank, 1966). The most common muscular sites for such complications are in the brachialis and quadriceps groups (Booth and Westers, 1989). The injury is usually caused by trauma to the muscular area. Calcification of the haematoma which forms, detachment of a periosteal flap, periosteal rupture, metaplasia of the intramuscular connective tissue and individual predisposition are possible theories which have been suggested in such an injury (Ellis and Frank, 1966).

Clinically, the player will complain of moderate to severe pain following trauma, and which has persisted for 10–14 days. The injury site is warm, tender and solid to palpation, with associated loss of active and passive movement. X-ray plates demonstrate the presence of a fibrous mass, often infiltrated with bony callus. Consideration should be given to more serious yet rarer pathologies such as neoplastic bone formation and osteomyelitis, when making the diagnosis of myositis. Rest and observation are important in the early stages. When rehabilitation commences, caution must be shown to prevent aggravation of the condition, with strengthening work only introduced in the final stages. Return to full competition is a slow process and the player is likely to be absent from football for several months, often up to a year in really bad cases. However, few individuals will be left with a functional impairment, with the correct conservative management (Booth and Westers, 1989).

Surgical intervention in the past has given poor results, though some individuals may insert a surgical drain to prevent such a complication from arising. Infection then becomes a possible danger.

An acute **compartment syndrome** can also develop very quickly following trauma in the quadriceps muscle group, with formation of an immediate and developing haematoma. This should be treated as a medical emergency, with regular observation and measurement of the trauma site. In acute, severe cases the insertion of a drain to draw off the excess blood, or surgical release or decompression of the fascia maybe necessary. A simple bruise to the thigh should not be treated lightly by player or physiotherapist.

Knee
The knee joint is the most commonly injured joint in soccer (Ekstrand and Gillquist, 1983a) and is the major cause of permanent total disablement in professional footballers in England and Wales (Windsor, 1997). This is in the main due to the anatomical configuration, for as a condylar joint there is no bony interlock between the femur or tibia, so there is a far greater dependancy on the meniscii, ligaments and muscular tissue to provide some form of structural support. Soccer, as with the majority of collision sports, requires the player to twist the upper body over a fixed foot, and this is a common description a player uses when describing how the injury occurred.

A **haematoma** to the knee joint can produce marked swelling and loss of function very quickly, but a thorough subjective and objective assessment should discount any major injury which may have been suspected from the immediate inflammatory symptoms.

Severe trauma to the patella can produce a **fracture**, which may require surgery to fixate the injury. Immobilization and rehabilitation can be a lengthy procedure, and the injury often requires constant monitoring on returning to full function to reduce the possibility of long-term complications.

Patellofemoral pain is one of the most common symptoms arising from the knee joint (Tria *et al.*, 1992), particularly in the adolescent player and numerous causes involving malalignment of the patella have been suggested. These include:

1. Patella alta (Insall *et al.*, 1976)
2. Patella glide (McConnell, 1986)
3. Patella tilt (McConnell, 1986)
4. Patella rotation (McConnell, 1986)
5. Antero-posterior tilt of the patella (Arno, 1990).

Chondromalacia patellae and growing pains are diagnostic labels given to individuals with such problems, but fail to directly influence the injury. More commonly the symptoms are due to abnormalities of patella tracking or an increase in retropatellar pressure. Arthroscopic surgery may show no evidence of joint damage in many cases (Bentley and Dowd, 1983). Those that have positive findings may not be relevant to the pathology of the injury (Bentley and Dowd, 1983). Treatment is dependent on an accurate and thorough examination. Rest and anti-inflammatory medication, with relevant strengthening, mobilizing or flexibility work, can only be prescribed after such an assessment.

Trauma to the articular cartilage and subchondral bone will produce different variations of osteochondral injuries. **Osteochondral fractures** occur most commonly around the lateral femoral condyle, particularly in adolescents. Acute trauma with a rotational component is the most common mechanism of such an injury. Radiographic views will confirm such a diagnosis.

Osteochondritis Dessicans must be differentiated from the osteochondral fracture as this is a more gradual process which involves diseased, ischaemic bone. Trauma is thought to initiate such a process, but other contributory factors include genetics, anomalies of ossification, excessive stress to the area and repeated microtrauma. The most common sites are on the condylar surfaces of the femur, particularly the medial, at its outer surface. As the stages of ischaemia and avascular necrosis occur, symptoms depend on whether the osteochondral fragment becomes detached. If the fragment remains attached symptoms may include:

- Generalized dull, aching pain
- Pain worse on activity and after exercise
- Effusion after activity
- Positive radiographs, MRI scans.

If a bony fragment becomes detatched from the condylar site, the symptoms may differ and include:

- Intermittent periods of pain
- Constant effusion

- Locking or giving way of the joint
- Positive radiographs, particularly tunnel or intercondylar views.

Management is dependent on the severity of the problem. Acute cases will often settle with rest and non weightbearing rehabilitation, with a gradual increase in the degree of stress as the symptoms improve. Stubborn or more chronic cases may require arthroscopic surgery to remove the loose bony fragment. Standard chondroplasty or abrasion chondroplasty techniques attempt to smooth over the damaged surface of bone, and the underlying bone may then be drilled to allow bone marrow cells to infiltrate the area. These cells then produce fibrocartilage, which can fill the defect but is inferior to normal articular cartilage. It may also be possible to drill through the lesion and fixate the area with wires or pins, particularly if a large segment of bone is involved. Further advances in surgical procedures for osteochondritic conditions are imminent, and tissue implantation using the player's own tissues cultured in the laboratory, a process known as autologous chondrocyte implantation (Brittberg *et al.*, 1994), is developing, although such surgical techniques and rehabilitation programmes are in their early stages.

Osteochondromatosis is another variation of degenerative changes in the adolescent sportsperson. This is a benign tumour which affects the synovial membrane. Cartilage and bone tissue will form in the synovial fronds, and on arthroscopy, 'snow storm' symptoms can be seen.

All of these degenerative disorders may be precursors to **osteoarthritis** of the knee, a common long-term problem in soccer players (Klunder *et al.*, 1980). Surgical intervention to remove torn menisci, and trauma to ligamentous tissue can also lead to degenerative changes in either the patellofemoral joint or either compartment of the knee joint. Rest, anti-inflammatory medication and physiotherapy will help in the short-term. Surgery is indicated in individuals who loose mobility due to the pain and stiffness produced. Arthroscopic debridement of the joint, osteotomy or knee replacement may be necessary, depending on the severity of the symptoms.

Danger

Osteoarthritis is a common problem that develops in sports people secondary to sports injury. The initial changes that occur are often painless and show none of the other symptoms such as swelling or bony deformity that are consistent with such a condition. It tends to occur initially at the periphery of the joint, in the non-weightbearing areas. Over time this then extends into the weightbearing areas, appearing as small cavities of erosion between the layers of cartilage fibres which will extend to the articular surface. Loose fragments may become detached and enter the joint space. Such changes will irritate the synovial membrane, and it is at this point that a player may be conscious of the onset of injury. The cartilage tissue becomes weaker due to the reduction in quality of proteoglycan and collagen cells, and it is affected by compression and tension forces. Radiographs will show a reduction in joint space. Necrosis of the subchondral bone cells encourages cyst formation, and osteophytes form at the periphery of the joint. As these develop, symptoms may arise due to irritation of the joint space or surrounding soft tissues. Thickening of the synovial membrane and joint capsule produce the more common signs of inflammation, with a resultant loss of active function in the diseased joint.

Radiographs and scans of many players involved in collision sports may show bone and soft tissue changes due to degeneration. It is only when subjective and objective symptoms develop which affect normal activity, that they are of any functional relevance. Early recognition of such problems, however, does allow the physiotherapist to introduce rehabilitation work which will reduce the possibility of the symptoms becoming more severe. Individual schedules may be necessary to avoid aggravation of the symptoms caused by training surfaces and certain exercise drills which increase the stress on the area. Soccer players are prone to such problems in the hip, knee and ankle joints (Vingard *et al.*, 1993; Klunder *et al.*, 1980).

Soft tissue injury to the knee joint is very rarely isolated to one particular tissue and constant reassessment is necessary as the acute symptoms subside. An injury to this area may include any combination of the following:

1. *Medial Meniscus*
2. *Lateral Meniscus*

Meniscal injuries produce a wide variety of isolated and complex knee injuries in the soccer player. Injury usually occurs due to lateral rotation of the flexed knee in a weightbearing position. Associated symptoms include pain (which becomes more localized to the joint line as the acute symptoms subside) swelling, locking or clicking of the joint, instability and positive signs on various manual tests such as McMurray or Apley.

In the acute and swollen knee neither manual test is possible due to the degree of pain and oedema.

Assessment notes

With McMurray's test, the hip and knee need to be placed into full passive hip and knee flexion with the player lying supine. The tibia is then rotated, depending on which meniscus is being investigated. To test the medial meniscus, the tibia is laterally rotated and abducted; the lateral meniscus is tested by placing the tibia into a medially rotated and adducted starting position. The physiotherapist places the fingers over the appropriate medial or lateral joint line, and the knee is then slowly extended. A positive test is suggested in the presence of an audible or palpable painful click over the joint line.

With Apley's test, the player is placed lying prone, and the offending knee flexed to 90°. Downwards compression and rotation of the knee is applied by the physiotherapist; pain on testing suggests a meniscal tear. In the same position, upwards traction and rotation can then be applied; pain on testing suggests a ligamentous strain.

Anatomically it is suggested that most tears should occur in the medial meniscus, as it is far more rigid and is anchored by the associated collateral ligament, unlike the lateral menisus. In soccer, however, lateral meniscus injuries tend to be as common due to emphasis of both medial and lateral rotation in performing the skills of the game. Associated cyst lesions and the complication of degenerative changes in the lateral compartment encourage a longer rehabilitation period than more orthodox medial tears. In the adolescent,

ANTERIOR

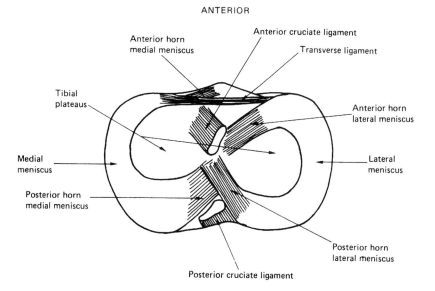

a

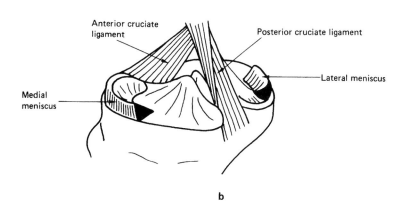

b

Reproduced with permission
from Palastanga *et al.*, 1994

symptoms may develop from the congenital malformation of the meniscii, usually the lateral meniscus, which is discoid in shape instead of the normal crescent shape. The adult male is more prone to meniscal problems between the ages of 21–40, with associated anterior cruciate injury between the ages of 21–30 years (Pochling *et al.*, 1990); females have a peak incidence between the ages of 11–20 years (Pochling *et al.*, 1990). Various types of tears can occur in the meniscus – peripheral, radial, horizontal, longitudinal, transverse, degenerative – and treatment and recovery is based totally on the surgical examination via the arthroscope.

Surgical notes   Total meniscectomies can produce short- and long-term complications such as instability and osteoarthritis, which may be avoided if only a partial meniscectomy is possible. Assessment and treatment with the more modern arthroscope is therefore preferred to the older open arthrotomy (Muckle, 1988) or arthrogram, which were invasive and often inaccurate in their findings. Magnetic resonance imaging (MRI) is a more popular procedure, but much debate exists about the use of MRI as opposed to arthroscopy and examination under anaesthetic (EUA). The former is noninvasive, quick, and can diagnose other pathology, yet only has an accuracy of 72–92% (Fischer et al., 1991). It is a purely diagnostic tool and is not available in some medical establishments. Arthroscopy is approximately twice as expensive as MRI scanning and carries the disadvantages associated with any operative procedure. It does, however, provide the surgeon with an accurate, objective, diagnostic and surgical instrument.

In terms of its diagnostic use, an arthroscopic examination has become an important adjunct to the clinical and radiological examination procedure in the diagnosis of relevant joint conditions. Once the patient has been anaesthetized, an initial EUA allows the surgeon to apply certain test procedures without any conscious resistance from the patient, who may give a false physical response under normal conditions. The arthroscopic procedure involves filling the joint cavity with saline solution, and a cannula and telescope are entered at the appropriate anatomical site. By correctly manoeuvring the telescope and using different sites of entry, the surgeon is able to gain an almost three-dimensional view of the internal aspect of the joint. The information gained from any visual indications can be further enhanced by probing any bone or soft tissue structures with an instrument introduced to the joint via another site. In surgical arthroscopy, the surgeon is able to perform a vast array of intra-articular procedures due to the array of power shavers, probes, punches, scissors and hooks which can be introduced.

A repair is possible if the damage is within 3 mm of the meniscosynovial junction, particularly if there is an associated anterior cruciate rupture, as this is the most vascular portion of the meniscus (Barber and Stone, 1985; Arnoczky and Warren, 1982). This decreases the possibility of degeneration in the articular cartilage (Graf et al., 1987). Rehabilitation will vary from four to eight weeks, depending on the nature of the tear, other associated problems and the age of the player. Success rates have been reported in some cases to be as high as 90% (DeHaven et al., 1989) and with an associated reconstruction of the ACL, the rate of meniscal healing has reached 94% (Buseck and Noyas, 1991). This higher success rate in what is a far more serious joint injury is thought to be due to the haemarthrosis caused by the reconstruction, which acts as a large 'fibrin clot' and thereby improves the ability of the meniscus to heal.

Meniscal transplantation has been used in individuals whose menisci have been damaged through trauma or who have undergone a previous meniscectomy. The short-term functional results are optimistic, with good or satisfactory results in 85–95% of patients (Veltri et al., 1994; Milachowski et al., 1989). The long-term success of this procedure will be based upon the effects of the degenerative process seen in post-meniscectomy comparatives.

3. Anterior Cruciate Ligament (ACL)

Any player who suffers disruption to the ACL may suffer instability of the knee joint, which prevents them from training or playing due to interference in functional activities by 'giving way' of the joint. The history of onset tends to be one of the knee collapsing, with a combination of abduction and rotation of the tibia on the femur. This mechanism of injury can also injure other medial and lateral structures, with associated complete tears of the medial collateral ligament and the medial meniscus labelled as **O'Donoghues triad**. Diagnosis can be made from a subjective and objective assessment and reinforced by more direct investigations, such as MRI scans or arthroscopy. The two most reliable manual tests are:

(a) The Lachman test (Cross and Crichton, 1987)
     This has been shown to be highly reliable (Donaldson *et al.*, 1985) and is performed with the player lying supine. The knee is held in 20° of knee flexion by the assessor (Iversen *et al.*, 1988), with one hand stabilizing the femur and the other applying an anterior force to the proximal and posterior aspect of the tibia. If anterior movement, as compared to that of the non-injured leg, is felt then the test is positive.

Case study	*In practice, I much prefer to perform a modified version of this test, referred to as the 'Reverse' Lachman test (Rebman, 1988). In this test, the player is put into prone lying and the knee is moved to 20° of flexion. By positioning both index fingers over the tibial tubercle and both thumbs around the back of the calf to hold the tibia, an anterior force can then be applied by the physiotherapist to the joint to assess the degree of forward displacement. The advantage of this position is that players are able to completely relax their hamstrings and so prevent resistance on examination, which may give a false sensation of stability to the injury site (Iversen et al., 1989). Also, the player with extremely large muscular legs or the examiner with small hands may have practical difficulties in performing the classical Lachman's test, and this modification provides an alternative method of testing.*

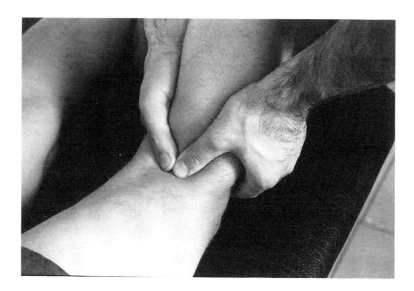

Figure 6.8 Reverse Lachman's procedure.

(b) The pivot shift test

   In order to produce a valid result, the pivot shift test needs to be performed with the player under a general anaesthetic, so that protective muscle spasm can be eliminated (Donaldson et al., 1985). The injured leg is placed in full extension, and the examiner grasps the ankle with one hand and applies a valgus force to the lower lateral aspect of the femur with the other. The tibia is positioned into maximum medial rotation with the distal hand and the knee is slowly flexed with the valgus force applied through the proximal hand. A positive result applies if sudden subluxation of the lateral tibiofemoral compartment is seen or felt as the tibia is reduced by the tension in the iliotibial band.

Other symptoms that tend to present themselves with such an injury include swelling, which may be a haemarthrosis (72%, DeHaven, 1980), temperature and loss of function.

Surgical notes

The ACL ligament provides 86% of the ligamentous restraint to anterior-posterior draw and 30% to medial displacement in the human knee (Palastanga et al., 1994). From this it has been recognized that the ACL is the most common cause of knee instability, although it must be remembered that not all individuals with ACL-deficient knees will develop functional instability. Primary repair of the acute ACL rupture has been attempted, but produced inconsistent static and functional results (Feagin and Curl, 1976; Feagin et al., 1972). In many acute cases such a procedure is not possible, as the ligament shreds in its substance. In the chronic ACL-deficient knee, numerous intra-articular substitution or extra-articular tenodesis procedures have been used. The object of these procedures is to prevent anterior subluxation of the tibia on the femur and to return functional stability to the knee joint. The intra-articular substitutions have utilized the patella tendon, semitendonosis, gracilis, tensa fascia lata, cadaveric allografts, Dacron, Goretex and carbon grafts (O'Brien et al., 1991; Zoltan et al., 1988; Warren-Smith and Forster, 1987; Butler et al., 1980, 1979; Eriksson, 1976). The extra-articular procedures consist of some form of tenodesis using the tensa fascia-iliotibial tract, often described as a MacIntosh procedure (Wilson et al., 1990). Some reconstructive approaches combine the two procedures, though it is suggested that there is limited indication for an extra-articular associated procedure if a strong intra-articular graft with firm fixation is used (Aglietti et al., 1992). Arthroscopically-assisted ACL reconstructions provide significant advantages over open techniques because of reduced surgical trauma, better visibility for the surgeon and more accurate tunnel placement for insertion of the graft (Raab et al., 1993; Jackson and Jennings, 1988). Player cooperation is vital if the whole procedure is to be a success. Players who do not exhibit instability or only suffer a partial tear of the ACL (anteromedial band) may make a good recovery with a functional rehabilitation programme, but statistics show that very few ever return to an equivalent level of competition with such care (Bonamo et al., 1990).

Treatment notes

A suggested rehabilitation programme for the ACL-reconstructed knee is included in Chapter 8, 'Lower limb variables'.

4. *Posterior Cruciate Ligament (PCL)*

This is the strongest ligament about the knee joint and, as such, ruptures are relatively uncommon when compared to those of the ACL. The most common mode of injury is a direct blow to the anterior aspect of the shin with the knee flexed, causing posterior movement of the tibia. The player may continue to play, but following the incident will complain of pain at the posterior aspect of the knee with very minimal swelling of the joint. Chronic cases will often demonstrate hyperextension of the knee, though the pain and effusion present in acute cases reduces the reliability in every instance. Manual examination tests include:

(a) Posterior 'sag'
    A positive finding is demonstrated when lateral inspection of the 90 degree, flexed knee produces an apparent disappearence of the tibial tubercle due to the gravity assisted posterior displacement of the tibia on the femur (Clancy, 1989).
(b) Posterior draw sign
    With the knee flexed to 90°, posterior movement of the tibia on the femur when compared to the non injured knee indicates a positive result. The test should be repeated with the foot in a neutral, externally and internally rotated position. A positive test occurs when posterior displacement and lateral rotation is evident in the externally rotated position, but is extinguished in the internally rotated position. Great care must be taken not to misinterpret the results of this test, as a positive anterior draw may point to an ACL rupture rather than a PCL problem, when anterior movement is only possible due to the gravity produced sag.

Surgical notes It has been reported that the PCL is responsible for 95% of the total resisting force to posterior displacement of the tibia (Butler *et al.*, 1980). The player with a chronic PCL rupture more often complains of disability rather than a true instability. A state of pseudo-instability often arises in that they suffer from a sudden sharp pain on making contact with an area of erosion on the medial femoral condyle.

Treatment very much depends on the clinical findings. In dislocated bony avulsions, reduction and internal fixation is required (Barton *et al.*, 1984) with immobilization for up to six weeks before commencing rehabilitation. Non displaced avulsions will often recover with conservative care. Isolated ruptures of the PCL are treated conservatively in the early stages, as instability tends to be unidirectional. Muscle strength is of great importance in such individuals, as the majority will make a full recovery with the appropriate rehabilitation schedule (Parolie and Bergfield, 1986).

As with ACL ruptures, various intra- and extra-articular surgical procedures have been used to rectify the ruptured PCL ligament. This is particularly so in PCL ruptures which are associated with additional soft tissue damage and which produce a multidirectional instability. These have involved using gracilis, semitendonosis, semimembranosis, iliotibial band, popliteus, the medial head of gastrocnemius, or the medial one third of the patella tendon (Eriksson *et al.*, 1986, Clancy *et al.*, 1983; Ogata, 1980; Trickey, 1980; McCormick *et al.*, 1976).

Various synthetic materials have also been used, but the theoretical advantages still outweigh the objective postoperative data available (Zoltan *et al.*, 1988).

5. *Medial Collateral Ligament (MCL)*
A valgus force to the flexed or extended knee with associated lateral rotation is one of the most frequent mechanisms of injury in soccer, resulting in damage to the medial structures. Injuries to the MCL can be divided into three grades:

(a) Grade 1 – valgus testing on a flexed knee (30°) produces pain, but no laxity.
(b) Grade 2 – identical testing produces 0–5 mm (mild) or 6–10 mm (moderate) opening of the medial joint line, with pain throughout. Some resistance will be felt at the end of range.
(c) Grade 3 – very little pain may be felt due to the completeness of the tear, with a degree of laxity greater than 10 mm. No resistance, or a 'soft' endpoint, may be felt.

Isolated grade 1 and 2 injuries are treated conservatively, with a removable brace to temporarily immobilize the injury and yet allow access for acute care (Ballmer and Jakob, 1988). More active rehabilitation can commence as the pain subsides, and the brace can be discarded as soon as good muscle control is obtained. Recovery time will vary from two to six weeks, during which time a full functional rehabilitation programme should have been completed successfully before returning to full competition.

Surgical notes

Ossification of the femoral attatchment of the MCL, **Pelligrini-Steida syndrome**, can occur following such a grade of injury. Much controversy exists regarding the operative and conservative approaches for a third degree tear. The advantages of early motion on preventing adverse articular cartilage changes and on limiting muscle atrophy is significant, particularly when one considers the fact that figures of up to 35% thigh muscle atrophy have been recorded following a third degree sprain of the MCL (Kannus, 1988). Older studies advocate surgery (Marshall and Rubin, 1977; Hughtson and Eilers, 1973), whereas more recent studies suggest conservative care may be the best option (Indelicato, 1983; Hastings, 1980). In sportspersons, however, surgery tends to be the choice of treatment, as a more thorough investigation of other relevant soft tissue structures is possible and the medial ligament and capsule can be tightened, which should reduce any instability in the joint long-term. Also the individual can be more positive in terms of the rehabilitation programme than if a period of immobilization is necessary before activity can begin.

6. *Lateral Collateral Ligament (LCL)*
The LCL injury can again be graded as the MCL, and tends to occur due to a varus force associated with internal rotation. Associated direct damage to the lateral meniscus is uncommon as the two structures are not connected, unlike in the medial aspect. Grade 1 and 2 injuries are treated in the same way as such strains of the MCL, with conservative care being the best approach. The most common site of a grade 3 rupture is from the fibular head attachment, and treatment can again be either conservative (Kannus, 1989) or surgical.

7. *Arcuate Complex (AC)*

Injury to the lateral compartment to produce posterolateral instability of the knee joint is rare, but it should be considered on examination (DeLee *et al.*, 1983b), particularly if there is no indication of ACL, MCL or PCL injury. The AC consists of the arcuate ligament, lateral collateral ligament, lateral head of gastrocnemius and the popliteus tendon. These structures can be tested using external rotational or posterolateral draw procedures.

Very little evidence exists for a surgical approach in this situation, with the bulk of the literature encouraging functional rehabilitation. Any operative procedure that has been used involves primary repair of the relevant structures, with moderate success (Hughtson and Jacobson, 1985; DeLee *et al.*, 1983b).

Inflammation of the patella tendon, **patella tendinitis**, can often result from a sudden increase in the intensity of training, or from using a different playing surface to the norm. Rest – that dreaded word to a player – physiotherapy and corticosteroid injection are the normal courses of treatment. Chronic cases may require surgery, and even though the external scar is small, recovery time is never less than eight weeks in order to give this weightbearing injury the chance to make a full recovery.

Shin

Fracture of the tibia and/or **fibula** are common major fractures in soccer players, which may be further complicated if the bone ends pierce the skin to create an open, unstable fracture. Good bony alignment is necessary to prevent long-term complications, and may require internal fixation or bone grafting in severe cases. A thorough rehabilitation programme is essential both physically and mentally following such an injury, and it may take up to 12 months for a full physical recovery. Confidence in the solid state of the fracture site is essential if the player is to make a full functional recovery.

Anterior, posterior and **lateral compartment syndromes** involve pain on exercise due to a build up of fluid in the relevant muscle groups, which gradually increases the intramuscular compartment pressure (Gershuni *et al.*, 1982). Hard training surfaces, change in footwear or a large increase in training workload are possible causes of such an injury. On examination, the affected group of muscles may be tight and swollen, with pain on active or passive movement of the ankle

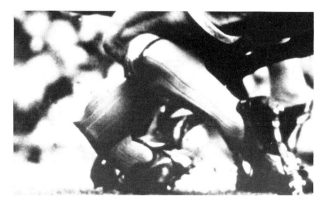

Figure 6.9 Fractured tibia and fibula.

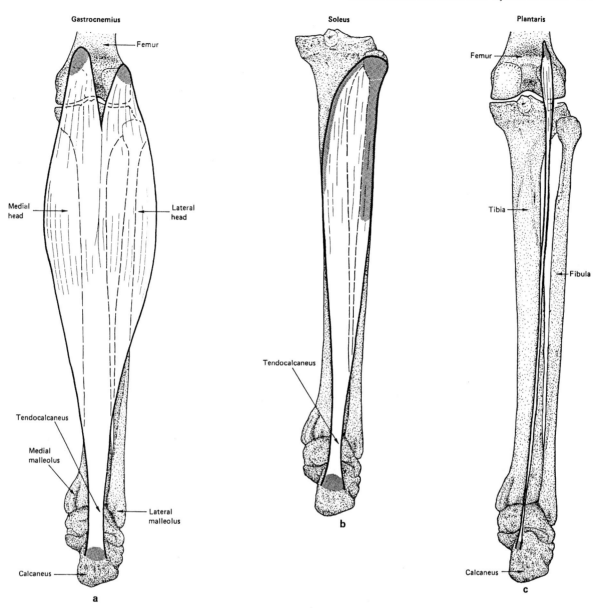

Gastrocnemius

Femur

Medial head

Lateral head

Tendocalcaneus

Medial malleolus

Lateral malleolus

Calcaneus

a

Soleus

Tendocalcaneus

b

Plantaris

Femur

Tibia

Fibula

Calcaneus

c

Reproduced with permission from Palastanga *et al.*, 1994

joint. If neurovascular structures are affected, the symptoms may include numbness to the distal parts of the toes, cramping of the particular muscles, or in rare cases a dropped foot. Involvement of the popliteal artery should always be considered in the differential diagnosis of such players, as embolization and occlusion may produce severe consequences. Rest, flexibility work and the use of orthotics may provide sufficient relief. In the more chronic cases, Doppler testing will demonstrate how much pressure is being created and will determine the need for surgical intervention. Acute cases of compartment syndrome which are caused by the development of a haematoma following a blow to the relevant muscle group should be treated as a medical emergency, and may require fascial release or decompression.

Tibial and fibular **stress fractures** are the final stages of an overuse injury, and occur due to poor biomechanics, excessive training loads, improper footwear, or changes in ground reaction forces if training or playing on an unaccustomed surface. Subjectively, the player will describe a history of increased pain on weightbearing exercise which improves with rest, although there is no initial history of significant trauma. Physical findings may include pinpoint tenderness, soft tissue swelling and a painless active and resisted range of movement. Radiographs, tomography and bone scans may be positive only after a certain time period post-injury, so a thorough examination is necessary in the early stages. Conservative treatment programmes are very successful, with a progressive weightbearing rehabilitation programme. Follow-up radiographs or bone scans will show when the lesion has healed, although a physical and functional assessment may give a more realistic picture of the stage of healing.

Muscle sprains, strains and **ruptures** of the calf occur on a fairly regular basis and need to be treated with appropriate acute and chronic modalities. A full functional rehabilitation programme is necessary to prevent a recurrent problem, particularly in the over enthusiastic player.

Injuries occurring in the Achilles tendon range from **peritendinitis** to total **rupture**. Diagnosis of the severity of the tendinitis can be made from the subjective and objective histories. A history of pain in the morning which eases throughout the day or with exercise, and fails to resolve with rest, is classified as **peritendinitis**. This involves trauma to both the paratendon as well as the tendon. Should the symptoms worsen over the day and on exercising, **tendinitis**, where the damage is isolated to the tendon itself, is the diagnosis. These two conditions are often initiated by a number of factors which need to be addressed before any treatment regime is going to be effective. A sudden increase in training load, different footwear or chronic repetitive exercise are all situations which can create excessive loading on the tendon. Excessive pronation of the foot can be a contributing factor as the excessive transverse plane movements produced can cause damage in the tendon fibres which are plaited, as opposed to those that interdigitate. Corrective orthoses may help in such an individual (Clement *et al.*, 1984). Alternative treatments include various physiotherapy modalities, active rehabilitation related to the rate of tissue healing, anti inflammatories or surgery. Injection of corticosteroids is avoided as there have been numerous reports of a link between injection and **total rupture** (Halpern *et al.*, 1977; Unverferth and Olix, 1973). Tendon degeneration, peritendinous adhesions, diminished blood supply or previous partial rupture may well be precipitating causes of complete rupture. Clinical symptoms include immediate pain, with the player stating that it 'felt as though I had been shot by a sniper in the crowd'. A positive squeeze test (player in prone lying with foot over the edge of the bed, 'squeeze' the calf muscle and test is positive if there is no movement of the foot), acute inflammatory signs, loss of function (unable to perform a calf raise, or hop in a weightbearing position on the injured leg) and a palpable gap at the site of the lesion, are all clinical symptoms of which to be aware. Surgical repair or immobilization are the immediate treatment regimes available, and full rehabilitation may well take up to a year.

Ankle injuries are mainly of the **soft tissue** type, 85% of them being sprains and 80% of those involving the lateral ligament (Adams, 1981). These injuries have been categorized into 3 grades of injury (Cass and Norrey, 1984):

Ankle

1. Grade 1 – a mild stretch of the lateral ligaments with no instability and mild functional incapacity.
2. Grade 2 – a moderate but incomplete tear of the ligaments with minimal instability and moderate functional incapacity.
3. Grade 3 – a complete tear of the ligaments with objective instability and a loss of function.

Ligamentous rupture with instability will require radiological stress testing before any decision is made as to the necessity of surgery to reduce the instability. It is recommended that the physical examination and specific diagnosis be delayed until four to five days after the initial injury, as the range of movement in the joint is in the main determined initially by the degree of pain, rather than any specific soft tissue damage (Van Dijk et al., 1996).

The lateral ligament complex is the most common site of injury due to the mechanics involved in the classical ankle sprain of plantar flexion combined with inversion. Immobilization and/or internal fixation will be necessary in the unstable ankle, with the rate of recovery very much dependent on good bony alignment and soft tissue repair, as well as a full functional rehabilitation programme. Minor ligamentous injuries will obviously recover far more quickly, but avoid a tunnel vision approach to such injuries. Assessment of knee, subtalar and midtarsal structures is essential at the initial and all follow up assessments, as other pathology can easily be missed with the obvious injuries to the soft tissues of the talocrural joint.

A combination of mechanical and functional instability in the ankle joint is the most commonly reported indication for surgical intervention. These reconstruction procedures involve two different approaches:

Surgical notes

1. *Anatomical*
Anatomical reconstructions involve use of the damaged ligamentous tissue in the repair procedure. This can occur many years after the initial injury (Brostrom, 1966), with good reports of successful recoveries (Althoff et al., 1988).

2. *Non-anatomical*
These techniques involve using other soft tissue structures of the body, such as the tensa fascia lata or peroneal tendon structures, to act as secondary ligament tissue at the injury site. The most common approaches include the Watson-Jones, Evans and Chrisman-Snook. Short-term results are excellent, but in the long-term the failure rate has been reported to be in excess of 50% (Karlsson et al., 1988). This may well be due to the fact that these procedures do not restore the normal biomechanical movement pattern of the joint.

The tendency is for this type of approach to be used following failure of an anatomical approach, in the presence of moderate arthritis or excessively lax joint structures, as stability following surgery has been recorded at greater than 95% (Chrisman amd Snook, 1969). A criticism of this approach is that it often results in restricted subtalar movement.

Danger

Following certain surgical procedures a neuroma can occasionally develop at the operation site, delaying a full recovery of the injury. In non-anatomical reconstructions of the lateral complex of the ankle joint, the development of a neuroma occurred in 16% of the patients (Chrisman and Snook, 1969).

Various sites of injury could be affected should a **fracture** occur in and around the ankle joint. These may include the following:

1. Displacement of the malleoli, which will disturb the joint mortice
2. Fracture dislocations
3. Fracture of the talus
4. Fracture of the calcaneus
5. Diastasis of the inferior tibiofibular joint
6. Avulsion fractures
7. Stress fractures
8. Undisplaced fractures.

Examination and X-ray investigations will usually confirm the problem. The stubborn soft tissue injury that fails to resolve after a number of weeks may need repeat views or more powerful scanning. Callus formation at the site of pain may be the first positive radiological indication of an undisplaced crack fracture. If the player has been weightbearing and the fracture is stable, a greater length of recovery time than first expected is the only step necessary. More routine fractures will require a period of immobilization, although this will be kept to a minimum to prevent unnecessary complications arising.

Traction or avulsion **osteophytes** on the anterior margins of the tibial/talus articulation arise due to the quick and forceful dorsi- and plantar-flexion of the ankle joint, which is a basic functional requirement of any soccer player. Commonly known as 'footballers ankle', the player will complain of chronic aching pain, stiffness in the morning and will have a limited range of movement, particularly dorsi-flexion. Normal gait pattern is usually unaffected and symptoms only become apparent on an increase in activity. Lateral and mortice X-ray films often confirm the situation and arthroscopic surgery can be performed to remove the osteophytic bone (Hawkins, 1988) and so eliminate any joint impingement which is occurring due to the bony growths. A short period of immobilization is followed by a full rehabilitation schedule and recovery is usually complete within six to eight weeks.

Articular cartilage lesions can occur on the medial and lateral aspects of the talar dome, following a combination of rotational and dorsi- or plantar-flexion forces at the ankle joint.

Surgical notes

Laterally based lesions tend to be fairly superficial, involving only the articular cartilage, and hence rarely heal, whilst the medially-based lesions tend to be deeper, often extending down to the subchondral bone, and because of this have a higher chance of going on to satisfactory union. In view of the small amount of clearance between the joint surfaces in the ankle, players with such lesions very rarely present with locking and usually present simply with pain or just mild discomfort, swelling or occasional giving way of the ankle joint. The diagnosis tends to be made on clinical grounds, as neither bone, CT or MRI scans can be relied upon to pick up the articular cartilage lesions, although they are more successful in picking up the combined osteochondral lesions. The site and nature of the lesions will determine whether or not they can be fixed back in position, preferably arthroscopically, with or without a transmalleolar approach, or whether the articular fragment alone needs to be removed and the surrounding surface smoothed.

With the high frequency of ankle injuries or 'sprains' sustained not only in collision sports but in normal daily activities, it is not surprising that a wide range of other soft tissue pathologies can result, and although they can cause significant morbidity they often remain undiagnosed. Arthroscopic assessment and/or surgery is often the desired approach in such instances.

In the ankle, as in the knee, congenital or traumatic **plicae** can develop and cause soft tissue impingement. Perhaps the most common lesion is the so-called 'meniscoid lesion' which commonly forms in the anterolateral gutter of the ankle between the lateral side of the talus and the articular surface of the malleolus. This lesion commonly follows a forced inversion injury with resulting capsular tear and/or lateral ligament damage. In the healing process, whilst the foot is rested and immobilized, the lining may become over-active and on subsequent mobilization of the ankle joint, the hypertrophied lining may become trapped between the lateral dome of the talus and the lateral malleolus. This condition frequently presents with pain and discomfort over the anterolateral part of the ankle, just in front of the lateral malleolus. The terminology 'meniscoid lesion' is a poor one, as this is not related at all to meniscal tissue but simply consists of fibrous tissue and overactive synovium. Resection of this lesion followed by active mobilization of the ankle is highly successful in resolving the symptoms. Impingement may also occur following damage to the syndesmosis of the inferior tibiofibula joint, or indeed from the anterior or posterior tibiofibular ligaments.

Bursitis around the malleoli and in the posterior aspect of the joint can arise in players and is usually due to repetitive friction over the area. Bursae vary in size and can repeatedly flare up once aggravated. Pressure-relieving pads, anti-inflammatories and physiotherapy are immediate choices of treatment, though aspiration and steroid injection may be necessary. Excision may be required in chronic cases, but care is needed in the recovery phase to prevent complications such as the development of a seroma (collection of fluid) and ultimately a bursa or even draining fistula. Most players will be able to carry on until the close season for such surgery.

Pain in the posterior region of the ankle joint can be caused by soft tissue impingement due to an **os trigonum** or **Stieda's process** (McDougall, 1955). This is an enlarged bony prominence on the posterior surface of the talus, which in many individuals is present as an asymptomatic structure. It has been reported to appear in 5% of the normal population (Helal and Wilson, 1988), but in soccer players this figure rises to 15.9% (Massada, 1991). Injury is caused by repeated minor trauma or an acute fracture due to forced plantar flexion, an ankle movement common in soccer. On examination, pain is present on forced passive plantar flexion and on palpation of the posterolateral aspect of the talus between the Achilles tendon and the peroneals. Lateral X-ray views and bone scans will confirm the diagnosis. Temporary immobilization, anti-inflammatories, physiotherapy, corticosteroid injection and (in severe cases) surgery to remove the excess bone, are the treatment modalities available. Recovery from surgery varies from four to eight weeks, the player with indications of other degenerative changes in the articular areas being advised to proceed more slowly with the appropriate rehabilitation programme.

It should not be forgotten that the ankle, as with any other joint, can be the prime area of manifestation of a generalized joint pathology such as rheumatoid arthritis, synovial chondromatosis, gout, bacterial, viral or fungal infections or synovitis.

Foot

Genetic conditions such as **talipes equinus, hallux valgus/varus/rigidus and pes cavus/planus** appear to different degrees in players of all ages, and may require orthotic control at some stage in a player's career. Initial assessment of such conditions may suggest taping, padding, passive mobilizations or active exercise in the early stages, but in the more chronic cases surgical choices such as soft tissue release, osteotomy or arthroplasty may be necessary.

Morton's toe is recognized by a shortened first metatarsal, a hypermobile first ray and a longer second toe. This may create problems in selecting the correct footwear in terms of size to prevent injury.

Case study

After a particular game, a player complained of a pain which had developed over the base of his second metatarsal whilst playing. The match was played in very heavy and slippery conditions, so the player had put on a pair of boots half a size smaller than normal to ensure that they didn't slip off in the game. On examining his foot after the game, he had a Morton's toe, and this had been aggravated by the smaller boot. When he put on his normal boots, I asked him how he chose the size of boots to wear. 'When I was a child, my mum used to prod the bottom end of the shoe to see how much room there was for my big toe and I still do that now' he replied. When we placed his foot on the top of his normal boot the second toe was still hanging over the edge, and really he needed another half to full size up to accommodate this digit. Size of footwear should therefore be made on the longest toe, not necessarily on the position of the big toe.

A **Morton's neuroma** may develop due to the use of narrow-fitting boots. Pressure on the interdigital nerve between the third and fourth metatarsal heads can produce 'electric shock' type symptoms along the sensory pathway. Acute cases are easily resolved by using a wider fitting boot. Chronic cases may require corticosteroid injection or surgical excision to remove the neuroma.

The most common sites for **stress fractures** in the foot are the second and third metatarsal shafts (Taunton and Clement, 1981). Preseason is the prime time for such problems to arise, often in individuals who have hypermobility of

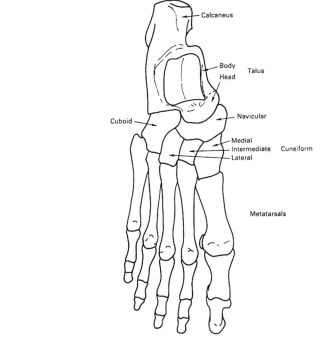

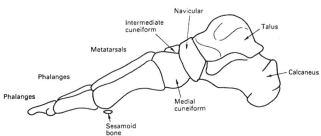

Reproduced with permission
from Palastanga *et al.*, 1994

the first metatarsal which increases weight transference to the second metatarsal head. Also, the base of the second metatarsal is the most stable and so has the least amount of motion compared to the others. Conservative care with a gradually increasing weightbearing rehabilitation programme is required, with orthotic control if necessary. In contrast to this, stress fractures of the fifth metatarsal (DeLee *et al.*, 1983a) and navicular (McBryde, 1985) will require immobilization for six to eight weeks in order to prevent displacement before commencing a similar recovery programme.

Fractures can occur around the foot region and those around the base of the fifth metatarsal can be very slow in recovery. If consolidation fails to occur, bone graft or internal fixation may be necessary to prevent a recurring problem. Immobilization and a full rehabilitation programme are necessary following such an injury.

Inflammation of the plantar fascia, **plantar fasciitis**, is most likely to occur during preseason training and is caused by a combination of factors. Hard training surfaces, poor footwear, biomechanical factors and hallux rigidus of the big toe are possible causes of this problem, with the most common site of pain being on the medial aspect of the fascia at the calcaneal attachment. Treatment consists of physiotherapy and corticosteroid injection (though related rupture may be a contraindication), and if a **heel spur** develops, surgery. Recovery is slow, and this is often a condition that an individual will continue to play with for many months.

Inflammation of the numerous tendon sheaths around the foot can produce **tenovaginitis**, where scarring is present throughout the whole tendon sheath, or **tenosynovitis**, where the lesion is present on the outside of the tendon and the inside of the sheath. Such conditions are most commonly seen in the preseason period when too drastic an increase in workload produces such overuse injuries. Symptoms include pain, crepitus, swelling and development of scarring over the site of the injury. Treatment modalities include immobilization, anti-inflammatories, physiotherapy, and a gradually progressive rehabilitation programme.

Within the foot, secondary ossification centres may produce numerous asymptomatic **accessory ossicles**, which can be seen as bony protrusions. Occasionally, any overlying bursae may also be involved. This is particularly common on the navicular, an os tibial externum, or on the posterior aspect of the talus, an os trigonum (See Chapter 6, 'Ankle'). Any symptoms produced occur due to pressure on the prominence, particulary from standard footwear. Conservatively, pressure pads and remoulding of the standard shape of the boot is often sufficient in the early stages. Should symptoms persist, then excision may be necessary. With large navicular prominences, the amount of bone that can be removed is limited by the involvement of the talonavicular joint. It is not uncommon for a degree of pain to remain for up to 18 months postoperatively.

Bony **exostoses** may develop on the bony surfaces following trauma. These are particularly common wherever a joint develops significant osteophytes. The most common sites are:

1. Distal phalanx, big toe
   A subungual exostosis is a bony growth on the dorsal surface of the distal phalanx to the big toe. Any relative symptoms are due to the pressure created when wearing certain footwear. In the early stages, padding and modifications to the footwear may relieve the symptoms. Surgical excision may be necessary in chronic cases
2. Navicular
3. Medial/lateral cuneiform of the foot.

Blisters often occur on the plantar aspect of the foot due to friction created within the shoe. Seams of socks or movement of the foot within the shoe create such problems, and treatment initially should be aimed at prevention Fitted insoles, talcum powder to reduce the collection of moisture and seamless socks are various preventative measures which can be used. Once the blister has formed and remained intact, removal of the fluid with a sterile syringe or needle and injection of compound benzoin tincture (friar's balsam) into the layer of epithelium is a painful yet very effective method of returning the player to training within 24 hours of the injury. If the blister has burst during activity, clean the wound, apply a dry iodine spray and a sterile dressing to prevent infection. The hygiene standards of the player will be tested as the wound must be kept clean and dry over the next few days. Level of activity will depend on the site and size of the blister.

References

Adams, I. D. (1981). Injuries to the ankle. *Sports Fitness and Sports Injuries.* pp. 241–244. London: Faber and Faber.

Aglietti, P., Buzzi, P. D., Andria, S. *et al.* (1992). Long-term study of anterior cruciate ligament reconstruction for chronic instability using the central one-third patellar tendon and a lateral extra-articular tenodesis. *Am. J. Sports Med.,* **20(1)**, 38–45.

Althoff, B., Peterson, L. and Renstrom, P. (1988). A simple reconstructive procedure of chronic ligament injuries of the ankle. *Lakertidningen,* **78**, 2857–2861.

Arno, S. (1990). The A-angle: A quantitative measurement of patella alignment and realignment. *J. Sports Phys. Ther.,* **12(6)**, 237–242.

Arnoczky, S. P. and Warren, R. F. (1982). Microvasculature of the human meniscus. *Am. J. Sports Med.,* **10**, 90–95.

Backous, D. D., Friedl, K. E., Smith, N. J. *et al.* (1988). Soccer injuries and their relation to physical maturity. *Am. J. Dis. Child,* **142**, 839–842.

Ballmer, P. M. and Jakob, R. P. (1988). The nonoperative treatment of isolated complete tears of the medial collateral ligament of the knee. A prospective study. *Arch. Orthop. Trauma. Surg.,* **107**, 273–276.

Barber, F. A. and Stone, R. G. (1985). Meniscal repair: An arthroscopic technique. *J. Bone Joint Surg.,* **67B**, 39–41.

Barton, T. M., Torg, J. S. and Das. M. (1984). Posterior cruciate ligament insufficiency. *Sports Med.,* **1**, 419–430.

Beer, E. (1924). Periostitis of symphysis and descending rami of pubes. *Int. J. Med. Surg.,* **37**, 224–225.

Bentley, G. and Dowd, G. (1983). Current concepts of etiology and treatment of chondromalacia patellae. *Clin. Orthop. Rel. Res.,* **189**, 209–228.

Berbig, R. and Biener, K. (1983). Sportunfalle bei Fussballtorhuettern. *Schweiz Zeitschr. Sports Med.,* **31**, 73–79.

Bigos, S. J. and Davis, G. E. (1996). Scientific application of sports medicine principles for acute low back problems. *J. Sports Phys. Ther.,* **24(4)**, 192–207.

Booth, D. W. and Westers, B. M. (1989). The management of athletes with myositis ossificans traumatica. *Can. J. Sport Sci.,* **14(1)**, 10–16.

Brittberg, M., Lindahl, A., Nilsson, A. *et al.* (1994). Treatment of deep cartilage defects in the knee with autologous chonrocyte transplantation. *New Eng. J. Med.,* **331**, 889–895.

Brostrom, L. (1966). Sprained ankles V-treatment and prognosis in recent ligament ruptures. *Acta Chir. Scand.,* **135**, 537–550.

Brynhildsen, J., Ekstrand, J., Jeppson, A. *et al.* (1990). Previous injuries and persisting symptoms in female soccer players. *Int. J. Sports Med.,* **11**, 489–492.

Burkett, L. (1970). Causative factors of hamstring strains. *Med. Sci. Sports Excs.*, **2**, 39–42.

Buseck, M. S. and Noyes, F. R. (1991). Arthroscopic evaluation of meniscal repairs after anterior cruciate ligament reconstruction and immediate motion. *Am. J. Sports Med.*, **19**, 489–494.

Butler, D. L., Noyes, F. R., Grood, E. S. *et al.* (1979). Mechanical properties of transplants for the ACL. *Orthop. Trans.*, **3**, 180–181.

Butler, D. L., Noyes, F. R. and Grood, E. S. (1980). Ligamentous restraints to anterior-posterior drawer in the human knee. A biomechanical study. *J. Bone Joint Surg.*, **62A**, 259–270.

Cass, J. R. and Morrey, B. F. (1984). Ankle instability: current concepts, diagnosis and treatment. *Mayo Clin. Proc.*, **59**, 165–170.

Chrisman, O. D. and Snook, G. A. (1969). Reconstruction of lateral ligament tears of the ankle. *Am. J. Bone Joint Surg.*, **51**, 904–912.

Clancy, W. G. (1989). Repair and reconstruction of the posterior cruciate ligament. Instructional course, AOSSM Annual Meeting, Traverse City, Michigan, pp. 141–155.

Clancy, W. G., Shelburne, K. D., Zoellner, G. B. *et al.* (1983). Treatment of knee joint instability secondary to rupture of the posterior cruciate ligament: Report of a new procedure. *J. Bone Joint Surg.*, **65A**, 310–322.

Clement, D. B., Taunton, J. E. and Smart, G. W. (1984). Achilles tendinitis and peritendinitis-etiology and treatment. *Am. J. Sports Med.*, **12(3)**, 179–185.

Connor, J. M. (1983). *Soft Tissue Ossification*. New York: Springer-Verlag.

Cross, M. J. and Crichton. K. J. (1987). *Clinical Examination of the Injured Knee*. London: Gower Medical Publishing.

DeHaven, K. E. (1980). Diagnosis of acute knee injuries with haemarthrosis. *Am. J. Sports Med.*, **8**, 9–14.

DeHaven, K. E., Black, K. P. and Griffith, H. J. (1989). Open meniscus repair: technique and two to nine year results. *Am. J. Sports Med.*, **17**, 788.

DeLee, J. C., Evans, J. P. *et al.* (1983a). Stress fracture of the fifth metatarsal. *Am. J. Sports Med.*, **11**, 349.

DeLee, J. C., Riley, M. B. and Rockwood, C. A. (1983b). Acute posterolateral rotatory instability of the knee. *Am. J. Sports Med.*, **11(4)**, 199–207.

Diamond, D. L. (1989). Sports-related abdominal trauma. *Clin. Sports Med.*, **8(1)**, 91–98.

Donaldson, W. F., Warren, R. F. and Wickiewicz, T. (1985). A comparison of acute anterior cruciate ligament examinations. *Am. J. Sports Med.*, **13**, 5–10.

Dorman, P. (1971). A report on 140 hamstring injuries. *Aust. J. Sports Med.*, **4**, 30–36.

Ekberg, O., Persson, N. M., Abrahamson, P., Westlin, N. E. *et al.* (1988). Longstanding groin pain in athletes. *Sports Med.*, **6**, 56–61.

Ekblom, B. (1986). Applied physiology of soccer. *Sports Med.*, **3**, 50–60.

Ekstrand, J. and Gillquist, J. (1983a). Soccer injuries and their mechanisms: a prospective study. *Med. Sci. Sports Exerc.*, **15(3)**, 267–270.

Ekstrand, J. and Gillquist, J. (1983b). The avoidability of soccer injuries. *Int. J. Sports Med.*, **4**, 124–128.

Ekstrand, J. and Tropp, H. (1990). Incidence of ankle sprains in soccer. *Foot Ankle*, **11(1)**, 41–43.

Ekstrand, J., Gillquist, J., Moller, M. *et al.* (1983). Incidence of soccer injuries and their relation to team success. *Am. J. Sports Med.*, **11(2)**, 101–105.

Ellis, M. and Frank, H. G. (1966). Myositis ossificans traumatica: With special reference to the quadriceps femoris muscle. *J. Trauma*, **6**, 724–738.

Engstrom, B., Forssblad, M. and Johansson, C. (1990). Does a major knee injury definitely sideline an elite soccer player? *Am. J. Sports Med.*, **18**, 101–105.

Engstrom, B., Johansson, C. and Tornkvist, H. (1991). Soccer injuries among elite female players. *Am. J. Sports Med.*, **19**, 273–275.

Eriksson, E. (1976). Reconstruction of the anterior cruciate ligament. *Orthop. Clin. North Am.*, **7**, 167-179.

Eriksson, E., Haggmark, T. and Johnson, R. J. (1986). Reconstruction of the posterior cruciate ligament. *Orthop.*, **9**, 217–220.

Feagin, J. A., Abbott, H. G. and Rokus, J. R. (1972). The isolated tear of the anterior cruciate ligament. *J. Bone. Joint Surg.*, **54A**, 1340–1341.

Feagin, J. A. and Curl, W. W. (1976). Isolated tear of the anterior cruciate ligament. Five year follow up study. *Am. J. Sports Med.*, **4**, 95–100.

Fischer, S. P., Fox, J. M., Del Pizzo, W. *et al.* (1991). Accuracy of diagnosis from magnetic resonance imaging of the knee. *J. Bone Joint Surg.*, **73A**, 2–10.

Gamble, J. G., Simmons, S. C. and Freedman, M. (1986). The symphysis pubis: Anatomic and pathological considerations. *Clin. Orthop. Rel. Res.*, **203**, 261–272.

Gershuni, D. H., Gosink, B. B. *et al.* (1982). Ultrasound evaluation of the anterior musculo-fascial compartment of the leg following exercise. *Clin. Orthop. Rel. Res.*, **167**, 185–190.

Gilmer, W. J., Anderson, D. L. (1959). Reaction of soft somatic tissue which may progress to bone formation. *South Med. J.*, **52**, 1432–1448.

Graf, B., Docter, T. and Clancy, W. Jr. (1987). Arthroscopic meniscal repair. *Clin. Sports Med.*, **6**, 525.

Gross, R. H. (1984). Hip problems in children: aids to early recognition. *Postgrad. Med.*, **76**, 97–105.

Halpern, A., Horowitz, B. and Nagel, D. (1977). Tendon ruptures associated with corticosteroid therapy. *West. J. Med.*, **127**, 378–382.

Hastings, D. E. (1980). The non-operative management of collateral ligament injuries of the knee joint. *Clin. Orthop.*, **147**, 22–28.

Hawkins, R. B. (1988). Arthroscopic treatment of sports related anterior osteophytes in the ankle. *Foot and Ankle*, **9(2)**, 87–90.

Heiser, T., Weber, J., Sullivan, G. *et al.* (1984). Prophylaxis and management of hamstring muscle injuries in intercollegiate football players. *Am. J. Sports Med.*, **12**, 368–370.

Helal, B. and Wilson, D. (1988). *The Foot.* pp. 567. London: Churchill Livingstone.

Hopkinson, W. J., Mitchell, W. A. and Curl, W. W. (1985). Chondral fractures of the knee: cause for confusion. *Am. J. Sports Med.*, **13**, 309.

Hoy, K., Lindblad, B., Terkelsen, C. *et al.* (1992). European soccer injuries a prospective epidemiologic and socioeconomic study. *Am. J. Sports Med.*, **20(3)**, 318–322.

Hughtson, J. C. and Eilers, A. F. (1973). The role of the posterior oblique ligament in repairs of the medial collateral ligament tears of the knee. *J. Bone Joint Surg.*, **55A**, 923–940.

Hughtson, J. C. and Jacobson, K. E. (1985). Chronic posterolateral rotatory instability of the knee. *Am. J. Bone Jt. Surg.*, **67(3)**, 351–359.

Indelicato, P. A. (1983). Nonoperative treatment of complete tears of the medial collateral ligament of the knee. *J. Bone Joint Surg.*, **65A**, 323–329.

Inklaar, H. (1994). Soccer injuries 1: incidence and severity. *Sports Med.*, **18(1)**, 55–73.

Insall, J., Falvo, K. A. and Wise, D. W. (1976). Chondromalacia patellae. *J. Sports Phys. Ther.*, **58A(1)**, 1–8.

Iverson, B. F., Sturup, J. and Jacobsen, K. (1988). Quantification of antero-posterior laxity in normal and anterior cruciate ligament repaired knees. Application of the data on clinical tests. *Ital. J. Sports Traumatol.*, **10**, 77–82.

Iversen, B. F., Sturup, J., Jacobsen, K, *et al.* (1989). Implications of muscular defense in testing for the anterior drawer sign in the knee. *Am. J. Sports Med.*, **17(3)**, 409–413.

Jackson, D. W. and Jennings, L. D. (1988). Arthroscopic assisted reconstruction of the anterior cruciate ligament using a patellar tendon bone autograft. *Clin. Sports Med.*, **7**, 785–800.

Julsrud, M. E. (1988). Osteochondrosis. In: *Conquering Athletic Injuries* (P. M. Taylor and D. K. Taylor, eds), pp. 292–293. Champaign: Leisure Press.

Kannus, P. (1988). Long-term results of conservatively treated medial collateral ligament injuries of the knee joint. *Clin. Orthop.*, **226**, 103–112.

Kannus, P. (1989). Non-operative treatment of grade 2 and 3 sprains of the lateral ligament compartment of the knee. *Am. J. Sports Med.*, **17**, 83–88.

Karlsson, J., Bergsten, T., Lansinger, O. *et al.* (1988). Reconstruction of the lateral ligaments of the ankle for chronic lateral stability. *Am. J. Bone Joint Surg.*, **70**, 581–588.

Keller, C., Noyes, F. and Buncher, R. (1987). The medical aspects of soccer injury epidemiology. *Am. J. Sports Med.*, **15(3)**, 230–237.

Klunder, K. B., Rud, B. and Hansen, J. (1980). Osteoartritis of the hip and knee joint in retired football players. *Acta Orthop. Scand.*, **51**, 925–927.

Leather. M. (1989). A torn external oblique aponeurosis with hidden inguinal hernia in a young professional footballer. *Physio. Sport*, **12(2)**, 3–5.

Leighton, J. R. (1956). Flexibility characteristics of males ten to eighteen years of age. *J. Arch. Phys. Med. Rehab.*, **37**, 494–499.

Leighton, J. R. (1964). Flexibility characteristics of males six to ten years of age. *J. Arch. Phys. Med. Rehab.*, **18**, 19–25.

Lewin, G. (1989). The incidence of injury in an English professional soccer club during one competitive season. *Physiotherapy*, **75(10)**, 601–605.

Lysens, R. J. J. (1987). Epidemiological study of soccer injuries in the 18 teams of the first division of the Royal Belgium Soccer Association (RBSA) during the season 1980–1981. In: *Proceedings 2nd Meeting Council of Europe: Sports injuries and their prevention* (C. R. van der Togt, A. B. A. Kemper and M. Koornneef, eds), pp. 16–17. Osterbeek: National Institute for Sports Health Care.

Mackay, G. M. and Hillis, W. S. (1996). Pre-season injuries in Scottish football: a prospective study. *Sp. Excse. Inj.*, **2**, 100–102.

Maehlum, S. and Daljord, O. A. (1984). Football injuries in Oslo: A one year study. *Br. J. Sports Med.*, **18**, 186–190.

Maelhum, S., Dahl, E. and Daljord, O. A. (1986). Frequency of injuries in a youth soccer tournament. *Physician Sportsmed.*, **14(7)**, 73–79.

Malycha, P. and Lovell, G. (1992). Inguinal surgery in athletes with chronic groin pain: The 'sportsman's' hernia. *Aust. N. Z. J. Surg.*, **62**, 123–125.

Marshall, J. L. and Rubin, R. M. (1977). Knee ligament injuries: a diagnostic and therapeutic approach. *Orthop. Clin. North Am.*, **8**, 641–668.

Massada, J. L. (1991). Ankle overuse injuries in soccer players. *J. Sports Med. Phys. Fit.*, **31(3)**, 447–451.

Mayhew, S. R. and Wenger, H. A. (1985). Time-motion analysis of professional soccer. *J. Hum. Move. Stud.*, **11**, 49–52.

McBryde, A. M. (1985). Stress fractures in runners. *Clin. Sports Med.*, **4**, 737.

McConnell, J. (1986). The management of chondromalacia patellae: A long term solution. *Aust. J. Physio.*, **32(14)**, 215–223.

McCormick, W. C., Bagg, R. J., Kennedy, C. W. Jr. *et al.* (1976). Reconstruction of the posterior cruciate ligament: preliminary report of a new procedure. *Clin. Orthop.*, **118**, 30–34.

McDougall, A. (1955). The os trigonum. *J. Bone Joint Surg. (Br.)*, **37**, 257.

Micheli, L. J. (1983). Overuse injuries in childrens sport: The growth factor. *Orthop. Clin. North Am.*, **14**, 337–360.

Milachowski, K. A., Weismeier, K. and Wirth, C. J. (1989). Homologous meniscal transplantation: Experimental and clinical results. *Int. Orthop.*, **13(1)**, 1–11.

Minarovjech, V. (1980). Knowledge of anti-injury in the league football soccer in Czechoslovakia. In: *Proceedings 1st International Congress on Sports Medicine Applied to Football* (L. Vecchiet, ed.), vol. 2, pp. 871–878. ROM NUM. Rome: D Guanella.

Moller-Nielsen, J. and Hammar, N. (1989). Women's soccer injuries in relation to the menstrual cycle and oral contraceptive use. *Med. Sci. Sports Exerc.*, **21(2)**, 126–129.

Mozes, M., Papa, M. Z., Zweig, A. *et al.* (1985). Iliopsoas injury in soccer players. *Br. J. Sports Med.*, **19(3)**, 168–169.

Muckle, D. S. (1988). Meniscal repair in athletes. *Sports Med.*, **5**, 1–5.

Murphy, C. P. and Drez. D. (1987). Jejunal rupture in a football player. *Am. J. Sports Med.*, **15**, 184–185.

Napravnik, C. (1980). Prevention of accidents in football. In: *Proceedings of 1st International Congress on Sports Medicine Applied to Football* (L. Vecchiet, ed.), vol 2, pp. 879–882. ROM NUM. Rome: D Guanella.

Nielsen, A. B. and Yde. J. (1989). Epidemiology and traumatology of injuries in soccer. *Am. J. Sports Med.*, **17**, 803–807.

Nyhus, M. L. (1994). A *Textbook of Hernia* Philadelphia: Lippincott.

O'Brien, S. J., Warren, R. F., Pavlov, H, *et al.* (1991). Reconstruction of the chronically insufficient anterior cruciate ligament with the central third of the patellar ligament. *J. Bone Joint Surg.*, **73**, 278–286.

Ogata, K. (1980). Posterior cruciate reconstruction using iliotibial band: preliminary report of a new procedure. *Arch. Orthop. Trauma. Surg.*, **51**, 547–550.

Palastanga, N., Field, D. and Soames, R. (1994). *Anatomy and Human Movement*. Oxford: Butterworth-Heinemann.

Panner, J. H. (1929). A peculiar affection of the capitellum humeri resembling Calve-Perthes disease of the hip. *Acta Radiol (Stockh.)*, **10**, 234.

Parolie, J. M. and Bergfield, J. A. (1986). Long-term results of nonoperative treatment of isolated posterior cruciate ligament injuries in the athlete. *Am. J. Sports Med.*, **14**, 53–58.

Pochling, G. G., Ruch, D. S. and Chabon, S. J. (1990). The landscape of meniscal injuries. *Clin. Sports Med.*, **9(3)**, 539–549.

Raab, D. J., Fisher, D. A., Smith, J. *et al.* (1993). Comparison of arthroscopic and open reconstruction of the anterior cruciate ligament. *Am. J. Sports Med.*, **21**, 680–683.

Rebman, L. W. (1988). Lachman's Test: An alternative method. *J. Orthop. Sp. Phys. Ther.*, **9(11)**, 381–382.

Reilly, T. and Thomas, V. (1976). A motion analysis of work-rate in different positional roles in professional football matchplay. *J. Hum. Mov. Stud.*, **2**, 87–97.

Renstrom, P. and Peterson, L. (1980). Groin injuries in athletes. *Br. J. Sports Med.*, **14**, 30-36.

Saal, J. A. and Saal, J. S. (1989). Nonoperative treatment of herniated lumbar intervertebral disc with radiculotherapy. *Spine*, **14**, 431–437.

Sadat-Ali, M. and Sankaran-Kutty, M. (1987). Soccer injuries in Saudi Arabia. *Am. J. Sports Med.*, **15(5)**, 500–502.

Safran, M., Garrett, W., Seaber, A. *et al.* (1988). The role of warm up in muscular injury prevention. *Am. J. Sports Med.*, **16**, 123–128.

Schmidt-Olsen, S., Bunemann, L. K. H., Lade, V. *et al.* (1985). Soccer injuries of youth. *Int. J. Sports Med.*, **19(3)**, 161–164.

Schmidt-Olsen, S., Jorgensen, U., Kaalund, S. *et al.* (1991). Injuries among young soccer players. *Am. J. Sports Med.*, **19**, 273–275.

Taunton, J. E. and Clement, D. B. (1981). Lower extremity stress fractures in athletes. *Phys. Sportsmed*, **9**, 77–86.

Tria, J., Palumbo, R. C. and Alicea, J. A. (1983). Conservative care for patellofemoral pain. *Orthop. Clin. North Am.*, **23(4)**, 545–554.

Trickey, E. L. (1980). Injuries to the posterior cruciate ligament. Diagnosis and treatment of early injuries and reconstruction of late instability. *Clin. Orthop.*, **147**, 76–81.

Tropp, M., Askling, C. and Gillquist, J. (1985). Prevention of ankle sprains. *Am. J. Sports Med.*, **13**, 259–262.

Tysvaer, A. and Storli, O. (1981). Association football injuries to the brain, preliminary report. *Br. J. Sports Med.*, **15(3)**, 163–166.

Unverferth, L. J. and Olix. M. L. (1973). The effect of local steroid injections on tendons. *J. Sports Med.*, **1**, 31–37.

Van Dijk, C. N., Lim, L. S. L., Bossuyt, P. M. M. *et al.* (1996). Physical examination is suffcient for the diagnosis of sprained ankles. *J. Bone Joint Surg. (Br.)*, **78**, 958–962.

Veltri, D. M., Warren, R. F., Wickiewicz, T. L. *et al.* (1994). Current status of allographic meniscal transplantation. *Clin. Orthop.*, **306**, 155–162.

Vingard, E., Alfredsson, L., Goldie, I. *et al.* (1993). Sports and osteoarthritis of the hip. An epidemiologic study. *Am. J. Sports Med.*, **18**, 694–697.

Walter, S. D., Sutton, J. R., McIntosh, J. M. *et al.* (1985). The aetiology of sports injuries. A review of methodologies. *Sports Med*, **2**, 47–58.

Warren-Smith, C. D. and Forster, F. W. (1987). Anterior cruciate ligament deficiency. Results of quadriceps/patellar tendon reconstruction and early results of Gortex replacement. *J. Bone Joint Surg.*, **69B**, 161.

Weber, H. (1983). Lumbar disc with a K heniation: A controlled perspective study with ten years of observation. *Spine*, **8**, 131–140.

Williams, P. E. and Goldspink, G. (1971). Longitudinal growth of striated muscle fibres. *J. Cell. Sci.*, **9**, 751–767.

Wilson, W. J., Lewis, F. and Scranton, P. E. (1990). Combined reconstruction of the anterior cruciate ligament in competitive athletes. *J. Bone Joint Surg.*, **72A(5)**, 742–748.

Windsor Sports Insurance Brokers (1997). *Investigation into career ending incidents to Professional Footballers in England and Wales, from 1987/88 to 1994/95.*

Worrell, T. W. and Perrin, D. H. (1992). Hamstring muscle injury: the influence of strength, flexibility, warm-up and fatigue. *J. Orthop. Sports Phys. Ther.*, **16**, 12–18.

Worrell, T. W., Perrin, D. H., Gansender, B., *et al.* (1991). Comparison of isokinetic strength and flexibility measures between hamstring injured and non-injured athletes. *J. Orthop. Sports Phys. Ther.*, **13**, 118–125.

Zoltan, D. J., Reinecke, C. and Indelicato, P. A. (1988). Synthetic and allograft anterior cruciate reconstruction. *Clin. Sports Med.*, **7**, 4.

7

Related issues and upper limb injuries in rugby

International rugby football is supposed to have originated at Rugby School, where William Webb Ellis created chaos over 170 years ago when he picked up and ran with the ball in the middle of a soccer match. It is unusual for a sport to trace its beginnings so accurately, and the Ellis legend is probably a mixture of fact and fiction.

Today there are two kinds of rugby – league and union. Rugby in the south of England was the game of the upper classes and the public schools. In the north and Wales it became the game of the workers. So when rugby teams in the north travelled south to play, it meant a loss of earnings. Those in the south could afford it, those in the north could not and wanted to be compensated for their loss of earnings. The Rugby Football Union, the governing body, insisted the game remain on an amateur status and would not meet the north's monetary demands. A split followed and the Northern Union was set up in 1893 over what had become known as 'broken-time' payments. That game very quickly became professional and formed what is the basis of rugby league today.

Rugby union is played in more than 100 countries and is the national game of Wales, New Zealand and South Africa. Each team has 15 players, and the game involves certain phases – rucks, mauls, lineouts, scrums, tackles – where collisions occur between the players. These are the prime stages of the game and are where the majority of injuries occur.

Rugby league is played mainly in Australia, New Zealand, France, the north of England and Papua New Guinea. The game is presently developing in smaller countries such as Fiji and Tonga, and attempts continue to be made to establish the game in the south of England. It is played by teams of 13 players, but has less various close contact phases. Rucks, mauls and lineouts do not exist in rugby league but tackling and, to a lesser degree, scrummaging predominate the collision phases of the game. However, there is a good deal of similarity and in this age of professionalism in both codes, players can transfer quite readily from one game to another. Obviously certain techniques and skills need to be adapted to switch from one code to another, but each game has developed new ideas with this crossover.

Definitions

As mentioned in the introduction, the game of rugby league has evolved from rugby union. In order to appreciate the differences between the two games with regard to the contact phases involved, a summary explanation is given.

	Rugby league	Rugby union
Scrums	✓	✓
Line outs	✗	✓
Rucks	✗	✓
Mauls	✗	✓
Tackling	✓	✓

Table 7.1 *Variations in phases of the game, rugby league to rugby union*

1. *The scrum*

This phase is used to restart the game after a certain offence has occurred. The forwards from each side bind together, the ball is thrown into the tunnel created and the players in the middle of the front row of the two opposing teams, the hookers (not the ones found on street corners!), attempt to divert the ball back. Collapsing and wheeling of the scrum are dangerous situations which can occur, deliberately or accidently, with the opposing forces being directed towards the ground or in a rotational plane, respectively. The rugby union scrum consists of eight players; the rugby league scrum of six.

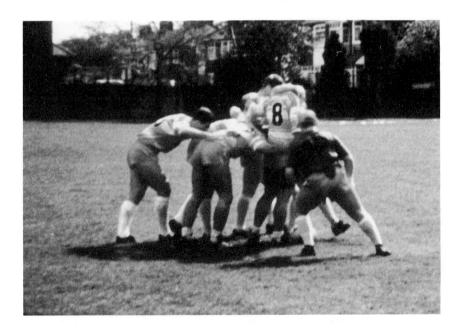

Figure 7.1 The scrum.

2. *Line outs*

A line out occurs when the ball leaves the field of play. A line of between two to seven players from each team stand perpendicular to the touch line and the ball is thrown between them. This phase only arises in rugby union. In rugby league, when the ball crosses the touchline play recommences with either a scrum or a tapped penalty.

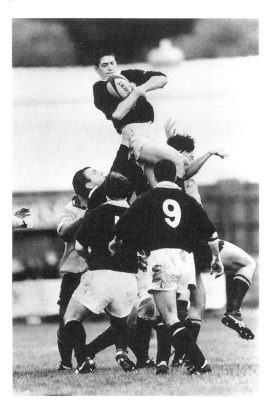

Figure 7.2 The line out.

3. Ruck

This occurs when a player is grounded with the ball and players from each team try to drive over the player and the ball, so it is available for other team members. This phase is only present in rugby union.

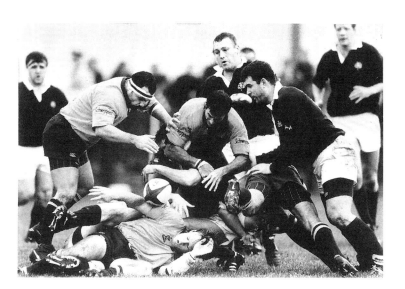

Figure 7.3 The ruck.

4. *Maul*

When a player with the ball is stopped and is still standing, this is classified as a maul. Opposing players then attempt to recover the ball, drive the opposition backwards and give clean possession to the other team members not involved. This phase also only occurs in rugby union.

5. *Tackling*

This phase of the game occurs in both codes. In rugby union, rucks and mauls develop once a player has been stopped by a tackle; in rugby league, once a tackle has been made play is restarted by a 'play the ball', with the tackled player being allowed to stand erect, back-heeling the ball between the legs to another team member.

In terms of research comparing rugby league to union, very little exists.

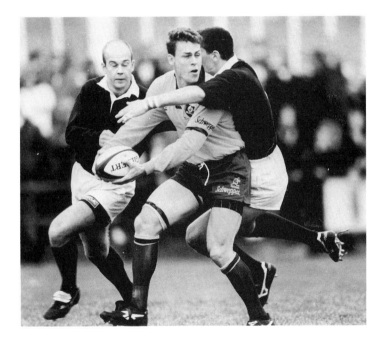

Figure 7.4 The tackle.

In order to attempt to rectify this, the following data is that collected from August 1987–April 1989 (two complete seasons) whilst I was chartered physiotherapist to Leigh Rugby League Football Club (Lancashire, England). All injuries sustained during a match involving players from the club were recorded and then classified as either minor or severe. An injury was classified as severe if the player had to be removed from the field of play, required medical attention and needed a minimum recovery period of ten days (Walkden, 1978; Durkin, 1977)

Case study

Results

During the two seasons studied 65 matches were played, giving a total of 845 appearances. From these, 167 injuries were documented, representing an overall injury incidence of 1:5.1 appearances. The incidence of severe injury was 1:26.4 appearences, with 71 players requiring removal from the field of play and examination by the match doctor. Of these, there were six fractures and one dislocation. The remaining 160 injuries required first aid care, including wound toileting, suturing, ice therapy and supportive strapping, with daily physiotherapy being available from the day after. The more serious soft tissue injuries were referred to the club's orthopaedic surgeon as soon as it was deemed necessary.

1. Total number of injuries recorded

All injuries sustained in the match situation were recorded. This included all lesions such as sutured cuts, lacerations and haematomas as well as the more serious injuries which were reported during or immediately after the game. The majority of these injuries tended to be damage to soft tissues.

Table 7.2 *Review of injury frequency according to anatomical site*

Head	28.1%
Neck	4.2%
Shoulder	5.4%
Upper limb	7.9%
Thorax/abdomen/back	6%
Pelvis/hip	3%
Knee	7.8%
Ankle	9%
Remainder of lower limb	28.6%

2. Total number of severe injuries

Thirty-three serious injuries in the match situation were recorded and were classified accordingly. These included head injuries requiring an overnight stay in hospital, dislocations, fractures and joint disorders which required further orthopaedic management.

Of the serious injuries, six were fractures (four facial, one thorax, one hand) and one was a dislocation (thumb). The remaining 26 included four joint disorders

Table 7.3 *Review of severe injury frequency related to anatomical site*

Head	12.5%
Neck	0%
Shoulder	15.5%
Upper limb	6.1%
Thorax/abdomen/back	12.5%
Pelvis/hip	12.5%
Knee	18.8%
Ankle	9.4%
Remainder of lower limb	12.5%

which required surgical intervention and 22 soft tissue injuries which responded to rest, appropriate physiotherapy and physical rehabilitation.

3. Injury incidence related to the players position

Injuries were correlated according to a player's position. A rugby league team consists of thirteen players – two wingers, two centres, two prop forwards, two second row forwards and one each of the remaining positions.

The total number of injuries for each position was adjusted to account for the number of players in the respective positions, e.g. the total number of injuries sustained by the prop forwards was divided by two, whereas for the scrum half no division of the figures was needed.

Position	%
1. Second row	14.8
2. Stand off	13.9
3. Hooker	12.3
4. Scrum half	12.2
5. Winger	10.4
6. Prop forward	10.4
7. Centre	9.5
8. Lock forward	8.7
9. Full back	7.8

Table 7.4 *Injury incidence related to playing position*

4. Injury incidence related to the phase of play

Injuries were recorded in regard to the various phases of play which occur during a game. Considering rugby union, only certain game situations arise in both codes – tackling, being tackled, running, scrummaging and collision.

Three other categories were included in this study which were felt to be missing from similar rugby union research:

(a) Environment – injuries produced by the condition of the playing surface.
(b) Equipment – injuries produced by the use of certain equipment.
(c) Violent play – injuries produced by foul play.

Phase of play	%
1. Tackled	39.7
2. Tackling	31.2
3. Running	16.2
4. Violent play	4.2
5. Scrummage	3.5
6. Environment	2.3
7. Collision	1.7
8. Equipment	1.2

Table 7.5 *Injury incidence related to the phase of play*

Injury comparison

Using this data and the other articles available on rugby league injuries, a comparison can be made with rugby union.

1. *Total number of injuries recorded*
When comparing the two codes, two methods of comparison exist:

(a) Incidence of injury per 10 000 player hours

	Incidence of injury (per 10 000 player hours)	Performance level	Reference
Rugby union	197.7	Schoolboy	Sparks, 1981
	194	Schoolboy	Sparks, 1985
	538.5	Senior club	Addley, 1988
Rugby league	582	Professional	Walker, 1985
	1485	Professional	Fevre, this volume

(b) Incidence of injury per appearances

	Incidence of injury (per appearances)	Performance level	Reference
Rugby union	1 per 14	Senior club	Addley, 1988
Rugby league	1 per 4.3	Professional	Gissane et al., 1993
Rugby league	1 per 5.06	Professional	Fevre, this volume

2. *Total number of injuries related to anatomical site*

	Anatomical site									References
	Head/ neck	Shoulder	Upper limb	Thorax/ abdomen	Back	Pelvis	Knee	Ankle	Lower limb	
Rugby union	13	32	5	11	8	0	13	8	10	Micheli and Risborough, 1974
Rugby league	32	5	8	6	3	0	8	9	29	Fevre, this volume

	Anatomical site				References
	Head/ neck	Upper limb	Thorax/ back	Lower limb	
Rugby union	16.1	32.3	11.2	40.4	Adams, 1977
Rugby league	32.3	13.3	9	45.4	Fevre, this volume
Rugby league	5.7	22	19.1	53.2	Gibbs, 1993
Rugby league	23	18.5	13	45	Alexander, et al., 1980

Table 7.9 *Comparison of the total number of injuries related to anatomical site (B)*

	Anatomical site							References
	Head	Neck	Shoulder	Upper limb	Thorax/ back	Knee	Lower limb	
Rugby union	19.5	5	13	9	11	9.9	33.1	Davies and Gibson, 1978
Rugby league	28.1	4.2	5.4	7.9	6	7.8	37.6	Fevre, this volume

Table 7.10 *Comparison of the total number of injuries related to anatomical site (C)*

	Anatomical site					References
	Head	Neck	Arm	Trunk	Leg	
Rugby union	16	7	27	14	36	Addley, 1988
Rugby league	28.1	4.2	13.3	9	45.4	Fevre, this volume

Table 7.11 *Comparison of the total number of injuries related to anatomical site (D)*

3. Total number of severe injuries

Incidence of severe injury			References
Rugby union	17%	Senior/international	Walkden, 1975
Rugby union	22%	Schoolboy	Sparks, 1981
Rugby league	21%	Professional	Walker, 1985
Rugby league	19.2%	Professional	Fevre, this volume

Table 7.12 *Comparison of the total number of injuries related to severe injury*

4. *Injury incidence related to playing position (rank order)*

Table 7.13 *Incidence of injury related to playing position*

	Position										References
	Full back	Wing	Centre	Stand off	Scrum half	Prop	Hooker	Second row	Wing forward	Lock	
Rugby union	1	4	2	6	9	7	8	10	4	2	Durkin, 1977
Rugby union	6	5	7	9	10	7	2	2	2	1	Roy, 1974
Rugby union	3	2	3	10	1	8	6	8	5	7	Van Heerden, 1976
Rugby union	3	6	9	3	10	2	3	6	1	6	Addley, 1988
Rugby league	9	5	7	2	4	5	3	1	N/A	8	Fevre, this volume

Table 7.14 *Incidence of injury related to the phase of play*

Phase of play	Rugby union	Rugby league
Tackled	18	39.7
Tackling	16	31.2
Running	13	16.2
Violence	Not recorded	4.2
Scrum	8	3.5
Environment	Not recorded	2.3
Collision	6	1.7
Equipment	Not recorded	1.2
	Addley, 1988	Fevre, this volume

Discussion

Despite the differences between the two games, the high injury incidence in both these sports is not surprising. When comparing the two different codes, the balance of injuries would appear to lean towards rugby league. This may partly be explained by the different demands of each sport. Larder (1988) quotes that in rugby union, the New Zealand All Blacks camp calculated that the ball is very rarely in play for more than 25 minutes out of the allotted 80; in rugby league, Larder states that the ball is in play for approximately 50 minutes of each game. He also states that a rugby union wing forward, the specialist tackler, will make on average 20 tackles a game, with the backs seldom being asked to make more than 10. In rugby league, the tackle count for each player will vary from a minimum of 20 up to a maximum of 50.

When comparing the total number of injuries recorded, rugby league would appear to produce a larger number of injuries than rugby union and this is supported by several other studies (Gissane et al., 1993; Alexander et al., 1979). Walker (1985) came to the same end result, but compared schoolboy figures in rugby union (Sparks, 1981) with his own figures in professional rugby league.

The difference in the total number of injuries may be due to the different methodologies used in research, a problem noted in the majority of papers concerning injuries in rugby (Silver, 1994). Sparks (1981, 1985) does not state his method of recording injuries, but Addley (1988) relied on voluntary reporting of injuries by the players. They both acknowledge that certain injuries may not have been reported, with the level of cooperation seeming to be influenced by the team performance and the importance of the match.

When relating injury incidence to anatomical position, both codes produce a large percentage of injuries in the lower limb, as expected in collision sports with a large bias on running. Rugby union produces a larger number of injuries in the shoulder/upper limb area of the body, but in rugby league, the head and neck region suffers the majority of all other injuries. These findings are supported by similar rugby league research (Stephenson et al., 1996; Gissane et al., 1993; Alexander et al., 1980). However, Gibbs (1993) reported that only five injuries out of a total of 141 involved the head region in his report from 1989–1991 seasons in Australian rugby league (Stephenson et al., 1996, and Gissane et al. 1993, collected their data from English rugby league). This was at a time when the Australian rugby league was having a purge on high tackles and giving out lengthy bans to offending players. It would appear therefore that head and neck injuries remain prevalent in rugby league.

In the majority of cases the head and neck regions experience mainly lacerations, concussion and, to a lesser extent, haematomas and fractures. Patel et al. (1984) reported that between 1956 and 1983, 13 rugby league players were admitted to the regional spinal unit at Pinderfields General Hospital, Wakefield; 8 of the 13 had been admitted in the last three years of the study. In rugby union, there was a large increase in the number of spinal injuries in the mid 1970s (Scher, 1987; Silver, 1984). Sparks (1985), in his schoolboy study, stated that 'injuries to the head and neck have been relatively commoner in the last four seasons (1980–1983) than in the previous thirty'. This increase occurred at the same time as the ruck and maul phases of the game were allowed to continue in an attempt to make the game faster, with a resultant epidemic of spinal injuries. In 1986 there was a change in the laws to shorten the time involved in the rucks and mauls, with a virtual elimination in the number of spinal injuries associated with these two phases of the game (Silver, 1993).

Patel et al. (1984) also states that 84% of the cervical injuries occurred in the tackling/tackled phase of the game. In rugby union, 68% (Silver and Gill, 1988) and 55% (Williams and McKibbin, 1978) occurred in the rucking, mauling and scrummaging phases of the game. In New Zealand between 1973 and 1978, 20 cervical spine injuries occurred in rugby union in the scrummaging situation; between 1980 and 1984, this fell to 15; during 1985 and 1986, instead of the predicted nine, only one occurred, which involved playing an inexperienced player in the front row (Burry and Calcinai, 1988). This decrease may well have came about due to two law changes which reduced the chances of the scrum collapsing and preventing the scrum from 'wheeling' (turning of the scrum to try and disrupt the quality of possession once the strike has been decided). In what is obviously a major phase of the union game so far as injury is concerned, slight rule changes appear drastically to have reduced the danger factor without affecting the fundamental nature of the game. Due to these different prevalent phases in each game, the variation in the mechanical causes of injury related to the neck would appear to be self-explanatory.

Severe injuries account for approximately 20% of the total number of injuries in both codes. Of the six fractures that occurred in my own study, four involved the facial, mandibular and zygomatic bones; only one of the four players was wearing a gumshield. Chapman (1985) stated that 67% of the 1984 Great Britain rugby league team in Australia suffered orofacial injuries; only 25% (seven) of the players used a gumshield. Myers (1980) also produced much higher figures for rugby union at international compared to club level for the incidence of orofacial injuries. Much evidence exists therefore that severe facial injuries are common in both codes. Evidence also exists that a gumshield reduces the transmission of impact forces to the skull, brain and cervical spine (Hayward, 1978; Hickey et al., 1967), and reduces the incidence of fractures to the mandible (Clegg, 1969). The problem would therefore appear in demonstrating the benefits of such use to the player.

Until recent years the role of the player in each code varied considerably. In rugby union the forwards were mostly involved in scrums, rucks, mauls and lineouts, with some use of ball and tackling skills. The backs were the ball handlers and made relatively few tackles compared with league players. Both codes have now moved away from specialization with regard to the players' roles in the team. Wingers and centres are expected to share the work load far more, while the forwards have become much more mobile and faster. All players are required to tackle, handle and run with the ball. Variations in the rank order results in rugby union over the years, relating injury to playing position, has undoubtedly a lot to do with recent tactical developments and law innovations. In this and other rugby league studies (Stephenson et al., 1996; Gissane et al., 1993; Alexander et al., 1979) the forwards, whose game is one of repeatedly driving with the ball, tackling and scrummaging, collect the majority of injuries. Worth noting is the rise up the injury table of the rugby league wingers, particularly as their role in the modern day game has altered greatly over the last 20 years. This is supported by other research into rugby league injuries (Lovell and Rostron, 1996).

The tackling/tackled phase of play produces the greatest number of injuries in both codes, with rugby league (70.9%) having virtually twice as many as union (34%). As a similar ratio exists between the number of tackles made in each game, this may explain such findings. A study of injuries by the Scottish Rugby Football Union (Scottish Rugby Union, Edinburgh, 1985) in 1984/85 found that six out of ten injuries resulted from a tackle and they concluded that the tackle was by far the most dangerous phase of the game. Scrummaging also produced several injuries in this comparative study of rugby union (8%) and league (3.5%). Larder (1988) produced figures regarding the average number of scrums in each code per match, 30 in rugby union, 19.4 in rugby league. When coupled with the difference in the number of players involved in this phase of the game

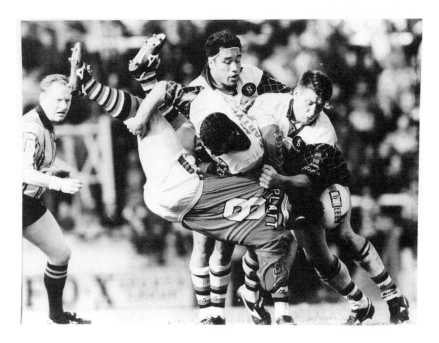

Figure 7.5 The most dangerous phase of both codes – the tackle.

– eight in union, six in league – the greater percentage of injuries in union compared to league could well be explained. This figure of 8% would still appear to be a small number of injuries in a situation where the inherent danger of serious neck and back injuries is always present.

In the light of these results it is suggested that professional rugby league produces a larger number of injuries than rugby union, with severe injury being equally likely in both codes. The demands of each player's position brings about different injury levels. This is constantly changing as the games themselves change. Game requirements produce different levels of injury. Constant reassessment by the governing bodies of each code should help alleviate any obvious problems and reduce the chances of severe injury. Regardless of these results, it would be unfair to suggest that rugby union is a safer alternative to rugby league, particularly at school level. Further similar research into school rugby league and its injuries is necessary and other studies are required to give a wider view of injury patterns in rugby league before being able to make any concrete conclusions.

Injuries

As already stated in the previous chapter, this section will only cover injuries from the pelvis upwards, as these are far more common in rugby than in soccer. This is not to say that soccer players never injure themselves above the waist, but reference to this section for such players will not be on a daily basis.

Childrens' rugby begins at around the age of eight, and there is certainly a great need to have some knowledge of young peoples' injury problems. It is true to say in the present day and age that fractures, dislocations, haematomas and sprains are as common in a child's play activity and in unsupervized sport as they are in organized sport. However, the chronic injuries that have been common in the adult sportsperson are now more frequently documented in the younger age group and it is suggested that the growing, softer skeleton of the child is more susceptible to this type of injury (Micheli, 1983). Reference should be made to Chapter 6, 'Children', with regard to the basic rules that should be applied to the injured youngster.

Skull

The acute effects of **concussion** and the appropriate treatment has already been discussed in Chapter 3, 'Concussion'. Once the initial life threatening state has been averted the continued playing career of the player may still be in question if the injury has been very severe initially (Grade 3), or a Grade 1 or 2 state of concussion becomes a regular occurrence. Referral to a spinal or neurosurgeon in order to investigate the recurring problem is often required. CT and MRI scans of the brain and cervical spine may well be necessary. Myelograms, where a dye is injected into the cerebrospinal fluid, can be used, but are not fashionable these days. The consultant may also feel it is relevant to assess the blood supply to the brain and cervical spine, and Doppler studies of the subclavian arteries are possible. Concussion in the young player should be looked at even more seriously than in the adult and an early medical opinion may be needed.

Lacerations are far commoner, and both codes now require players with wounds to be removed from the field of play, so the injury can be assessed and the necessary repairs carried out. Most facial lacerations require suturing, whilst many to the top and back of the skull may be stapled using a medical stapler. Minor lacerations and grazes can be sealed temporarily with petroleum jelly (Vaseline). Clotting times can also be reduced by using seaweed-impregnated dressings, as used in plastic surgery, and this type of dressing can be strapped to the skin in order to allow a player to carry on until the end of the game, when a more thorough repair is possible.

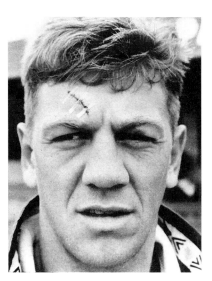

Figure 7.6 Laceration to the head.

Head injury is a medical state that should never be solely determined by the external appearance of the player. One of the best examples I have seen to support this statement came at a lecture given by Dr I. Adams, the former Leeds United F.C. and Leeds R.L. doctor. Initially he put a slide on the screen of a child with a three pin electrical plug stuck in the centre of his forehead, who had been brought into casualty. All the audience were shocked by this slide, as visually it appeared to be a very serious injury. He then told everybody that after removing the plug, the wounds were very superficial and required only basic medical care. He then put up a slide of a boy of a similar age, with a bruise the size of a ten pence piece on his forehead. This young lad died within the hour. The moral of the story is that all head injuries need to be assessed properly regardless of the obvious visual appearance, in order to eliminate the possibility of any internal bleeding.

Case study

In collision sports such as rugby, the skills of a good dentist are often called upon. Players quite readily lose teeth, particularly when associated with fractures around the skull area and require urgent attention after the game to prevent the complete loss.

Players will also develop the common problems such as **abcesses, erupting wisdom teeth, gingivitis, loss of fillings** and **decay**. Regular six-monthly checkups will reduce the risk of such problems arising before important games.

Dental injuries

A **'cauliflower' ear** is a haematoma in the connective tissue between the cartilage and the skin of the ear. It is caused by a direct blow or by the grinding impact of scrummaging, so is most prevalent in the front five forwards. In acute cases any inflammation is left to nature, but in severe cases aspiration of the haematoma is necessary followed by compression with a sterile bandage. Recurrent symptoms are not unusual in such cases.

Ear injuries

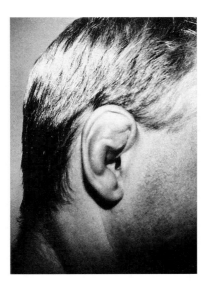

Figure 7.7 A cauliflower ear.

Infection of the inner and middle ear is usually caused by a bacterial, chemical or allergic reaction, and is treated in the acute stages with the appropriate antibiotics. The excess secretions can then be removed by using ear drops to soften the wax, followed by syringing of the ear passage. Chronic cases may well require surgery, and players may need several months away from the game to give the operation any chance of working.

Eye injuries

Eye injuries tend to occur due to the physical clashes which occur in the competitive situation, such as a stray or, occasionally, deliberate elbow or finger passing directly into the eye socket. In the United Kingdom, soccer has been found to generate more eye injuries than any other sport (MacEwen, 1987), with an unfortunate rise in the number of deliberate injuries which in some cases have led to a successful prosecution (Grayson, 1990). The management of a severe eye injury under the ophthamologist may only be able to offer a degree of damage limitation. Fortunately the penetrating type of injury to the eyeball is rare, particularly as the possibility of intraocular infection can have a devastating effect. The presence of foreign matter may necessitate a surgical approach to remove the offending particles.

The more common blunt injury to the anterior portion of the eye tends to produce a **subconjunctival haematoma** or painful **corneal abrasion**. The resultant increase in intraocular pressure may produce temporary or permanent damage to important internal structures such as the lens, blood vessels or nerve pathways. In the posterior segment of the eye, **retinal detatchment** may present later following an initial blow to the eye and requires immediate surgical intervention. Less damaging **retinal tears** may also present themselves and can be treated prophylactically with an argon laser to prevent full detachment from arising at a later date.

Conjunctivitis may be caused by trauma, or by other causes such as infection or an allergic reaction. Antibiotic cream from the player's GP is often prescribed, although mild cases can be helped by eye wash (Optrex). Players who use contact lenses can also develop this problem, so encourage a good standard of hygiene in these individuals.

Facial fractures

The most common **fracture** sites in the facial area are the zygomatic arch and the lower mandible. The healing ability of such fractures is good and a player will normally be able to return to playing after bone consolidation, which is usually about six weeks later. Complex surgery and internal fixation may be necessary, and constant monitoring is required as infection is a possible complication. Psychologically the injury may prevent the player from total commitment on their return to playing for several weeks, until they have confidence that the fracture site can take a blow without refracturing.

Around the eye the bony orbital margins are very strong, yet the internal walls are very thin, leaving this area exposed to a 'blow-out' following trauma to the anterior aspect of the eye. Direct sudden pressure to the inferior orbital margin can also buckle the orbital floor and cause a snap fracture, thus simulating a 'blow-out' displacement. A player will often complain of numbness over the cheek and upper teeth due to damage to the infraorbital nerve. Cosmetically the eye may appear initially to protrude more prominently. Due to the lack of support, however, the eyeball may sink downwards and backwards, with an unacceptable cosmetic appearance. In such situations a false silastic orbital floor may need to be inserted to alter this appearance and to enlarge the field of binocular vision. Should the orbital rim fracture, surgical repositioning may be necessary under the guidance of a maxillofacial surgeon.

Lacerations to the mouth and tongue produce plenty of blood, but tend to heal quickly due to the dense capillary network. Appropriate first aid care and the use of an antiseptic mouth wash (Oraldene) will help to prevent any problems.

Mouth injuries

A **broken nose** is a common problem in rugby players and requires specialist, immediate reduction if a reasonable alignment is to be achieved. Such an injury may prevent air from entering the nasal passages and some players have taken to wearing a nasal strapping (Breathe easy strips) to try and enlarge the nostrils. Isolated case studies recommend this choice of treatment, though more scientific proof is required if any objective benefits are to be believed.

Nasal injuries

Nose bleeds require good first aid care and should cause little long-term concern, except in a more serious cases where the conscious state of the player will suggest the severity of the problem. Packing of the nasal cavity should be loose so that the bleeding stops gradually, rather than completely blocking the airway.

Infection of the sinuses can be a chronic, recurrent problem, particularly in players who play in the cold, damp climate of a British winter. Nasal sprays, antibiotics and, in extreme cases, surgery may be necessary, with continuing inhalation and washouts to prevent the possibility of recurrence.

Major spinal injuries occur when the spinal cord is directly involved, and further damage is possible due to the instability of the spinal column. The role of the medical team and the first aid procedures used to immobilize, transfer and be aware of developing complications is never under greater scrutiny than in this situation. Even though major spinal injury is among the most serious of sports injuries, it only constitutes 3% of such injuries (Leidholt, 1963). In South Africa, it has been recorded that rugby has the highest incidence of spinal cord injury of all organized sports (Scher, 1981).

Spine

Lesser spinal injuries within the normal population as well as the sporting community can cause many problems in the daily routine of any individual. The players' occupations, as well as their playing careers, may well be affected by an injury to the spinal column. This can be an even greater problem with a professional player, whose whole life is centred around their ability to perform on the pitch. If an X-ray or MRI/CT scan were to be taken of the cervical and lumbar regions of all the players involved in collision sports, a large proportion would have signs of spinal disease or trauma. The important thing to remember is that information gained from such tests must be considered in relation to any symptoms the player is complaining of. Scans and radiographs are very useful but can sometimes provide misleading information to the medical team as to the diagnosis of a problem. Many players will have played for years with a spinal pathology, yet have been symptom free. This can sometimes make it hard for players to understand why spinal conditions take a time to settle and often recur. Certain injuries within the spine are common to all the main regions, cervical,

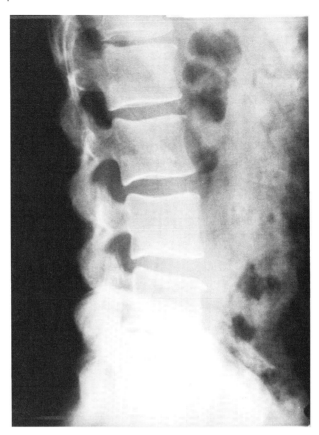

Figure 7.8 Major narrowing of the L5-S1 disc space in a 50 year old ex-professional soccer player. Note the virtual perfect joint spaces and definition at all other lumbar levels. His first relevant symptoms from the lumbar spine started at the age of 49.

thoracic and lumbar. Details of more specific injuries to the lumbar spine can be found in Chapter 6, 'Lumbar spine'.

Fractured vertebrae may vary greatly in severity, some occurring without symptoms at the time of injury. The fracture itself is sometimes accompanied by a dislocation, and can produce either a stable or an unstable injury.

1. Stable injury

Thankfully the majority of fractures of vertebrae are stable ones, with most occurring at the bony prominences present on the vertebral body. Fractures within the vertebral body itself are often termed 'compression' or 'wedge', depending on the direction of force and the resultant damage. These heal most often by fibrous union and seldom create problems after sufficient rest. If the fracture occurs in the vertebral body, the same type of healing process takes place but there is a greater possibility of complications due to the role of the vertebra in transmitting weight and allowing movement.

2. Unstable injury

This is defined as 'loss of ability of the spine to move without damage or irritation of the spinal cord or nerve roots and without the development of deformity' (White *et al.*, 1976).

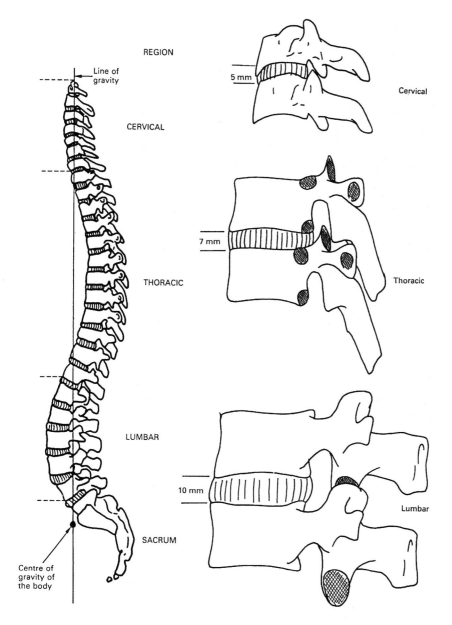

REGION

Line of gravity

5 mm

Cervical

CERVICAL

7 mm

THORACIC

Thoracic

LUMBAR

10 mm

Lumbar

SACRUM

Centre of gravity of the body

Reproduced with permission from Palastanga *et al.*, 1994.

Obviously, to classify this type of injury a meticulous clinical examination is necessary along with the appropriate investigative tests. The first aid care of such an injury is described in Chapter 3, 'Spinal injuries'. In the long-term, the vast majority of fractures can be treated quite well conservatively with orthotic support and encouragement. Ligamentous disruptions causing instability are an entirely different group and these almost invariably need surgical treatment.

Prolapsed intervertebral discs can be a primary or secondary problem in the injured spine. In such a situation, the nucleus pulposus pushes through the outer annulus fibrosis of the disc, with pain and spasm produced by inflammatory pressure on the surrounding muscular, ligamentous and nervous tissue, as well as by the disc itself. This will obviously cause symptoms of pain, weakness, disturbed sensory patterns or loss of function to the affected spinal section and relative limbs. Surgery may be necessary in cases that refuse to settle with conservative care, or where the bulge is so great that further trauma could cause more serious problems. Referral to Chapter 6, 'Lumbar spine – surgical notes' is recommended for more detailed notes on this subject.

In the older player or the younger player who has been subjected to excessive physical stresses in their early years, **degeneration of the spine** can produce chronic episodes of pain and loss of function. In the elderly non-athletic individual, surgery may be considered to allow a better quality of life. Unfortunately, in the active sportsperson such surgery will produce a reduction in the level of pain experienced, but will also reduce the possibility of continuing to play at the standard they are used to. Individuals often panic when an arthritic label is attached to their particular injury, but it is a problem that develops in everybody to a certain degree as the years go by, some more quickly than others, depending on the stress that has been applied to the affected area. Many individuals who have a much more sedentary lifestyle such as those in clerical or driving jobs are just as likely to develop similar problems due to lack of movement and exercise, so what is the happy medium? This type of problem will require intermittent periods of physiotherapy and postural advice depending on the symptoms, and only in very severe cases is surgery necessary. Even then it is only used as a salvage procedure.

Ankylosing spondylitis is a rheumatic disorder that is common in males under the age of 30 and should never be discounted as a differential diagnosis in players with chronic episodes of spinal and systemic joint symptoms. Once diagnosis has been confirmed by an HLA-B27 test – the antigen which is present in some 90% of patients with ankylosing spondylitis – a strict spinal exercise programme is necessary to help maintain and improve mobility. Such individuals can continue to play, but have a tendency to take longer to recover from other injuries than other players due to the inflammatory nature of this systemic problem. This is also true with players who have associated conditions, e.g. diabetes.

Cervical spine

The cervical spine is particularly vulnerable to injury because of its extreme mobility and poor stability, which is due to the shape of the vertebra. The injuries that occur in this region depend on the magnitude and direction of the applied force, the stability of the vertebral segments and the integrity of the discs and surrounding soft tissues. All injuries to this area should be treated as serious until proven otherwise.

Tetraplegia, which in the worst cases can mean paralysis of all four limbs plus loss of bowel, bladder and sexual function, is fortunately not a common problem in rugby, but even one incident per season is enough to spell out the possible dangers of playing such a sport. The death rate in such individuals can be as high as 30% (Scher, 1977), and the possible long-term complications of pressure sores and infection add to the high morbidity rate. More common problems are **cervical spondylosis, prolapsed intervertebral discs** and **soft tissue injuries** to the cervical structures. Surgery for such conditions is only advised in extreme cases, and often signals the beginning of the downward slope in an individual's playing career.

Radiographs, MRI and CT scans are normal investigative procedures, followed by intensive physiotherapy and prescription anti-inflammatories.

In the thoracic spine, **spinal cord damage** due to playing rugby is very rare, with Silver and Gill (1988) quoting only one case out of 19 recorded at Stoke Mandeville Hospital, England, between 1983 and 1987.

Thoracic spine

In the adolescent, **Scheurman's Disease** is a spinal condition which can limit the progress of an individual player. This osteochondritic-related problem mainly affects the lower thoracic and upper lumbar vertebral segments (Greene *et al.*, 1985), with disturbance of the two secondary ossifying centres, the ring epiphyses, in the cartilage end plates. On X-ray investigation, discal material can often be seen entering the vertebral body through the cartilage endplate, which is labelled as a Schmorl's node. An active mobilizing and strengthening programme is required, with particular emphasis on hamstring flexibility and lumbar extension.

A **fractured sternum** is not the most common of injuries, but is probably one of the most painful. Radiographs will confirm such a problem and recovery is slow, as the player needs to be completely pain-free and fully functional before returning to play.

Thorax

Bruised, cracked or **fractured ribs** are very common injuries in rugby, which often take up to eight weeks to heal. This very much depends on the clinical picture exhibited by the player on functional testing. The most common sites of injury are at the rib angle or close to the sternocostal joints. The pain is usually due to damage in the surrounding intercostal muscles rather than the fracture, though crepitus may be felt over the fracture site on deep inhalation. Strapping of this area tends to be avoided as it often inhibits the player from using that area of lung tissue to breathe, which may encourage infection or collapse.

Drug taking and its detection is a major part of sport in the modern-day society. This can lead to injury and raise its head in unusual circumstances. A colleague of mine told me of a bodybuilder he was treating who developed a sharp pain over a rib angle which developed whilst bench pressing with excessive weight and low repetitions. As there was no history of direct trauma, he examined the area and diagnosed an intercostal muscle strain which he treated accordingly. Four weeks on, the injury had failed to respond, so he referred the patient to an orthopaedic consultant who X-rayed the rib cage, which showed a fracture. On further questioning the bodybuilder admitted to taking anabolic steroids, which was felt to be a predisposing factor to the injury due to the adverse effect steroids have on hormonal balance and subsequent bone density.

Case study

Intercostal **muscle strains** produce very similar symptoms to a fracture, but with rest and physiotherapy make a full recovery within six weeks. Exercising of the rib cage to regain mobility using breathing and spinal exercises will help to stretch the area.

Injury to the **ligamentous tissue** and **rib cartilages** at the sternocostal and costochondral joints is also a common injury to the thorax. This tends to occur in the close contact phases of the game – mauling and scrummaging – and has a limiting effect on the ability of the player to train on the weights due to the pressure increases created in the thorax.

Sternal costoclavicular hyperostosis is typified radiologically by an increase in bone density of the clavicle and sternum, ossification of the first costal cartilage and synostosis of the sternoclavicular joint. The individual will tend to complain of dull aching sensation at the inflammatory site, often demonstrating bilateral chronic painful swelling of the clavicle, sternum and first rib. Blood tests may demonstrate a raised erythrocyte sedimentation rate (ESR) and hyper-gammaglobulin level. Symptoms often respond to non-steroidal anti-inflammatory medication.

In severe cases, a fractured rib may encourage air to enter into the pleural lining to produce a **pneumothorax**. This state requires urgent admission to hospital and insertion of a chest drain to alleviate the symptoms. Any reduced breath sounds over the area using a stethoscope, with resonance on percussion may well suggest such a problem. Should blood enter the unwanted air pocket, this is called a **haemopneumothorax**.

Rupture of the pectoralis major muscle is a very disabling and disfiguring injury for any player who suffers such a problem. The player will complain of a short sharp pain, possibly followed by a sensation of burning, which then disappears. The individual may well try to carry on playing, but will soon realize that something serious is wrong when trying to use the arm as normal. On examination, there will be a marked hollow over the lateral aspect of the pectoralis muscle with bruising around the site of injury. This may well become widespread as the injury settles and the bleeding gravitates. Always check the biceps muscle as well, as there may be an associated rupture in this muscle group. Initial immobilization is followed by a graduated rehabilitation programme. Care must be taken when devising a weights programme to ensure further damage is avoided. Returning to play can take up to six months in severe cases, depending on the severity of injury and position of the player in the team – front row forwards may well find great difficulty in scrummaging initially.

| Case study | *In one particular rugby league match, the prop forward of the team I was looking after suffered a severe rupture of his pectoralis major. On this particular day his opposite number happened to be the heaviest player in the league, which is no problem in fast open play, but when scrummaging or trying to tackle can create problems. Our prop forward was no weakling, as his full time job was doorman at the local nightclub, but this was to be a totally new experience for him. As the first scrum was being formed, the two front rows were trying to impose themselves on each other in order to gain early superiority in a vital area of the game with regards to possession of the ball. Unfortunately our team were not as big and strong as the opposition and the whole front row collapsed. As these three players were heading face first into the ground, the very large prop forward stood bolt upright with our prop forward's hand still gripping the back of his shirt. As you can imagine the only thing that could give way under the strain was the soft tissue over the anterior aspect of the glenohumeral joint, and so the rupture occurred.* |

Abdomen   Abdominal and groin injuries in rugby players tend to be very different in signs, symptoms and causes to those in soccer players, though this may change as union players become professional and are expected to train daily and league players ask more of their bodies in terms of playing back to back rugby in the two different codes or on the other side of the world. The common exceptions in rugby are the goalkickers, who tend to get identical problems to the soccer players due to more repetitive kicking than the other members of the team. Referral to Chapter 6, 'Abdomen', provides the appropriate information on groin disruption syndrome.

The typical history of the injured rugby player includes:

- A specific moment of trauma.
- Formation of a visible haematoma in the lower abdomen, genital and adductor region.
- Associated sharp pain, swelling, increased temperature, discoloration and loss of function.
- Constant pain.
- Muscular injury to the lower abdomen and adductor regions (often delayed awareness).
- Unilateral symptoms.

Treatment of the problem tends to be conservative initially, even though there are more external signs than in the degenerative 'sportsman's hernia' described

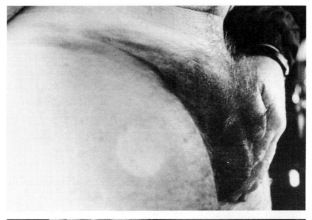

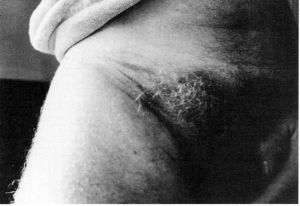

Figure 7.9/7.10 Traumatic injury to the abdominal wall and genitals in a professional rugby league player after kicking a ball.

in the previous chapter. This is to allow the acute symptoms time to settle. Surgery may well be necessary if the player fails to make sufficient functional progress within two to three weeks, with the appropriate medical and rehabilitative care. Abdominal repair and adductor release procedures are totally dependent on the symptoms of the individual.

Shoulder girdle

The clavicle acts as a strut over the front part of the chest wall and often suffers injury at either of the two end points, the acromioclavicular and sternoclavicular joints, or in the bone itself. The structural role of the clavicle and its role in the biomechanics of the upper limb is what makes this a very painful area to injure. A **fractured clavicle** is often a very disfiguring injury visually, yet once it has healed it will regain full function and strength. Only in very severe cases is internal fixation required, so most are immobilized in a full sling and mobilization begun as soon as possible. As healing occurs, callus formation may cause the fracture site to become more prominent, but apart from the player's vanity, this is irrelevant.

Complete or partial dislocation of the acromioclavicular joint is a common shoulder girdle problem, and the 'step' that is produced is often a worrying complication to the player. This is caused by the complete or partial rupture of the coracoclavicular ligament, which inserts into the inferior, distal end of the clavicle. Injury is usually due to falling onto the point of the shoulder with the force driving the scapula downwards. The resistance to this movement comes from the coracoclavicular ligament, which with excessive stress is partially or totally ruptured. In the short-term immobilization is necessary, and a pad placed over the acromioclavicular joint and held in place by zinc oxide tape which loops around the upper forearm is very useful. The whole arm can then be placed in a sling or collar and cuff. In the long-term, previous trauma may well speed up degenerative changes in the joint (Taft *et al.*, 1987), but in the short-term this will only give cosmetic problems to the player, providing they have gone through the necessary rehabilitation of six to eight weeks. Surgery is very rarely undertaken as no distinct advantage has been recorded in the long-term management of the patient (Dias and Gregg, 1991). Occasionally some dislocations produce a posterior displacement, buttonholing through the trapezius muscle tissue, or in the case of a severe upward displacement the end of the clavicle may lie just under the skin. Both situations may need surgical repair as they often produce prolonged symptoms.

Dislocation and **subluxation of the sternoclavicular joint** is not as common, but follows a similar pathology and treatment programme. A posterior dislocation could inhibit the normal respiratory pattern and quick, appropriate action must be taken in such a situation. Bony callus, particularly from an anterior subluxation, will often produce a long-lasting reminder of the injury, but functional rehabilitation is possible as soon as the pain subsides. Surgical internal fixation has been used, but complications appear to abound. Conservative management would appear to give good long-term care (Rockwood and Odor, 1989). Full rehabilitation and return to match fitness will take approximately six to eight weeks.

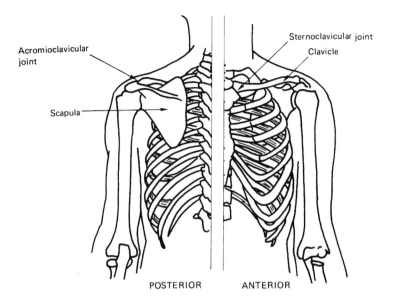

POSTERIOR   ANTERIOR

Acromioclavicular joint

Scapula

Sternoclavicular joint

Clavicle

Reproduced with permission from Palastanga *et al.*, 1994.

Danger

Following surgical intervention to internally fixate and stabilize any fracture site, there is always the possibility that any metalwork can loosen and move into other areas of the body. In internal fixation of the sternoclavicular joint, reports of migration of a Steinman pin or Kirchner wire into the heart have been recorded (Garrick and Webb, 1990).

A **fractured scapula** is not a common injury, and even when it does occur, it rarely displaces due to the extensive muscle attachments on the main body of the bone. Initial immobilization is followed with the appropriate rehabilitation programme.

Scapula

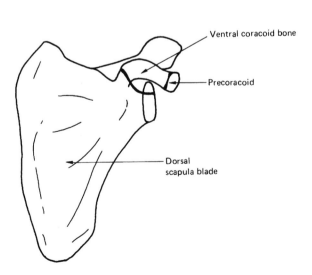

Ventral coracoid bone

Precoracoid

Dorsal scapula blade

Reproduced with permission from Palastanga *et al.*, 1994.

Glenohumeral joint

Dislocation and **subluxation of the glenohumeral joint** are common injuries amongst rugby players, and as with most of the shoulder girdle injuries occur due to the player falling onto an outstretched arm. The possibility of an associated **fracture** should never be ignored. Initially the player may well be advised to rehabilitate the shoulder after a period of immobilization, with particular emphasis on rotatory work in the shoulder, although lateral rotation combined with abduction and hyperextension should be avoided in the early stages.

Surgical notes

Recurrent dislocations or acute situations where an MRI scan is performed in the early stages may demonstrate a hole (Bankhart lesion) in the supporting capsular wall and glenoid labrum. Between these two categories, certain individuals will fall into an atraumatic group, with problems which are structural in nature and require surgery, whilst others will have habitual problems requiring solely rehabilitation. Diagnostically, arthroscopy can also be used in the evaluation of the unstable shoulder. With straightforward traumatic anterior dislocations, it is not usually necessary, as it does not provide any extra information. For subluxations and atraumatic dislocations it can be very useful in confirming a suspected diagnosis and information on the direction of instability. In the case of collision sports, dislocation of the glenohumeral joint is an extremely common injury. Surgery should be considered in the individual with appropriate pathology and an appreciation of the necessary rehabilitation, and should be relevant to the demands of the sport.

The recurrent instability a traumatic dislocation produces is, in the main, treated with open procedures, depending on the degree of damage. The initial priority is to repair any Bankhart lesion present within the capsular wall, the principal cause of instability in any traumatic glenohumeral instability (Braly and Tullas, 1985). An anterior repair using a closed arthroscopic approach is most effective in such players, with less than four to six redislocations. Surgical procedures such as a full or modified Bristow procedure (Schauder and Tullos,

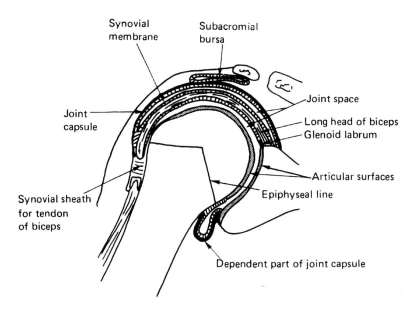

Reproduced with permission from Palastanga *et al.*, 1994.

1992; Braly and Tullos, 1985; Helfet, 1958) with transfer of the coracoid process produce long-term limitation of shoulder external rotation, a functional complication to any player whose role in the team involves throwing from overhead. This problem can now be avoided in most cases by repairing the defect using sutures through drill holes in the glenoid rim, or by using appropriate suture anchor techniques (Bayley, 1996). The capsule can then be repaired by overlapping methods. Excessive lateral rotation can be reduced at this stage if necessary. In worse situations, secondary stretching produces capsular instability on top of the labral defect (Bayley, 1996), which makes it more difficult to restore stability with closed techniques. In terms of rehabilitation, the major advantage of the arthroscopic approach is the preservation of joint proprioception.

The most common **fracture** sites are around the neck and midshaft of the humerus. Fractures around the humeral head and lip of the glenoid labrum are usually associated with a dislocation or subluxation of the joint. Treatment is determined by the presence of displacement at the fracture site, and the ability to immobilize the area without increasing the risk factor to the surrounding nerves and blood vessels.

Soft tissue injuries, such as **rotator cuff tears, partial tears, tendinitis, intra-** and **extra-articular bursitis** and **bicipital tendinitis** can occur due to trauma in the match situation but may also arise from weights work in the gymnasium. Determine the cause of the injury first. If it is from gym work – usually due to a poor lifting technique, a badly planned training programme, or inadequate equipment – try to make adjustments if possible before advising complete rest. If alterations to the player's weights programme and treatment make little difference to the injury then complete rest may be necessary, but many such injuries often settle with fine adjustments and this will reduce the possibility of recurrence. Rehabilitation programmes should take into account the possibility of reversed humeroscapula movement in the painful shoulder. It is also important to strengthen the agonist, synergic and fixator roles of each muscle used in the functional patterns needed for that players position.

Surgical notes

Stubborn cases may require the opinion of an orthopaedic surgeon, who has a choice of treatments available. A corticosteroid injection attempts to inhibit the inflammatory response and may reduce the possibility of myositis in the tissue (Molloy and McGuirk, 1976). Although steroids have a strong anti-inflammatory effect, they may also produce a catabolic response which may be detrimental to the healing process. Many case studies exist about the detrimental effects of repeated steroid injections into a particular injury site. A maximum of three injections is the present safety limit, and certainly the use of corticosteroids in the treatment of chronic sports injuries has decreased dramatically in the last ten years.

Should active rehabilitation fail to settle the injury, surgery may be necessary. Subacromial decompression can be performed much better, arthroscopically, with quicker recovery due to the less extensive exposure. This consists of division of the coracoacromial ligament and modest removal of the underside of the anterior aspect of the acromion to change its undersurface from being curved to flat. Often a player will complain of both pain and instability in the shoulder. It is important that the surgeon treats the primary abnormality first, usually the instability, before considering decompression for the pain. The arthroscopy also allows the surgeon to examine the relationship between the soft tissues and relevant bony structures. Many impingement syndromes involving the rotator cuff, synovium, head of the humerus, glenoid cavity and acromion exist, and can be identified and treated accordingly, in many cases nonoperatively.

Ruptures of the rotator cuff which involve only a small tear can also be treated via the arthroscopic camera, though many players often continue to play ignorant of such a problem and then present as chronic cases in later years. Total arthroscopic repair procedures are still in their infancy and are technically demanding of the surgeon. At present, such procedures do not rival open or arthroscopically assisted methods (Bayley, 1996).

Treatment notes

Reference should be made to Chapter 8, 'Upper Limb Variables', with regard to rehabilitation procedures following surgical intervention.

Calcification of the soft tissues around the glenohumeral joint may occur due to trauma or impingement of the tendon tissue decreasing an already limited blood supply, particularly around the attachment of supraspinatous. Steroid injection and surgery are useful tools in such chronic injuries.

Rupture of the biceps tendon may be an isolated problem, or associated with other soft tissue trauma. Surgery is very rarely recommended for such individuals, where the distal belly of the muscle rolls up to appear as a lump over the anterior aspect of the arm when the muscle contracts (the 'Popeye' sign). Rehabilitation following conservative management is important to regain full functional use in the upper limb. In those individuals where surgery is advocated, the distal tendon of the biceps muscle is reattached to the radial tuberosity. Rehabilitation consists of static splinting, controlled mobilization and muscle strengthening (Hurov, 1996).

Elbow

The elbow gives rise to both traumatic and chronic niggling injuries. Isolated **fractures** and **dislocations** do occur, but more commonly the injury is a combination of the two. The most common fracture sites are the olecranon, capitulum, head of radius and the two epicondyles of the humerus. Surgical fixation of the fracture may be necessary, but is avoided if possible due to the effect it may have on a full functional recovery. With a dislocation, reduction under anaesthetic is necessary in most cases as the pain from such an injury is usually very severe, producing protective spasm in the surrounding muscle tissue, and the arm will be grossly disfigured. Rehabilitation will initially be cautious in order to prevent any complications, though early mobilization is essential to have any hope of a full recovery. Care must be taken to prevent redislocation or calcification of the soft tissues and it is not unusual in the long-term for a player to lose full flexion or extension. Functionally, however, they should make a full recovery, and can return to playing when the fracture or dislocation is stable.

Due to direct trauma on the joint, **bursitis** and the production of **loose bodies** are chronic, niggling injuries that can develop. Loss of full extension with a marked effusion are common signs of the two conditions. In the acute stages, anti-inflammatories and physiotherapy can be used to settle the symptoms. More chronic problems may require arthroscopic surgery to assess and remove the offending bursa or bony fragment. This can be done during the close season, and most players will continue to play with such injuries. A corticosteroid injection may be used to allow the player to carry on until a convenient time for surgery can be arranged.

Epicondylitis at the medial and lateral epicondyle of the humerus (golfer's or tennis elbow) are not injuries that occur due to playing rugby directly, but more to training in the weights room. Poor lifting techniques, excess resistance, badly planned training programmes or having to grip the weights bars too tight are all possible causes of such an injury, and need rectifying before commencing any physical treatment. Physiotherapy and anti-inflammatories are direct treatment procedures. More chronic problems may respond to corticosteroid injection, or need surgery to remove the excess scar tissue deposits produced.

Danger

One of the possible complications at the elbow joint is a contracture following traumatic injury, most typically in children with supracondylar fractures. This is known as a **Volkman's ischaemic contracture**. It must be remembered that this may also occur due to trauma in the forearm, in crush injuries or if a plaster cast or bandage compresses the area too tightly. Symptoms include numbness, swelling and discoloration of the fingers with increasing pain. Early recognition of the problem allows the compartment syndrome to be treated appropriately.

Forearm

A **fracture** can occur to the radius or ulna in the midshaft due to direct trauma, or at the distal end close to the wrist (Smith or Colles' fracture) by falling onto an outstretched arm. X-ray investigations, reduction if necessary and immobilization are the normal treatment procedures, but in severe cases internal fixation may be necessary. In stubborn cases that refuse to fully consolidate or refracture, a bone graft may be an option.

Wrist

Around the wrist joint, various little **fractures** and **dislocations** can occur in the two rows of carpal bones which articulate with the radius, ulna and metacarpals. The most common and chronic injury is the **fractured scaphoid**. Unfortunately the initial radiographs may not show any sign of the problem (Garrick and Webb, 1990), but if repeat radiographs are taken weeks later, a fracture line may become more evident. This is because the bony configuration and soft tissue attachments virtually prevent the possibility of any displacement. The area should be immobilized for 6–12 weeks. Complications can develop as the bone itself has a very poor blood supply and non-union may occur. Various surgical techniques are often attempted at this stage – fixation with a screw, bone graft or excision – but the injury often tends to produce aggravation later on in life due to arthritic changes.

Dislocation or **subluxation** of the lunate or capitate may occur due to falling onto the outstretched hand. With the wrist held in flexion, a subluxed capitate is seen as a prominent bump on the back of the hand. Reduction is possible with manual traction. The lunate subluxes anteriorly, often with a complete rupture

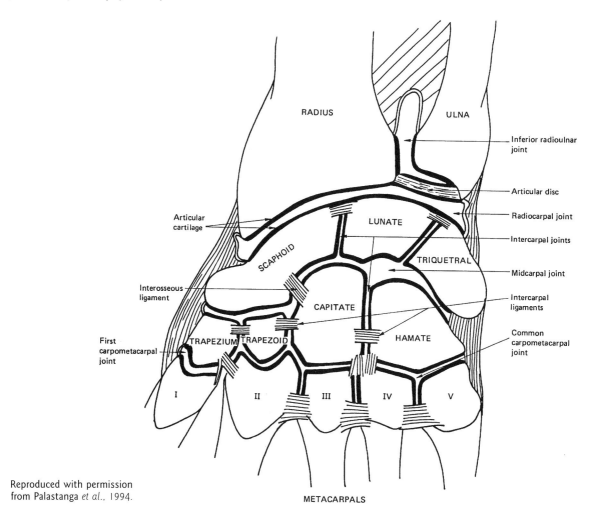

Reproduced with permission from Palastanga *et al.*, 1994.

of the scaphoid-lunate ligament, which allows the lunate to rotate. This will require reduction under anaesthetic and immobilization in slight flexion. Full extension will need to be limited on resuming normal sporting activities in order to reduce the possibility of recurrence.

Hand In the hand, **fractures, dislocations** and **ligamentous** injuries tend to occur in isolation or together. The thumb is a very vulnerable area. **Fracture** to the first metacarpal at the base of the thumb (Bennett's fracture) and **dislocation** of the saddle-shaped bony articulations often require reduction under anaesthetic. Fractures to this area may require internal fixation with pins or screws if the fracture line invades the joint surface, followed by immobilization in a plaster cast for 3–4 weeks. Complete or partial **rupture of the ulnar collateral ligament** of the thumb (Skier's thumb) can be an injury that has functional limitations for the rugby player. Laxity at this site will affect grip and the ability to pass the ball, and appropriate taping techniques are needed to limit extension and abduction of the thumb. Physiotherapy and taping will help in most cases, although chronic or severe problems may require surgery and/or immobilization.

The metacarpal bones are also subject to the risk of **fracturing**. Undisplaced fractures are well splinted by the surrounding bones, and a wool and crepe dressing is sufficient to immobilize in the initial stages. As the pain subsides, functional movements such as gripping can be started. Displaced fractures may need a more rigid immobilization, and in severe cases internal fixation may be necessary. Problems of this type tend to be very common amongst boxers, so the mode of injury should not be too hard to deduce! **Fractures** of the phalanges occur quite commonly, with immobilization limited to a simple splint or taping to the next digit. Should the fracture extend into the joint space then it may take longer to regain full mobility, if at all. **Dislocation** of the phalangeal bones can easily be reduced and the player may well be able to continue by splinting to the next finger. However, an X-ray should still be a routine procedure following such an injury to ensure that there has been no bony damage caused by the avulsion force. A thorough assessment should also be made of the flexor and extensor tendons in case of **partial** or **complete rupture**. Flexor tendon ruptures occur most commonly at the site of the flexor digitorum profundus insertion into the base of the distal phalanx. On examination no active flexion is possible at the distal interphalangeal joint, and immobilization in a finger splint is necessary before examination and possible surgery from the orthopaedic team. On the extensor aspect, rupture of the long extensor tendon into the distal phalanx produces the deformity known as 'mallet' finger. A flexion deformity at the distal joint and an inability to actively extend the flexed joint are classical signs. Splintage and an orthopaedic consultation as to the benefits of possible surgery are necessary immediately. If the rupture occurs in the middle of the tendon at the proximal interphalangeal joint, the deformity produced is one of hyperextension of the distal joint and the injury is classified as a Boutonnière deformity. Management is the same as for the other tendon ruptures. Early recognition of the problem gives the necessary surgery a chance to succeed, and the player a hope of full mobility. In terms of the digits, damage can occur to the collateral ligaments, which tends to produce a swollen, stiff joint unless mobilization occurs quickly. Complete ligamentous rupture may warrant surgical intervention, particularly if the damage occurs in the two most important fingers responsible for the gripping action, the index and little finger. Cosmetically the appearance may make little improvement from its initial state.

Case study

Whilst working with a rugby league team I was summoned onto the pitch by one of our players just after the opposing team had scored a try. As I approached him I could see he was cradling his hand. 'Dave, just wipe this white stuff off my hand. It must be the paint used to mark out the pitch.' What he hadn't noticed was the deformity at the distal end of the finger. The white paint was actually an open, fracture dislocation of the fourth digit at the proximal interphalangeal joint. As soon as he realized it was bone and not paint, he fainted and was stretchered off!

References

Adams, I. D. (1977). Rugby football injuries. *Br. J. Sports Med.*, April, 4–6.

Addley, K. and Farren, J. (1988). Irish rugby survey: Dungannon Football Club (1986–87). *Br. J. Sports Med.*, **22(1)**, 22–24.

Alexander, D., Kennedy, M. and Kennedy, J. (1979). Injuries in rugby league football. *Med. J. Aust.*, **2(7)**, 341–342.

Alexander, D., Kennedy, M. and Kennedy, J. (1980). Rugby league football injuries over two competition seasons (letter). *Med. J. Aust.*, **2(6)**, 334–335.

Bayley, I. (1996). Surgical management of the injured sporting shoulder. *Physio. Sport*, **11(1)**, 14–18.

Braly. W. G. and Tullos, H. S. (1985). A modification of the Bristow procedure for recurrent anterior shoulder dislocation and subluxation. *Am. J. Sports Med.*, **13**, 81–86.

Burry, H. C. and Calcinai, C. J. (1988). The need to make rugby safer (editorial). *Br. Med. J.*, **296(16)**, 149–150.

Chapman, P. J. (1985). Orofacial injuries and the use of mouthguards by the 1984 Great Britain rugby league touring team. *Br. J. Sports Med.*, **19(1)**, 34–36.

Clegg, J. H. (1969). Mouth protection for the rugby football player. *Br. Dent. J.*, **127**, 341–343.

Davies, J. E. and Gibson. T. (1978). Injuries in rugby union football. *Br. Med. J.*, **2(6154)**, 1759–1761.

Dias, J. J. and Gregg, P. J. (1991). Acromioclavicular joint injuries in sport. *Sports Med.*, **11(2)**, 125–132.

Durkin, T. E. (1977). A survey of injuries in a first class rugby union football club from 1972–1976. *Br. J. Sports Med.*, **11(1)**, 7–11.

Garrick, J. G. and Webb, D. R. (1990). *Sports Injuries: Diagnosis and Management.* London: W. B. Saunders.

Gibbs, N. (1993). Injuries in professional rugby league. *Am. J. Sports Med.*, **21(5)**, 696–700.

Gissane, C., Jennings, D. C. and Standing. P. (1993). Incidence of injury in rugby league football. *Physiotherapy*, **79(5)**, 305–310.

Grayson, E. (1990). Sports medicine and the law. In: *Medicine, Sport and the Law*, (S. D. W. Payne. ed.), Oxford: Blackwell.

Greene, T. L., Hensinger, R. N. and Hunter, L. Y. (1985). Back pain and vertebral changes simulating Scheurmann's disease. *J. Paed. Orthop.*, **5**, 1–7.

Haywood, J. R. (1978). Recent advances in the management of facial fractures. *Int. J. Oral Surg.*, **1**, 263–264.

Helfet, A. J. (1958). Coracoid transplantationfor recurring dislocation of the shoulder. *J. Bone Joint Surg.*, **40B**, 198–202.

Hickey, J. C., Morris, A. L., Carlson, L. D. *et al.* (1967). Relation of mouth protectors to cranial pressure and deformation. *J. Aust. Dental Assoc.*, **74**, 735–740.

Hurov, J. R. (1996). Controlled active mobilization following surgical repair of the avulsed radial attachment of the biceps brachii muscle: A case report. *J. Orthop. Sports. Phys. Ther.*, **23(6)**, 382–387.

Larder, P. (1988). *The Rugby League Coaching Manual.* London: Heinemann.

Leidholt, D. J. (1963). Spinal injury in sports. *Surg. Clin. North Am.*, **143**, 351–361.

Lovell, M. E. and Rostron, P. K. M. (1996). Referral of professional rugby league players to the orthopaedic service: a review of 447 injuries in 147 players. *Sports Excs. Inj.*, **2(2)**, 103–107.

MacEwen, C. J. (1987). Sport associated eye injury: a casualty department survey. *Br. J. Opthamol.*, **71**, 701–705.

Micheli, L. J. and Riseborough. E. M. (1974). The incidence of injuries in rugby football. *J. Sports Med.*, **2(2)**, 93–98.

Micheli, L. J. (1983). Overuse injuries in children's sport: The growth factor. *Orthop. Clin. North Am.*, **14**, 337–360.

Molloy, J. C. and McGuirk, R. A. (1976). Treatment of traumatic myositis ossificans circumscripta: use of aspiration and steroids. *J. Trauma*, **16**, 851–857.

Myers, P. T. (1980). Injuries presenting from rugby union football. *Med. J. Aust.*, **2(1)**, 17–20.

Palastanga, N., Field, D. and Soames, R. (1994). *Anatomy and Human Movement*. Oxford: Butterworth-Heinemann.

Patel, K., Burt, A. A. and Bradbury, J. A. (1984). Are spinal injuries more common in RU than in RL football. *Br. Med. J.*, **288(6426)**, 1308.

Rockwood, C. A. and Odor, J. M . (1989). Spontaneous atraumatic subluxation of the sternoclavicular joint. *J. Bone Joint Surg.*, **71A**, 1280–1288.

Roy, S. P. (1974). The nature and frequency of rugby injuries. A pilot study of 300 injuries at Stellenbosch. *S. Afr. Med. J.*, **48(56)**, 2321–2327.

Schauder, K. S. and Tullos, H. S. (1992). Role of the coracoid bone block in the modified Bristow procedure. *Am. J. Sports Med.*, **20(1)**, 31–34.

Scher, A. T. (1977). Rugby injuries to the cervical spinal cord. *S. Afr. Med. J.*, **51(14)**, 473–475.

Scher, A. T. (1981). Diving injuries to the cervical spinal cord. *S. Afr. Med. J.*, **59**, 603–605.

Scher, A. T. (1987). Rugby injuries of the spine and spinal cord. *Clin. Sports Med.*, **6(1)**, 87–99.

Scottish Rugby Union (1985). Significant injuries in rugby. 1984–1985. Edinburgh.

Silver, J. R. (1984). Injuries of the spine sustained in rugby. *Br. Med. J.*, **288**, 37–43.

Silver, J. R. and Gill, S. (1988). Injuries of the spine sustained during rugby. *Sports Med.*, **5(5)**, 328–334.

Silver, J. R. (1993). Spinal injuries in sports in the UK. *Br. J. Sports Med.*, **27(2)**, 115–120.

Silver, J. R. (1994). Methods of recording injury statistics in rugby football: the experience in the United Kingdom. *Sports Excs. Inj.*, **1(1)**, 46–51.

Sparks, J. P. (1981). Half a million hours of rugby football. The injuries. *Br. J. Sports Med.*, **15(1)**, 30-32.

Sparks, J. P. (1985). Rugby Football Injuries, 1980–1983. *Br. J. Sports Med.*, **19(2)**, 71–75.

Stephenson, S., Gissane, C. and Jennings, D. (1996). Injury in rugby league: a four year prospective survey. *Br. J. Sports Med.*, **30(4)**, 331–334.

Taft, J. N., Wilson, F. C. and Oglesby, J. W. (1987). Dislocation of the acromioclavicular ligament. *J. Bone Joint Surg.*, **69A**, 1045–1051.

Van Heerden, J. J. (1976). An analysis of rugby injuries. *S. Afr. Med. J.*, **5**, 1374–1379.

Walkden, L. (1978). Immediate post injury considerations in rugby football(proceedings). *Br. J. Sports Med.*, **12(1)**, 39–40.

Walker, R. D. (1985). Sports injuries; Rugby league may be less dangerous than union. *The Practitioner*, **229(1401)**, 205–206.

White, A. A., Southwick, W. O. and Payabi, M. M. (1976). Clinical instability in the lower cervical spine: a review of past and present concepts. *Spine*, **1**, 15–27.

Williams, J. P. R., McKibbin, B. (1978). Cervical spine injuries in rugby union football. *Br. Med. J.*, **2**, 23–30.

8

Functional rehabilitation of the injured player

This chapter is dedicated to physical rehabilitation and the various components of the injured player which must be fully rehabilitated before a return to sport. A full recovery will not happen naturally unless appropriate stimuli have been included in the physical programmes of such individuals. A player cannot be passed fit to play after ten minutes of electrotherapy, sitting on a treatment couch. Various functional and physical attributes are required, which will not be gained from a sedentary position in a nice warm treatment room. In designing a rehabilitation programme, the physiotherapist must always approach the format using his anatomical, pathological, physiological, functional and psychological skills. The schedule needs to be progressive throughout the recovery period in order to demonstrate improvement to both the player and the physiotherapist. At the same time, constant reassessment and adjustment is necessary if problems occur, to ensure that acute complications do not become chronic. Experience in such situations is an important factor for the physiotherapist involved, and this can only be gained by direct involvment in sports rehabilitation.

Unfortunately, the majority of injured players do not have direct access to medical advice and facilities, and will try and return to play once the acute inflammatory signs and symptoms have subsided. Most of these injuries will regress and players may become statistics on hospital waiting lists. In many cases, advice and help with regard to the appropriate rehabilitation is all that is necessary. At the end of the day, the player must also have the desire to return to full fitness.

Rest

It may seem strange to start a chapter on rehabilitation discussing the merits of rest in the recovery programme of the injured athlete, but it is a subject that should not be ignored. In order to gain the full benefits from a rehabilitation programme, sufficient rest and recovery are required. Energy systems, muscle groups or body parts need time to recover from the stress placed on them during the rehabilitation programme. It is during the rest period that the body 'rebuilds' itself in preparation for the next effort. If an individual continues to exercise the same energy system or muscle group daily, a plateau or decline in recovery is likely to take place. Symptoms to be aware of in regard to overtraining include:

Muscle soreness that lasts longer than 48 hours
Difficulty in recovering from a particularly demanding session
Chronic joint pain
Disrupted sleep pattern
Lethargy
Depression.

To counteract such signs adjustments are needed to the intensity, frequency and duration of the sessions, with extra rest periods introduced if necessary.

Overload principle

Any rehabilitation programme regardless of the physical parameter concerned, must utilize the variables stated in the overload principle if progression is to occur. This states that muscle improvement in strength, power and endurance and subsequent hypertrophy will only occur when the muscle performs for a given period of time at its maximal strength and endurance capacity. The three main contributary factors in this equation are:

Intensity
Frequency
Duration.

This principle was first quoted by Lange (1919), and has now been modified to produce the term progressive resistance exercise.
   Factors which should be considered when determining the type of rehabilitation required for the individual include:

1. Protection of the injury site
2. Reduction of inflammatory signs
3. Increase in the mobility of soft tissue and joint structures
4. Increase in the strength, power and endurance forces necessary for motion
5. Increase in muscle activity of the necessary functional type, depending on the particular requirements of the sport
6. Increase in joint proprioception
7. Increase in functional ability
8. Maintenance and improvement of the predominant energy systems of the sport
9. Correction complications or mechanical dysfunctions.

Mobility

Following injury, the normal active or passive range of movement of a joint may be affected due to damage of some or all of the relative structural components. Problems include:

1. Tightness of skin, superficial fascia or scar tissue
2. Muscular weakness or inefficiency
3. The formation of adhesions
4. The presence of a foreign body
5. Cartilaginous or bony destruction.

Limitation of movement impairs the functional capacity of a joint and its associated muscles. Different measures which can increase this mobility must go hand in hand with strengthening work to stabilize and control the movement and include the following:

1. Relaxation

If mobility is restricted by muscle spasm, then different relaxation techniques may be necessary before attempting any active or passive work. Ice or heat can be applied to the area, which will diminish the spasm (Scott, 1977). Hold-relax proprioceptive neuromuscular facilitation (PNF) techniques can also be used.

2. Passive movement

Various passive mobilizing and manipulative techniques are available to the physiotherapist, for both spinal and peripheral joints, which will aid in the recovery of full mobility.

Pendular movements using axial sling suspension render the injured limb gravity-free and can be used passively to promote relaxation and increase the range of movement.

3. Active exercise

Active assisted exercise can be performed with direct help from the players themselves, the physiotherapist, pendular sling suspension work or by utilizing the active assisted component offered by isokinetic equipment. Exercise which is assisted but involves a degree of active concentric work from the injured player is often successful in increasing the range of movement.

Free active exercises involve the player independently performing the necessary correct movement patterns. These may be non, partial or fully weightbearing, depending on the stage in rehabilitation, and active over pressure at the limit of range may be necessary to gain any improvement. In full weightbearing exercises, sufficient muscle strength is necessary in both agonist and antagonistic muscle groups to ensure stability of movement.

Resisted active exercise facilitates mobilization of stiff joints. Slow reversal and rhythmic stabilizations are PNF techniques which help to lengthen tight muscular structures and strengthen muscle tissue in the newly gained range of movement.

Strength

Support and stability provided by active muscle strength is an important ingredient in the recovery of any injured player. Maintenance and rehabilitation of muscle strength must begin from onset of injury and be progressed as the healing process goes through the various stages of recovery. In the first eight days following injury when a period of immobilization may be necessary, strength losses can vary between 2–6% per day depending on the individual (MacDougall et al., 1980; Muller, 1970). By this stage most players might consider swimming or other simple active work, yet could have lost between 16–48% of muscle strength. Fortunately this rate of wastage decelerates after eight days (Muller, 1970).

Sport requires various types of muscle strength and analysis of the necessary components of functional movement is a vital part of the physiotherapist's role in planning an appropriate rehabilitation programme.

Isometric exercise

This is a static contraction where no movement takes place, but muscle tension is produced. There is no change in the length of the muscle fibres. Such exercise can be used early in the rehabilitation programme in order to help reduce oedema, without fear of causing further joint irritation since there is no movement. Static muscle strength will increase, although any gains will be specific to the joint position at which the exercises are performed, with an approximate 10° physiological overflow either side of the set angle. Isometric muscle contractions will also help to stimulate the mechanoreceptor system in the joint capsule and maintain neural pathways in the area of contraction. Very little equipment is necessary, though biofeedback is only possible through the use of electromyographic machines or isokinetic graphical representation.

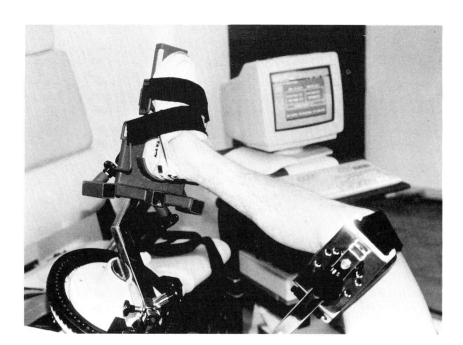

Figure 8.1 Isometric ankle inversion/eversion using an isokinetic ankle dynamometer.

Isometric work should involve a 10 second cycle for each repetition, with two seconds to build up to the desired tension (submaximal or maximal) in order to reduce the possibility of aggravating the injury. This contraction is then held for six seconds, with two seconds to gradually relax the contraction, again to prevent the sudden onset of pain. The six second contraction is necessary to produce maximal strength gains (Astrand and Rodahl, 1977; Hettinger, 1962).

Isotonic exercise

The muscle tissue shortens whilst lifting a constant load at a variable speed. Free weights, dumbells and barbells can be used to produce isotonic work in the muscle tissue. Such equipment allows movement throughout any particular

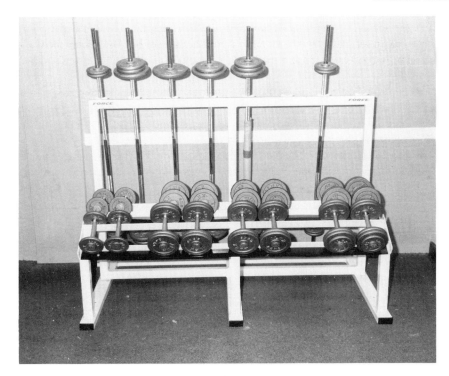

Figure 8.2 Free weights and bars provide variety, yet are cost effective for many physiotherapists.

plane with no restriction on speed. A wide selection of exercises with very little equipment is possible, at a relatively low cost for the variety of exercise possible. An element of muscular control is required, however, to control the direction of movement. Should the resistance be too heavy for the player, then further injury may occur unless training with a partner.

Individual exercise machines may use a selection of cables and pulleys to lift the weight stacks, or hydraulic units incorporated into the frame, which provide

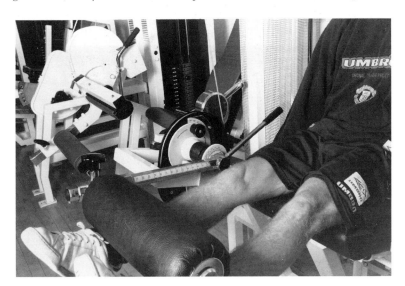

Figure 8.3 Isotonic leg extension using a cam operated unit.

the resistance. Older type multigyms with circular pulleys do not create uniform resistance, as once the inertia of the weight has been overcome and momentum has been established, the force required to move the selected resistance varies according to the degree of force the muscle can produce through the range of movement. Maximum resistance is greatest when the angle of pull is approximately 90° and gravitational effects are at their highest. In order to overcome this, conventional pulleys have been replaced by individually designed cams for each exercise unit. Each cam is designed to allow less resistance when the joint angle or muscle length is at a point of mechanical disadvantage, yet provides near maximal resistance in the 'easier' arcs of motion.

Concentric exercise

This involves shortening of the muscle tissue whilst lifting a load, whether it be a constant or variable resistance. Concentric work is possible in isotonic and isokinetic exercise, and is the most popular form of strength training.

Eccentric exercise

Muscle tissue lengthens whilst lowering a load, whether it be a constant or variable resistance. Eccentric work is possible in both isotonic and isokinetic exercise and is an important ingredient in the complete rehabilitation of an injured player.

Collision sport involves interaction of concentric and eccentric muscular activity during changes of momentum, independent of the linear, vertical or rotational plane of movement. Many physiological benefits can also be gained from using eccentric exercise (Dean, 1988), but tend to be neglected due to reported cases of muscular soreness following such work (Albert, 1991; Newham et al., 1983). Further work has shown, however, that it is the intensity of such work which causes the damage rather than the type of work being performed (Fitzgerald et al., 1991).

Eccentrically, the player also has the potential to produce a far greater muscular force than when performing exercises isometrically or concentrically (Cabri, 1991; Elftman, 1966). This pattern is consistent through all muscle groups. Generally, the difference between eccentric and concentric work increases as the speed of movement increases (Chandler and Duncan, 1988).

Different types of exercise which involve an eccentric component such as plyometrics can be included at the appropriate time in the rehabilitation programme. As well as developing muscular strength, the player will also benefit in other areas such as proprioception, neuromuscular stimulus, speed of movement and variable loadbearing on joints and muscles.

Case study

Eccentric exercise can be used in the rehabilitation of musculoskeletal injuries, particularly in chronic muscle and tendon conditions. Subjectively, a player will often inform you that they can feel pain when performing eccentrically-based movements, for example, coming downstairs or lowering themselves into a car seat. This is because the maximum load placed on a tissue lesion is during the eccentric phase of movement. As the injury progresses, it will start to irritate the player more during the concentric and isometric phases of movement. A rehabilitation protocol of warm-up, flexibility work, eccentric work, flexibility work again and the application of ice has been shown to have benefits in muscular (Stanton and Purdham, 1989) and tendon (Curwin and Stannish, 1984) injuries. Clinically I have used this treatment regime to good effect on hamstring muscle lesions and adductor, patella and Achilles tendon problems.

Isokinetics

The muscle tissue can produce either a concentric or eccentric contraction, but lifts or lowers a variable resistance at a constant speed. Maximal muscle tension can be produced throughout the full range of motion and is accommodated once the player achieves the preset angular velocity.

Commercially available isokinetic dynamometers are connected to the latest computer technology with software that allows the physiotherapist to analyse muscle function in various forms. Isokinetics has many uses in the sporting environment and can most easily be summed up by the use of the following schedule:

Individual rehabilitation programmes for the different injuries that occur.
Screening of the players, with baseline measurements for future reference.
Overlay of numerical and graphical data shows progression or regression.
Knee, shoulder, elbow, wrist, lumbar spine, hip and ankle joints can be tested.
Incentive from visual and auditory biofeedback on the computer monitor.
Numerical values and reports give quantification of torque and work values.
Early rehabilitation is possible using the continuous passive motion facility.
Time is needed by the physiotherapist to utilize the unit to the maximum.
Interpretation of the relevant data assists in the next stage of rehabilitation.
Computer knowledge and skills are needed to gain maximum benefit.
So many functional movement patterns are possible with some thought.

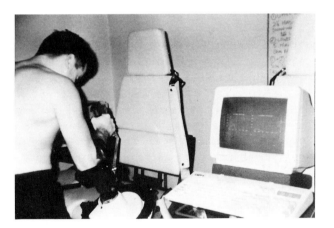

Figure 8.4 Isokinetic shoulder work, medial and lateral rotation in a modified standing position. This utilizes the large spinal, scapulothoracic and rotator muscles of the shoulder. It is *not* the optimum position for isolated shoulder work.

The numerical and graphical data that is produced gives information in many areas relative to muscle activity. These include:

Peak torque
Total work
Power
Strength

Endurance
Muscle ratios
Reproducibility
Range of movement
Functional capacity.

Isokinetic units also provide different forms of testing and exercise modalities:

Continuous passive movement
Active assisted
Isometric
Isotonic
Isokinetic
Concentric
Eccentric
Open kinetic chain
Close kinetic chain.

In practical terms the greatest problem for the physiotherapist is accessibility to such units, as the cost would swallow up a large if not the total percentage of funds available for new equipment. Also, in order to utilize the machine fully, physiotherapists need time to familiarize themselves with the unit and to learn how to interpret the data. The next stage is to develop functional patterns and rehabilitation schedules related to the sports they are involved with, information which cannot be gained from the company manual.

Isokinetic units have many more uses other than testing and rehabilitating the knee joint.

Agonists
The agonists are the primary muscles which initiate and maintain the force required to produce movement. They must be strong enough to overcome gravity, tissue resistance, inertia of the segment to be moved and any initial resistance offered from the antagonistic muscle group.

Antagonists
The antagonists directly oppose the action of the agonists, so must relax to control and allow any movement. Apart from an immediate variable burst of activity at initiation of the movement, the antagonists remain inactive until the final brief deceleration period. Agonist and antagonist strength ratios can be numerically quantified by using isokinetic testing equipment.

Synergists
These muscle groups work with the agonists to facilitate movement. They may also be required to modify the direction of pull of the agonist or to control joints not directly involved in the movement pattern.

Fixators
Occasionally the agonists and antagonists work together as fixators to stabilize the origin from which the agonist works. Contraction of both muscle groups also increases the transarticular compression, which further enhances the stability of the joint. Gravity or action of the agonist alone may provide such fixation, but this is not always the case and co-contraction of the two opposing groups may be necessary.

Following on from these definitions, a progressive strengthening programme can be drawn up which incorporates these variables at the appropriate stage of rehabilitation. This general approach was suggested by Davies (1992), but requires alteration to include all the necessary rehabilitation components of resistive exercise. The principles on which it is based are those of patient safety and overload, and involve varying the type of muscle work, the range of movement and the effort required. The first table only involves concentric work.

Muscle work	Range of movement	Effort required
Isometric	Variable angles	Submaximal
Isometric	Variable angles	Maximal
Isokinetic	Short arc ROM	Submaximal
Isotonic	Short arc ROM	Submaximal
Isokinetic	Short arc ROM	Maximal
Isokinetic	Full ROM	Submaximal
Isotonic	Full ROM	Submaximal
Isokinetic	Full ROM	Maximal
Isotonic	Full ROM	Maximal

Table 8.1 *A progressive strengthening programme using isometric and concentric work*

This can then be progressed to include eccentric exercise, within the different variable structure, with the obvious exclusion of isometric work.

Muscle work	Range of movement	Effort required
Isokinetics	Short arc ROM	Submaximal
Isotonics	Short arc ROM	Submaximal
Isokinetics	Short arc ROM	Maximal
Isokinetics	Full ROM	Submaximal
Isotonics	Full ROM	Submaximal
Isokinetics	Full ROM	Maximal
Isotonics	Full ROM	Maximal

Table 8.2 *A progressive strengthening programme using eccentric work*

Some individuals have questioned the use of the term 'submaximal' (Dvir, 1995), with regard to its effect on producing a training response and quantitative significance. Slow twitch muscle fibre recruitment and stimulus to the neurological pathways which control muscle function are important stages in rehabilitation which can commence early in the rehabilitation programme by using submaximal exercise. To produce a submaximal contraction, subjective use of the pain response of the player can be used as a guideline to determine the effort involved. The player needs to be educated about exercise pain and injury pain, and to have the ability to appreciate the symptoms felt on exercise. Another subjective method available is to use a modified Borg Rating Perceived Exertion (RPE) scale (Borg, 1982). This is used primarily for cardiovascular patients or in certain exercise testing situations, and is based on the numerical response of the individual to the sensation of exercise exertion:

1–6
7 - very, very light
8
9 - very light
10
11 - Fairly light
12
13 - Slightly hard
14
15 - Hard
16
17 - Very hard
18
19 - Very, very hard
20

The players exercise to the point of pain, and a numerical value is then applied to the type of individual sensation percieved. They are then instructed to exercise at a level just below that, which quantifies the level of submaximal exercise. As healing of the injury progresses, reassessment on such a scale is necessary. Objectively, submaximal work can be quantified by using isokinetic equipment, biofeedback or electromyographic (EMG) monitors, which can give numerical or visual responses to the degree of effort applied. Auditory or visual signals can then be introduced by the physiotherapist in order to ensure that the player can recognize when the effort level applied is too great for the healing state of the injury and so prevent aggravating the condition.

Practically, not all physiotherapists involved in sport have direct access to isokinetic equipment, but the majority will be able to incorporate isotonic and isometric exercises into the rehabilitation routine. In such instances, the progression of any strengthening rehabilitation can be modified to the following:

Table 8.3 *A progressive strengthening programme using isometric and isotonic work*

Muscle work	Range of movement	Effort required
Isometric	Variable angles	Submaximal
Isometric	Variable angles	Maximal
Isotonic	Short arc ROM	Submaximal
Isotonic	Full ROM	Submaximal
Isotonic	Full ROM	Maximal
Isotonic (eccentric)	Short arc ROM	Submaximal
Isotonic (eccentric)	Full ROM	Submaximal
Isotonic	Full ROM	Maximal

A variety of different training programmes exist in order to improve muscular strength. Early training programmes exist with very similar formats.

Set no.	Delorme and Wilkins (1951)	Oxford Technique (Zinovieff, 1951)	MacQueen (1954)
1	50%/10 RM (10 R)	100%/10 RM (10 R)	100%/10 RM (10 R)
2	75%/10 RM (10 R)	75%/10 RM (10 R)	100%/10 RM (10 R)
3	100%/10 RM (10 R)	50%/10 RM (10 R)	100%/10 RM (10 R)
4			100%/3 RM (3 R)
5			10%/3 RM (3 R)

Table 8.4 *Various weight training regimes*

RM - repetition maximum weight for the number of repetitions stated.
R - number of repetitions.

The concept of daily adjusted progressive resistance exercise (DAPRE) allows the player to adjust the resistance according to progress of the individual throughout the rehabilitation programme.

Set no.	Knight (1979)
1	50%/6 RM (10 R)
2	75%/6 RM (6 R)
3	100%/6 RM (Maximum)

Table 8.5a *The daily adjusted progressive resistance exercise (DAPRE)*

In the fourth set the weight is then adjusted depending on the number of repetitions performed in the third set.

No. of reps 3rd set	Adjusted weight for 4th set	Next exercise session
0–2	−5–10 lbs (−2.3–4.5 kg)	−5–10 lbs (−2.3–4.5 kg)
3–4	−0–5 lbs (−0–2.3 kg)	Same weight
5–6	Same weight	+5–10 lbs (+2.3–4.5 kg)
7–10	+5–10 lbs (+2.3–4.5 kg)	+5–15 lbs (+2.3–6.8 kg)
11+	+10–15 lbs (+4.5–6.8 kg)	+10–20 lbs (+4.5–9.1 kg)

Table 8.5b

Advanced rehabilitation strengthening regimes have also been designed (Sanders, 1990).

No. of sets	Amount of weight	Repetitions
4 (3x week)	100%/5 RM	5
4 (Day 1)	100%/5 RM	5
4 (Day 2)	100%/3 RM	5
1 (Day 3)	100%/5 RM	5
2 (Day 3)	100%/3 RM	5
2 (Day 3)	100%/2 RM	5

Instead of relying on trial and error for the initial weight resistances, starting weights were calculated from the body weight of the player (Sanders, 1990).

Exercise	% of body weight
Barbell squat	45
Barbell bench press	30
Leg extension	20
Upright rowing	20
Leg extension machine	20
Bench press machine	30
Leg curl machine	10–15
Leg press machine	50

Open kinetic chain

Open kinetic chain rehabilitation exercises are useful in developing strength and improving proprioceptive responses in specific muscles. Such isolated work occurs when the proximal bone segment in either upper or lower limb is fixed but the distal segment is free. The most obvious example in the lower limb is that of knee extension, which is specific to the quadriceps, easy to perform and is the most traditional of quadriceps rehabilitation exercises. It does, however, place an excessive strain on certain soft tissue structures. Knee extension exercises from 22° of knee flexion to full extension with a 20 lb(9 kg)-weight produced an anterior displacement of the tibia, with recorded values of 87–121% of an 80 lb (36.4 kg) Lachman test (Henning *et al.*, 1985). In the same study with 45° of knee flexion this figure dropped to 50%. Comparative close kinetic chain exercises, such as cycling and a half squat, produced results of 7 and 21%. This is supported by similar studies performed at 30° and 60° of knee flexion (Jenkins *et al.*, 1997).

The upper extremity is most functional in an open kinetic chain system, with stabilization of the proximal joint segments and free movement of the hand. The

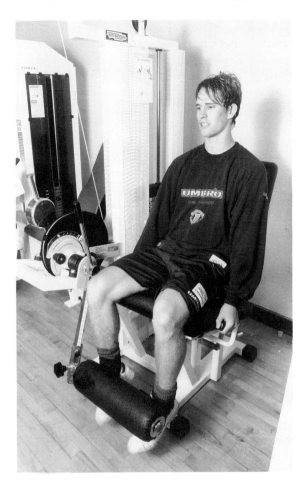

Figure 8.5 Open kinetic chain, leg extension.

only functional activity in the lower limb which is open chain work is kicking.

The link system associated with kinetic chain exercise was first proposed by mechanical engineers (Steindler, 1977), and has now been adopted as a more functional and beneficial form of rehabilitation in many upper and lower limb injuries. Close kinetic chain (CKC) work occurs when there is fixation of the proximal bone segment, as with the open kinetic work, coupled with stabilization or fixation of the distal segment. Functionally, this occurs in the lower limb when weightbearing. Much debate exists, however, in relation to the pure definition of an OKC or CKC exercise (Buckley, 1997), as variable factors such as the degree of proprioception and the changeable direction of the weightbearing force present technical difficulties in such statements.

CKC exercises are most commonly used in rehabilitation programmes involving injury and reconstruction of the ACL. The older approach of immobilization and non-weightbearing exercises has now been replaced with immediate

Close kinetic chain

Treatment notes

continuous passive movement and weightbearing as early as the second day. Quadriceps and hamstring co-contraction occurs with CKC exercise and reduces the unwanted shear forces which can aggravate the knee joint in anterior cruciate ligament (ACL) deficient players (Kaland *et al.*, 1990), or damage the graft site in players with an ACL reconstruction (Renstrom *et al.*, 1986; Arms *et al.*, 1984).

Even in the more active stages of rehabilitation, ideas have changed as knee rehabilitative exercises have been defined and redefined by clinical experience, mechanical analysis of movement and more thorough scientific research into exercise rehabilitation. The early exercise programmes of quadriceps strengthening with leg extension work and emphasis on full knee extension work has been shown to increase the strain on the ACL graft, due to the increases in anterior tibial translation produced (Renstrom *et al.*, 1986; Arms *et al.*, 1984). Such exercises have now been replaced by those that produce a co-contraction of both the hamstring and quadriceps muscles – CKC exercises. Hamstring co-contraction is an important rehabilitation consideration, particularly in ACL deficient players where different muscle firing patterns (with hamstring involvement being greater) has been shown to occur following rehabilitation (Cicotti *et al.*, 1993) and during functional activity (Tibone *et al.*, 1986).

Lower limb

The types of exercise in the lower limb that are classified as CKC include the following:

1. Mini squat
This exercise can be used very early in a CKC rehabilitation programme, as the range of movement allowed is only 0–40° in both the hip and knee. Hip extension and knee extension, which occur as the player rises from the squat position, produce simultaneous concentric and eccentric activity in the rectus femoris and hamstring muscle groups. This is known as a concurrent shift contraction and is essential during normal weightbearing activity.

2. Mini squat with increased flexion of the trunk
This exercise involves the same degree of movement as the mini squat, but with increased forward flexion of the upper body and trunk. This anterior movement of the centre of gravity helps to reduce the shear forces at the knee further, and decreases patellofemoral compression forces (Ohkoshi *et al.*, 1991).

3. Static bike
When using cycle ergometers for CKC activity, the defined kinetic chain only includes the lower limb, with the pelvis fixed on the seat and the foot on the pedal. It could be argued that this is an OKC activity if the whole body is included in the defined chain, as the head and neck, the proximal segments, are not fixed but open.

Aerobic and CKC work can be performed on a stationary bike and this is useful in the very early stages of rehabilitation when the degree of allowed loading on the joint needs to be limited. It also allows active assisted flexion work, with consideration of the height of the seat and the degree of help provided by the other leg or upper limbs, if using a Schwinn aerodyne bike.

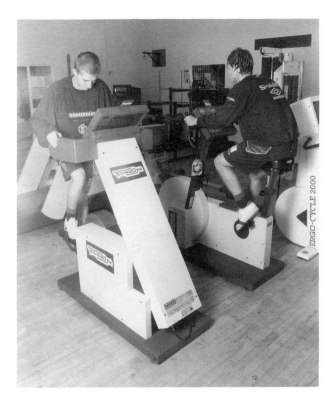

Figure 8.6 Static bike and step machine.

4. *Stepping machine*

Stair climbing machines can be used for CKC exercise work and to improve cardiovascular levels. In order to ensure it is pure CKC work, the foot of the player should never leave the footplate. A similar biomechanical pattern occurs as with that of the leg press.

This exercise does produce greater percentages of gastrocnemius activity (Cook *et al.*, 1992) than lateral step ups, which may result in increased strain on an ACL graft due to the posterior translation of the femur on the tibia. Fortunately, it has been shown that maximum quadriceps activity does not occur at the same stage in the exercise, as this would create a situation of maximum anterior shear force on the knee (Cook *et al.*, 1992).

5. *Leg press*

CKC work that can be performed on a horizontal leg press machine provides support for the lower back of the player, eliminates the effects of gravity and can provide resistance lower than body weight. In order to get the full benefit of hamstring co-contraction, certain adjustments are necessary for the standard leg press unit. Separate foot plates should move in an arc rather than a straight line in order to increase the hip flexion moment and decrease the knee moment of force. Full hip extension ensures maximum hamstring co-contraction at the knee (Palmitier *et al.*, 1991).

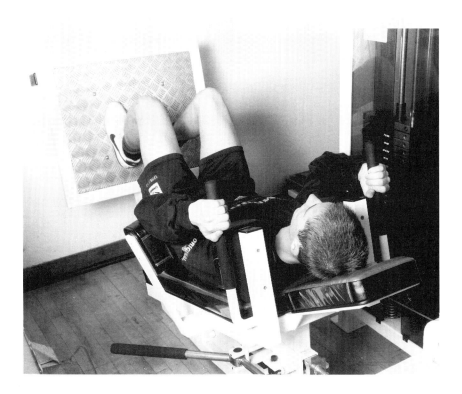

Figure 8.7 Leg press unit.

6. *Full squat*
In terms of safety, this is classified as movement to 90° of knee flexion, from the upright position. Recent research suggests caution with the use of this exercise following ACL graft, as EMG studies indicate only a maximum of 3% (semimembranosis) and 4% (biceps femoris) hamstring activity during a free squat exercise (Gryzlo *et al.*, 1994). Such figures suggest a lack of co-contraction with this exercise.

7. *Lateral step up*
Lateral step ups are often included in CKC rehabilitation programes, using blocks of various height to alter the work intensity. However, box heights greater than 20 cm (8 in) have been shown to reduce the effects of hamstring co-contraction and therefore increase the degree of anterior shear force (Brask *et al.*, 1984). This occurs due to the increasing amount of quadriceps EMG activity, caused by movement of the centre of gravity of the individual and low hamstring co-contraction activity (Cook *et al.*, 1992).

Upper limb   Upper limb CKC exercises are predominantly used to strengthen and improve neuromuscular control of the muscles that stabilize the shoulder girdle and glenohumeral joint.

1. Press ups
2. Seated push ups
3. Shoulder protraction (in standing).

CKC work in both the upper and lower limbs can be performed on isokinetic units. This gives numerical values for the torque produced, which can be used in both testing and rehabilitation schedules.

On assessing normal functional activity in sport, muscular contraction involves different stages of accelerating, concentric muscle activity coupled with decelerating, eccentric activity. This needs to be reproduced in the functional stages of rehabilitation, and is possible through exercise drills called plyometrics. These are a series of exercises that enable a muscle group to reach maximum strength and power, concentrically and eccentrically, in as short a time as possible, two important ingredients that are often lost after injury. Demands are placed on the stretch-shortening cycle, rather than just the concentric action used in many isotonic weights programmes. Stimulation of the elastic components – actin, myosin and tendon tissue – and the proprioceptive receptors of the muscle encourages the tension produced by rapid stretching to be stored briefly, producing a potential elastic energy. Also, the response of the stretch reflex to stimulation by sudden stretch produces an immediate, maximal, concentric muscle contraction, important factors in relating plyometrics to functional sports rehabilitation. Plyometric drills are effective for the upper and lower extremities as well as the spinal musculature (Voight and Dravitch, 1991).

The basis for all plyometric exercises developed from the concept that dynamic strength can be optimized by modelling the training programme on functional work which involves jumping activities. European countries developed the early protocols based on the 'shock' method advocated by Verkhoshanski (1969 and 1973), which consisted of rebound jumps from a height to develop the reactive neuromuscular centres of the player. These depth jumps varied in height from 0.8–3.2 m, with the optimal height being at the lower end of the scale and producing maximum speed in switching from eccentric to concentric work. One can understand why this type of work is described by the word 'shock', with a maximum height of 3.2 m!

The different exercises involve the use of various pieces of basic equipment, such as cones, boxes, blocks, hurdles and barriers of varying heights. To increase body weight or in upper body work, free weights and medicine balls can be utilized to progress the work. Single exercise stations such as a horizontal leg press can be used to avoid full body weightbearing and eliminate the effects of gravity in the eccentric phase of movement if required.

Many variations of exercise exist but all are based on various central exercises.

Plyometrics

1. *Depth jumps*
Gravity and body weight produce the resistance as the player steps off a box, drops to the ground and then immediately attempts to jump onto a box of equal height.

2. *Box drills*
These incorporate depth jumps with multiple hops, which can be low in intensity or extremely stressful, depending on the height of the boxes used.

3. *Bounding*
This involves exaggeration of the normal running stride pattern, covering distances longer than 30 m.

4. *Jumps (on the spot)*
Low intensity work with movement in the horizontal plane only.

5. *Jumps (standing)*
Standing jumps incorporate movement in a horizontal or vertical plane.

6. *Multiple hops and jumps*
Such drills combine the work performed in the previous two exercises to produce a specific programme. Hurdles, boxes and barriers can be incorporated into the routine.

As with all training programmes, the fundamental characteristics of the overload principle are essential if a progressive improvement is to take place. Intensity can be increased by raising the height of jumps or performing drills whilst holding weighted dumbbells. The type of exercise can determine the degree of work and has been rated from low to high intensity (Stone and O'Bryant, 1987).

LOW
Jumps (on the spot)
Jumps (standing)
Multiple hops and jumps
Box drills
Depth jumps
HIGH

Intensity of work can also be quantified by counting the number of foot or hand contacts, and can be increased as the player progresses, for example,

Table 8.7a *Progression of a plyometric training programme in the close season*

Level of fitness	Low intensity	Moderate intensity	No. of foot/hand contacts
Beginner	✓		60–100
Intermediate	✓		100–150
Advanced	✓	✓	150–250

Table 8.7b *Progression of a plyometric training programme during preseason*

Level of fitness	Moderate intensity	High intensity	No. of foot/hand contacts
Beginner	✓		100–250
Intermediate	✓		150–300
Advanced	✓	✓	150–450

Bounding-type plyometric activities can also be made harder by increasing the distance to be covered, up to a maximum of 100 m per repetition.

The stressful nature of plyometric drills necessitates two to three days between sessions in terms of frequency, although upper and lower body parts can be exercised on alternate days and still give 48 hours recovery.

Duration and recovery time between sets should be calculated at a ratio of 1:5–1:10 to ensure activity produces anaerobic effects. Too short a recovery time between sets does not allow for maximum recovery and makes the work more aerobically based.

Plyometrics, if used properly and progressively, are a very functional and useful method of rehabilitating the injured player. However, if used or performed incorrectly then an injured player may fail to make the expected progress. As with all exercise-based drills, thoughtful and planned preparation is essential.

Proprioception

From the start of the injury process, the most noted and dramatic losses in function tend to be associated with mobility and strength. Functional instability in the joint of an injured player can be helped by including more specific proprioceptive work in the rehabilitation phase. Proprioception is 'the awareness of posture, movement and changes in equilibrium and the knowledge of position, weight and resistance of objects in relation to the body' (*Taber's Cyclopedic Medical Dictionary*, 1977). Failure to rehabilitate the balance strategies of the injured player will result in a poor functional recovery, increase the possibility of re-injury or produce another injury situation.

The initiation of these forces comes from information supplied by receptors found in muscles (muscle spindles), tendons (Golgi tendon organs) and synovial joints (types 1–4). They all monitor changes in muscle and tendon tension, joint position, relative weight of body parts and joint movement, and have a modifying effect on the function of one another (Baxendale *et al.*, 1988). These afferent stimuli then pass to the spinal cord, where an appropriate efferent response is returned to the necessary muscle groups to stabilize the joints concerned and therefore realign the body. Proprioceptive deficits have been shown to exist in older individuals (Skinner *et al.*, 1984), injured athletes (Leach, 1982), joint arthrosis (Barrett *et al.*, 1991) and anterior cruciate disruption (Barrack *et al.*, 1989).

Commercially there are several devices available which assist the physiotherapist in implementing proprioceptive work:

1. Balance boards
The classical wobble board, a round piece of plywood on a central fulcrum, has many variations in size, materials and plane of movement. Balance activities can be performed on these various balance boards and cause changes in joint rotations and pressures, stimulating the various receptors and preparing the body for more vigorous activities. Numerous physical variables such as the degree of visual input or size of the base of support can be altered to change the intensity of the rehabilitation programme. Strengthening and functional activities can also be incorporated into the proprioceptive work. In response, the players must respond quickly and without conscious thought to changes in their centres of gravity.

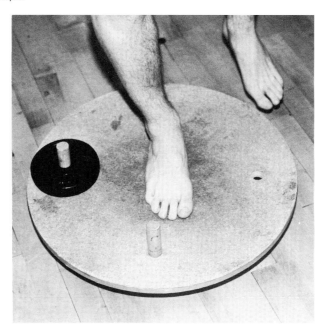

Figure 8.8 Balance board with variable weight resistance.

2. *Slide boards*

Plywood covered with a Formica surface allows a player to improve joint proprioception and lateral leg strength, and helps provide an aerobic stimulus with the correct programme (Boyle, 1991). The slide board lets the player perform a side-to-side slide, with friction minimized by wearing socks or plastic overshoes on the feet. Functionally, the ability to move laterally quickly is an important component of any player's rehabilitation. Good instruction and a base level of dynamic stability is necessary to get appropriate use out of this piece of equipment.

3. *Trampet*

Mini trampets can be used in a similar manner to wobble boards, providing an unstable surface on which to perform lower limb proprioceptive exercises.

4. *Medicine ball*

This can be used for both upper and lower limb proprioceptive exercises, usually in the advanced stages of rehabilitation when stability is at a good level.

Lower limb

Balance exercises provide stimulus to the various proprioceptive receptors of the body. Afferent information to the motor control area of the brainstem with regard to the posture and balance of the body is provided by the various joint proprioceptors, particularly important in the lower limb. At the same time it should be remembered that other systems, internal and external to the body, are necessary to maintain balance. These include:

Strength
Mobility

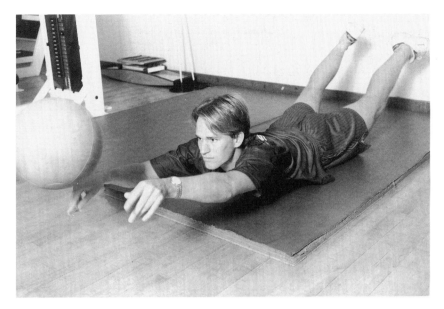

Figure 8.9 Upper limb proprioceptive work with medicine ball.

Vestibular factors
Visual factors
Auditory factors
Reaction time
Movement time
Level of motivation
Environmental factors.

In order to quantify balance, various static or dynamic tests are possible:

1. *Static*

(a) Single leg stance (Tropp *et al.*, 1984)
(b) Romberg test (Jansen *et al.*, 1982)
(c) Standing force plates, with computer attachments (Shimba, 1984).

2. *Dynamic*

(a) Hop test for distance (Noyes *et al.*, 1991)
(b) Functional reach test (Duncan *et al.*, 1990)
   Both these types of testing examine different aspects of the balance system in any injured player. Trial runs and clear instructions to the player are essential for viability of any test scores.
(c) Fastex movement reactor system (Cybex)
   The reactor assesses functional activities such as stability, agility, balance, coordination, reaction time and speed of movement. These measurements are possible through the functional response of the player to various visual cues on the screen monitor. This allows the physiotherapist to assess the quality of the functional movement produced, a factor often neglected following injury.

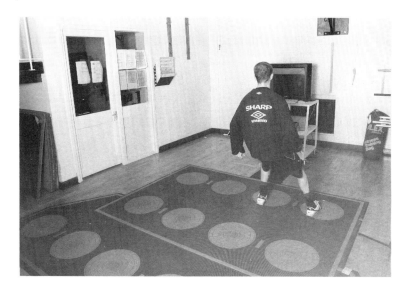

Figure 8.10 Fastex Movement Reactor System mat.

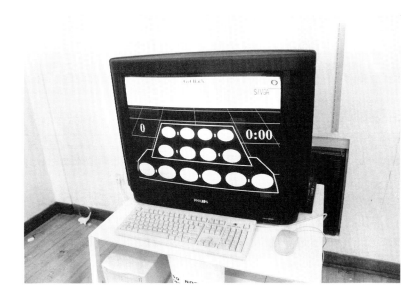

Figure 8.11 Fastex Movement Reactor System screen monitor.

Manually, the use of proprioceptive neuromuscular facilitation techniques (Knott and Voss, 1968) gives the physiotherapist a tool which can be adjusted to suit the individual requirements of each player where necessary. Electrical muscle stimulation may help to supplement these various exercises (Kennedy *et al.*, 1982).

Upper limb   In the upper limb, particularly where the glenohumeral joint is involved, static and dynamic control related to joint motion and position are important proprioceptive factors to be considered in the rehabilitation programme. Instability in the shoulder joint is most commonly attributed to the loss of static and dynamic mechanical restraints provided by the capsule, ligamentous and

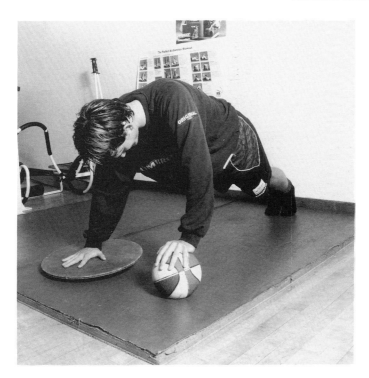

Figure 8.12 Glenohumeral joint stabilization using a close chain component with a wide base of support.

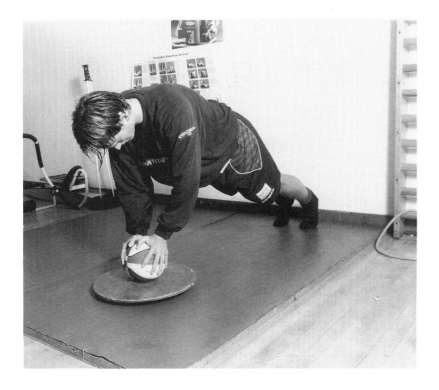

Figure 8.13 Glenohumeral joint stabilization using a close chain component, with a narrow base of support.

muscular structures. When injury occurs to these structures, partial de-afferentation occurs with loss of proprioceptive response. Such a deficit increases the possibility of further injury and greater functional instability (Borsa *et al.*, 1994), particularly where co-contraction of antagonistic and synergic muscle groups is required to provide good joint stability (Glousmann *et al.*, 1988). Motor control with regard to body position and movement can also be provided by the learned responses of the individual to changes in equilibrium, and must be considered in the recovery stage following disturbance of the proprioceptive system. Rehabilitation directly following injury therefore needs to be based upon the specific nature of the injury and any surgical procedures performed. Following surgical repair to the capsule, glenoid labrum and ligamentous tissue, proprioceptive response has been shown to return to near normal levels (Lephart *et al.*, 1994). Rehabilitation for joint stabilization must involve co-contraction of the relative muscle groups, so disturbance of the equilibrium is essential. This can be practised using manual techniques, such as PNF, providing open chain work, or using an unstable base of support such as a ball or wobble board, which involves a close chain component. Functional positions and activities must be considered throughout. Both open and closed chain proprioceptive exercises may be required by the injured player depending on their team position.

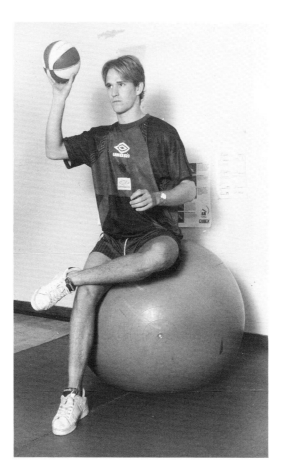

Figure 8.14 Open chain rehabilitation with throwing component.

Individuals who have a throwing component to their game – goalkeeper in soccer, quarterback in American football – may, however, need to concentrate on more open kinetic work. Rugby players, who incorporate both open and closed kinetic work in their game, will need progression from open to closed work. Proprioceptive rehabilitation work should also address the cognitive response to joint position, with motor skills progressing from conscious to unconscious control as recovery occurs. Functional active and passive joint repositioning work, with elimination of visual input and emphasis at the end of range, will stimulate the joint and muscle proprioceptive organs.

Knee

Proprioceptive factors in relation to the knee joint have centred mainly on anterior cruciate ligament (ACL) injury and reconstruction techniques. Reduction in proprioceptive response (Corrigan *et al.*, 1992) and slower hamstring reflex times (Beard *et al.*, 1993) following ACL injury have been recorded, with similar results after ACL reconstruction surgery compared to the norm (Barrett, 1991). Use of closed kinetic chain work in the player with an ACL deficient or ACL reconstructed knee increases the level of hamstring co-contraction, reduces shear force on the graft and so improves overall stability of the joint (Lutz *et al.*, 1993).

Ankle

Following injury to the ankle joint, two types of instability exist:

1. *Mechanical instability (MI)*
This occurs due to ligamentous laxity, with joint motion that exceeds normal physiological limits (Tropp, 1985).

2. *Functional instability (FI)*
This is caused by poor ankle proprioception, with joint motion beyond voluntary control (Tropp, 1985).

   The degree of FI is determined by the amount of damage to the afferent and efferent nerve supply of the joint and muscular structures. The degree of proprioceptive loss is determined by the severity of the articular deafferentation (Freeman *et al.*, 1965) and motor denervation, which will have a derogatory effect on reflex muscle response and voluntary muscle activation. The inability to maintain unilateral postural balance has been highly correlated with FI, and is often associated with individuals who have chronic instability, whether it be a predisposing factor or a direct result of the injury (Lentell *et al.*, 1990; Freeman *et al.*, 1965). In rehabilitation terms, proprioceptive exercises mainly involve balance work on a multitude of tilting boards or surfaces, which will stimulate the concentric and eccentric firing patterns of the muscle groups which act upon the ankle joint. All balance exercises, regardless of the degree of disturbance, that involve the lower limb produce activity at the ankle joint. Only when alteration in the centre of gravity is of a greater magnitude than the ankle can deal with do the receptors of the hip joint become involved (Horak and Naschner, 1986). Static balance work can begin as soon as the injured player is able to weightbear, and can readily be progressed from bilateral to unilateral

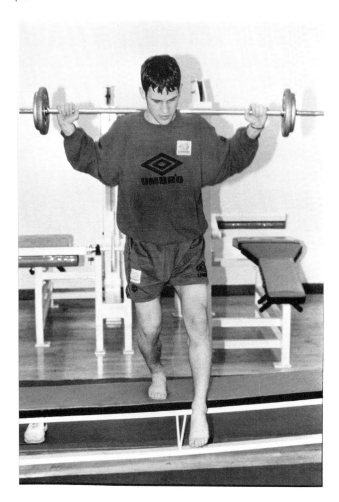

Figure 8.15 Slow step down from bench (with eyes closed to remove visual input) to stimulate right lower limb proprioceptors.

work, introducing the various physical variables at the appropriate time. Endurance and cognitively learned movement patterns must be included in the rehabilitation programme to ensure a full proprioceptive recovery.

Dynamic plyometric activities can be introduced to make the rehabilitation programme as functional as possible in both the upper and lower limbs.

Cardiovascular factors

With any injured player, strength, flexibility and a full functional recovery tend to be major priorities in the rehabilitation programme. Cardiorespiratory fitness is often neglected, yet is a very important factor for the injured player. The physiotherapist must therefore include alternative functional activities that help to maintain a cardiorespiratory endurance base whilst not impairing the healing process of the injury site. Consideration must be given to the energy systems a particular sport utilizes, in order to provide an appropriate training schedule which will be of benefit when the player returns to full fitness.

Oxygen transport throughout the body is essential in order to function correctly, and depends on coordination between the blood, blood vessels, heart

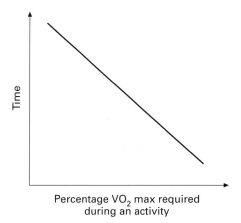

Time

Percentage VO$_2$ max required
during an activity

The greater the percentage of VO$_2$ max required during a physical
activity, the less time that activity can be performed

Figure 8.16 VO$_2$ max. required
during activity.

and lungs. The rate at which oxygen is taken in and used by the body during exercise is referred to as the **maximal oxygen consumption (VO$_2$ max.)**. This level is an individual characteristic and has a large bearing on the ability of the player to perform an activity. The greater the percentage of the VO$_2$ max. required during an activity, the less time the activity may be performed for (Figure 8.16).

This level of oxygen consumption is basically a genetically controlled factor, and is largely dependent on the metabolic and functional properties of the fast and slow twitch muscle fibre percentages which are present in the individual. Fast twitch fibres, which are important for speed and power activities, do not depend on the presence of oxygen and very quickly fatigue. Slow twitch fibres are more important for endurance activities, require oxygen to be functional and are more resistant to fatigue. The range of VO$_2$ max. is inherited, and the more active a player, the higher the level of VO$_2$ max. within that range (Weymans and Reybrouck, 1989).

Muscle tissue therefore has two energy systems available, which are necessary for the different types of activity necessary in most sports. Most collision sports involve short, sharp bursts of **anaerobic** work followed by an active **aerobic** 'recovery' period. Anaerobic metabolism involves rapid use of adenosine triphosphate (ATP), which is the energy store available to the muscle tissue produced from the breakdown of carbohydrates, fats, protein and muscle glycogen. No oxygen is necessary for this process to occur. Such intense exercise is only possible for a short period due to the production of the waste product, lactic acid.

As exercise continues, the aerobic energy system is needed. This does require oxygen, and involves metabolism of carbohydrates and fats to produce the required ATP. Lactic acid will again be produced, but obviously at a far slower rate than with anaerobic work.

The type of cardiovascular conditioning work that is possible is dependent on the site of injury and the dominant energy systems of the sport. Injuries to the upper limbs allow activities such as walking, running, the stairclimber or cycling.

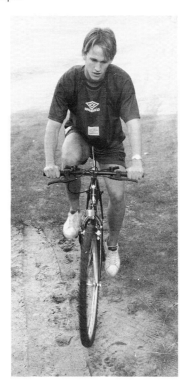

Figure 8.17 Cycling to maintain aerobic fitness.

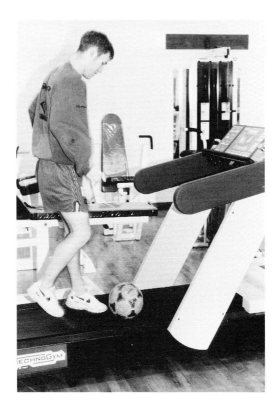

Figure 8.18 Functional treadmill running incorporating ball skills.

On the contrary, injuries to the lower limbs permit non-weightbearing activities such as swimming or rowing to try and maintain a cardiovascular base. Gradually, functional activities that increase the stress on the injury site can be introduced, but the physiotherapist must ensure that the time is right in order to prevent aggravation of the injury. Sports-related activities should be introduced as quickly as possible in order to achieve match fitness.

On returning from injury, a good aerobic base is essential before progressing to more specific conditioning work. Swimming, cycling and use of upper body ergometers are all activities that may help to provide a good aerobic base without aggravating the injury site. Jogging, stair climbing, skipping, circuit training and walking are all weightbearing activities that incorporate the extensor thrust mechanism necessary for running, and should be introduced as soon as the injury is strong enough to be able to absorb the increased stress. The intensity of work can be determined by various methods:

1. *Heart rate*
This can be recorded manually, or with the use of sophisticated heart monitors which are readily available. Target heart rates can only be calculated for the individual by determining the maximal heart rate (MHR). This can be estimated by using the following formula, which is age-related:

$$220 - age = MHR$$

In many athletic individuals, however, this gives a false measurement. More reliable scores can be obtained from a graduated maximal stress test, using a cycle ergometer or treadmill. Maximum heart rate levels are sports specific and will vary between sports. For example, swimmers tend to have a maximum heart rate 10–13 beats lower than that of runners. A minimum of three and a maximum of six exercise sessions per week is required, each lasting 20–60 minutes, with the heart rate elevated to desired training levels (Hage, 1982). Training intensity is judged mainly by the degree of stress placed on the cardiorespiratory system.

2. *Anaerobic threshold*
This can be calculated in two ways, both of which require laboratory equipment:

(a) Minute ventilation
The player to be tested runs at different, increasing speeds on a treadmill. After several minutes of running at each speed, minute ventilation is recorded and plotted on a graph (Figure 8.19).

This demonstrates a uniform increase initially, followed by an abrupt rise. The sudden change represents the exercise intensity at or slightly above the anaerobic threshold and this recorded running speed can be used as a baseline exercise intensity for the player during rehabilitation.
(b) Lactic acid
The onset of blood lactate accumulation (OBLA) is often used as a measurement to determine the endurance capacity of a player, with a figure

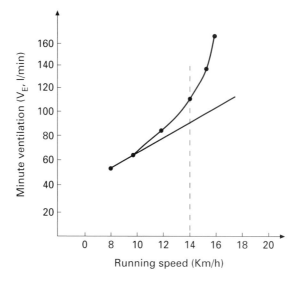

Figure 8.19 Minute ventilation and the anaerobic threshold.

Training intensity in this example = 14 km/h

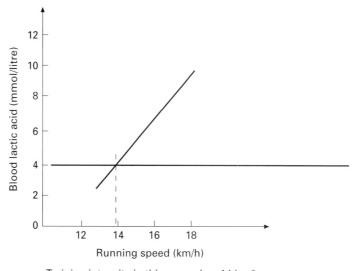

Figure 8.20 Blood lactic acid and the anaerobic threshold.

Training intensity in this example = 14 km/h

of 4 mmol/l being the suggested reference value, although this will vary amongst certain individuals (Spurway, 1992). The player again runs on a treadmill at varying increasing speeds until a level of 4 mmol/l of blood lactic acid is recorded. This information is then plotted on the appropriate graph (Figure 8.20).

Knowledge of the anaerobic threshold is very useful in recognizing when an injured player is nearing full cardiovascular fitness, and in planning the intensity of work required. In both tests, the intensity of exercise is determined by the stress placed on the metabolic system of the skeletal muscles.

3. Bleep test

A good baseline measurement of cardiovascular fitness is provided by the multistage fitness bleep test (Brewer *et al.*, 1988), and referral to previous scores will indicate if the player is making a good aerobic recovery.

Most collision sports require an element of speed-endurance work, which can be developed using interval-based running drills. These require a work load which intermittently, produces a heart rate in excess of 85% of the MHR, followed by less intense activity where the player is working at 60–70% of the MHR. The training session is determined by time or distance, with recovery periods throughout to ensure a player is able to work at these high heart rate levels over short periods of time. Game-related functional activities such as collisions or rising from the floor break up the momentum of continuous running, and ensure a more realistic approach to the necessary rehabilitation.

Plyometric drills and sprint work provide a purer anaerobic session, and can be used in the cardiovascular rehabilitation programme where necessary. Total rest periods between repetitions are vital to ensure aerobic work is kept to a minimum.

Careful planning is therefore needed when introducing cardiovascular work into the rehabilitation schedule. Identical sessions should never be repeated on consececutive days, as recovery is necessary to ensure maximum gains are made from quality work.

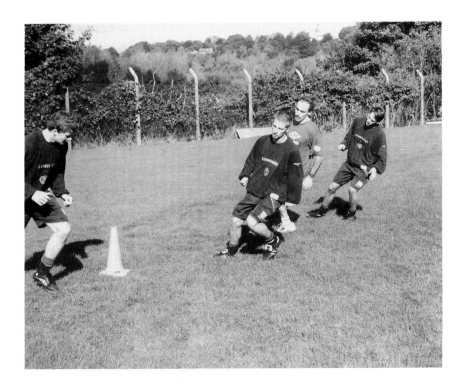

Figure 8.21 Turning . . .

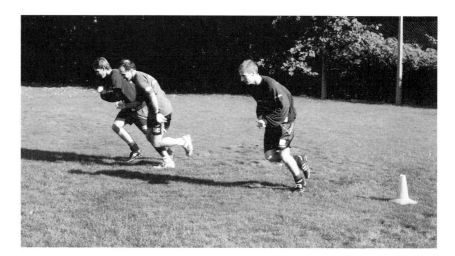

Figure 8.22 . . . and running to ensure cardiovascular recovery is functional.

Function

The physiotherapist involved in any particular sport must be prepared to look outside the realms of the medical textbook when dealing with sports-associated injuries The most important factor to the player is the length of time before they can return to competition. Before this final decision is made, the player must be able to demonstrate the ability to perform functional tasks at full intensity, at a functional speed, and with opposition from other players. The physiotherapist must therefore have a personal knowledge of the functional factors that make up that player's position in the team. From this, specific drills that test the physical or mental approach to the task required can be created. The player must be able to demonstrate that they can perform competently, even in pressure situations. Well planned drills will progress this stage of rehabilitation from simple to complex movements. Variety is important, as the use of a few favourite drills over and over again will only avoid testing the injury to the full and be very boring for both parties.

Different variables contribute to the intensity of the programme and should be altered as required. These include:

Size of playing area
Number of players
Use of equipment (tackle bags, shields, cones, markers, match balls)
Time in possession of the ball
Non-full contact
Degree of competition
Length of time
Functional components (jumping, falling, cutting).

It is also important to appreciate that drill work can test both technique and physical conditioning and demonstrate any relevance the injury may have to these two factors. Conditioning drills can still incorporate some sports specific skills, which add to the challenge, but less emphasis is necessary on perfect execution.

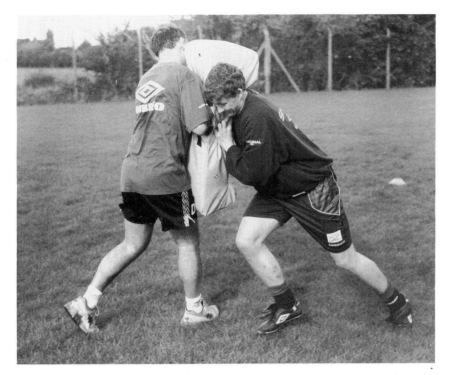

Figure 8.23 Increase intensity and reproduce collisions in outdoor rehabilitation work.

Case study

Skills from other sports can quite readily be incorporated into the rehabilitation programme of any injured player. These provide specific skill work, physical conditioning, variety and competition, yet by selecting the appropriate drill can still be relevant to the particular sport of that player. In relation to the rehabilitation of an injured soccer player, I regularly incorporate training routines and drills from the following sports:

Swimming
Basketball
Boxing
Rugby league
Rugby union
Handball
Volleyball
Cricket
Gymnastics
Cycling

These help the player in both the physical and mental recovery from injury, yet involve skill work that is necessary for soccer.

Most players hate having to perform specific sets and bouts of plyometric drills, yet if this involves the use of a basketball court and a ball and an element of competition, they tend to raise very little opposition. When you then inform the group they have just

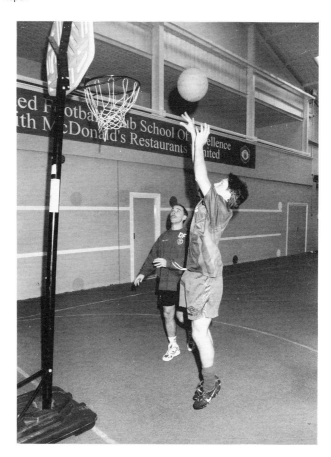

Figure 8.24 Plyometric work using basketball drills.

gone through 30 minutes of plyometric work without realizing it, using the various basketball skills of leaping, bounding, standing jumps, running and cutting, it's too late for them to register a valid protest.

Upper limb variables

With regard to rehabilitation programmes for the upper limb, structured planning is necessary in order to produce a safe yet progressive programme. Many of the muscles that influence upper limb function originate in the trunk, or are influenced by trunk stability. This proximal stability is necessary in order to produce increased distal mobility, and should be considered when planning the rehabilitation programme. Progression through the appropriate stages should be as follows:

Trunk muscles
↕
Scapulo-thoracic muscles
↕
Scapulo-humeral muscles
↕
Upper limb muscles

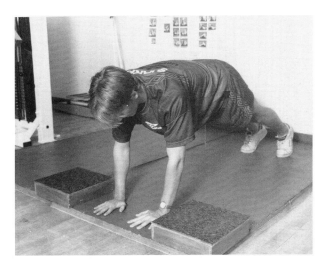

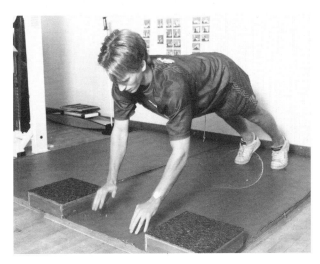

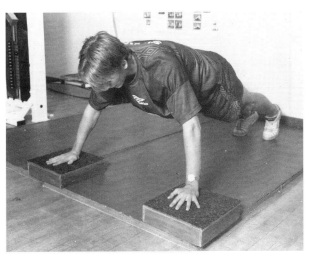

Figure 8.25a,b,c Plyometric abduction, lateral rotation and retraction drill, to maximally stimulate the appropriate humeral and scapular muscle groups.

Other functional objectives must be considered in upper limb rehabilitation, particularly around the glenohumeral joint. The dynamic stabilizers of the shoulder include the scapular muscles – serratus anterior, rhomboids and trapezius – which stabilize and rotate the scapula during activity, and the rotator cuff muscles, which fixate the humeral head in the glenoid fossa whilst having an effect on certain active movements. Both these groups require strength, power and endurance work to help stabilize the joint during continuous activity. In order to produce the desired active work, the two groups must work together to allow a smooth, controlled motion of the humerus on a stable scapula base. Exercises such as pressups, push ups and dumbbell work based on isolated shoulder patterns incorporating abduction, rotation and retraction have all been shown from electromyographic studies to maximally stimulate the appropriate humeral and scapular groups (Townsend *et al.*, 1991). Synergically, the larger, more superficial muscles – pectorals, biceps, triceps and latissimus dorsi – must be re-educated in providing strength and power for appropriate overhead functions.

Abdomen

Little consideration has been given to the rehabiliation protocol for the player who has undergone surgical repair to the abdominal wall. Many players with such injuries will have been unable to play or train to their maximum potential for weeks, months, or even years prior to a surgical repair. Physical atrophy, below average fitness levels and the poor psychological profile of the problem are common symptoms following surgery.

Treatment notes

The following protocol is primarily written for the professional soccer player from my own experience of working with such athletes. The reader must adapt this schedule in order to accommodate the sport they are involved with and the level of facilities available to them.

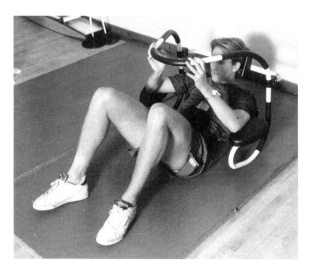

Figure 8.26 Use of abdominal frame to strengthen rectus abdominis.

Week	Procedure
1	Walk (1–2 days)
	Submaximal isometric abdominals/hip flexors, extensors, abductors, adductors, rotators
	Staples/stitches removed during the week
2	Increase walking using time as limiting factor, increasing by 5 minutes each day if no ill effects
	Continue isometrics, 10 reps/4 times per day
	Wound care/mobilization
	End of week commence active assisted cliniband/isokinetic work in functional position
3	Commence running programme, progressing from aerobic to anaerobic over the next 3 weeks
	Submaximal to maximal isometric hip work – isokinetics if available (20°/standing work). Bias towards presurgical isokinetic test results
	Once 25% (or lower) deficit between limbs, begin active concentric work, starting on fast speeds (240) progressing to slower (60) depending on daily reassessment
	Swimming if wound healed
	Cycling
	Neurological gymnastic ball work
	Flexibility work, active and passive
	Wound care
4	Return to active assisted work to re-educate concentric/eccentric work
	Structured isotonic adductor programme
	Functional work
	Running forwards/backwards
	Abdominal work with frame
5	Concentric/eccentric lower limb muscle patterns – manual/cliniband/isokinetics
	General weights work with abdominal belt/lumbar support
	Full functional programme
	RETURN TO PLAY ACCORDING TO FUNCTIONAL REASSESSMENT ONLY

Table 8.8 *Rehabilitation procedure following prolene mesh repair of abdominal wall disruption in a soccer player*

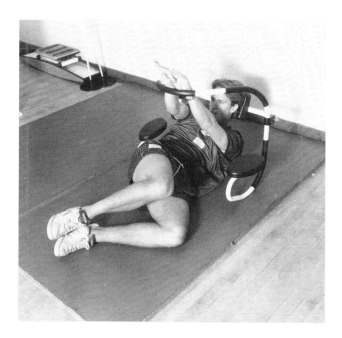

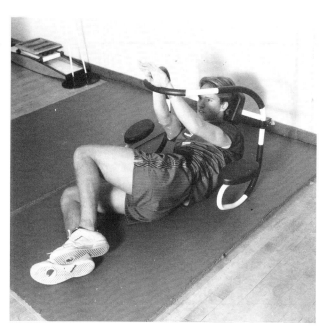

Figure 8.27a,b Use of abdominal frame to strengthen internal and external obliques.

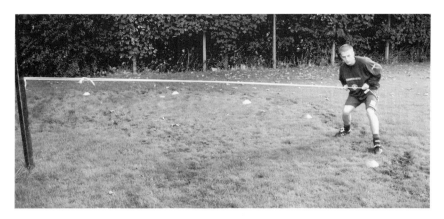

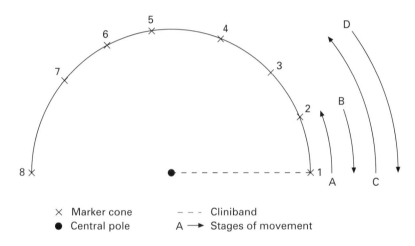

×	Marker cone	– – –	Cliniband
●	Central pole	A →	Stages of movement

Figure 8.28a,b A specific aerobic, plyometric and lower limb co-contraction drill for the adductor muscle group. The player faces the central pole with a loop of resistive Cliniband fastened to their waist and around the pole. The player must move in a sideways direction along path A from the first marker X1 to X2 and back (B). They then immediately move to X3 (C) and return (D). This pattern continues up to marker X8. At all times they must face the central pole and keep outside the semicircle even though the Cliniband is trying to pull them in. The target time limit to complete the drill is 45 seconds.

Rehabilitation after **anterior cruciate ligament reconstruction** (ACLR) involves many different postoperative routines, depending on the thoughts of the medical team involved.

The following schedule is one that I have compiled from personal experience and from the numerous research papers available on the subject. It is used purely as a base from which to work. ACLR is one of the few instances where a time and force restraint rehabilitation programme is recommended. Objective physical measurements, such as oedema, range of movement and muscle strength, do not indicate the degree of healing of ligamentous tissue. Fractures demonstrate clinical and radiological signs of healing, unlike ACLR where there is no accurate way to assess the strength of the reconstructed ligament other than time maturation.

Players are often given set dates at which they can increase their activity level, based purely on subjective assessment and manual testing of the knee. An important point in the rehabilitation programme is the 12 week stage, when

Lower limb variables

Treatment notes

Table 8.9 *Rehabilitation procedure following anterior cruciate ligament reconstruction of the knee*

Time scale	Activity level
Immediate post-op	Continuous passive motion (0–60°), increase 10° per day to 90° maximum
	Ice and elevation (avoid moisture on wound) Cryocuff
	Thackerey splint/or limiting brace
	Weightbearing with crutches as tolerated
	Ankle mobilizing exercises
	Patella mobilizations
	Static quadriceps/trophic stimulator if inhibited due to pain, 3–6 hours per day for slow oxidative fibres.
Weeks 1–6	Supervized knee mobilization work, flexion and full extension CPM 0–90°
	Prone lying, knee extended over bed (30 minutes per day)
	Weightbearing as tolerated with crutches
	Multi angle, submaximal isometrics (quads/hamstrings)
	Straight leg raises (4 planes)
	Mini squats (30° of lumbar flexion)
	Hamstring curls
	Patella mobilization
	Calf raises
	Pelvic and lower limb extensor thrust work, to simulate the mechanics of running
	Hamstring/calf flexibility work
	Early balance, weight transference and proprioceptive work
	Swelling control using ice and electrotherapy modalities
	Wound care.
Week 4	Bicycle for ROM and compression stimulus
	Pool walking programme (if wound completely healed)
	Submaximal quads eccentrics (40–90°)
	Hip extension/flexion (total hip machine)
	Leg press, 0–60° (2 leg)
	Mini squats (vertical).
Brace removed if	ROM 0–115
	Decreased effusion
	Quadriceps control of knee in lying and standing.

Table 8.9 *(Contd.)*

Time scale	Activity level
Week 6–8	Full weightbearing
	Leg press (1 leg), isokinetic if available
	Hamstring curl (1 leg)/hamstring re-education pattern
	Skipping
	Swimming programme (crawl kick only)
	Step ups, varying height and weight.
Week 9–14	Lateral step ups
	Knee extension (90–40°), 2 leg
	Hip abduction/adduction (total hip machine)
	Cycle work for aerobic exercise, using pulsemeter
	Pool running
	Step machine.
Week 12	Isokinetic test (See Tables 8.10 and 8.11)
	Begin running programme if satisfactory clinical, functional and isokinetic test
	Initially, increase intensity of running by time factor (15 minute plus 5 minutes, alternate days)
	Submaximal eccentric quadriceps work (40–90°).
Week 16	Leg press with jump (1 leg).
Week 18	Begin functional work, skill drills and plyometric work
	Increase intensity of running programme with cutting, backwards and functional patterns.
Week 24	Isokinetic test, full ROM, 60–180–300° per second.
Week 28	Isokinetic eccentrics, submaximal.
Week 32	Isokinetic eccentrics, maximal.
Week 36	Concentric/eccentric/endurance/functional test
	RETURN TO PLAY
Week 52	Isokinetic test, concentric/eccentric, quads/hamstrings
	BEWARE PATELLOFEMORAL/GRAFT SITE SYMPTOMS ADJUST PROGRAMME AS REQUIRED

(a)

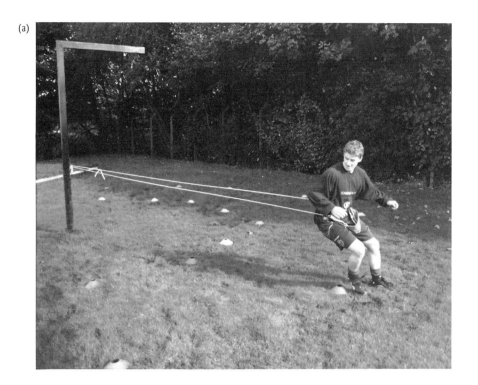

Figure 8.29a,b,c A specific aerobic, plyometric and lower limb co-contraction drill for all lower limb musculature, particularly useful in the final stages after ACL reconstruction surgery. The player faces away from the central pole with resistive Cliniband fastened to their waist. The player must run forwards from Xa to X1 (A), take short, shuffling steps around the marker and then run backwards from X1 to Xb (B). They then immediately move to X2 (C) and continue this process to X8, before returning to X1 in the same pattern. At all times they must face away from the pole (Fig. 8.29a). This process can be reversed by performing the same movement pattern facing the pole (Fig 8.29b). The time limit to complete the drill is 45 seconds.

(b)

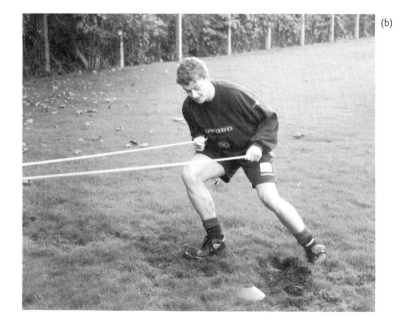

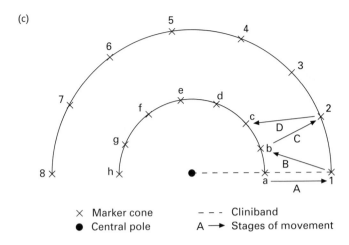

(c)

×	Marker cone	– – –	Cliniband
●	Central pole	A →	Stages of movement

Figure 8.29 Continued

more functional activities, such as running can commence. Two key factors which should be quantified at this stage are muscular strength and body weight. If a player's leg is not strong enough to carry body weight, or body weight has increased since the time of injury, the graft will come under extra stress with an increase in weightbearing activity. Before allowing a player to start running, a bilateral isokinetic test will assess both these parameters and give appropriate data on strength/body weight ratios. All players must perform an active warm-up prior to the test, which is then performed in the sitting position, avoiding the last 30° of extension in order to protect the graft from excessive anterior tibial translation. The following technical criteria are used:

Protocol for 12 week Isokinetic Test (Wilk, 1990)		
Angular velocity	*Warm-up reps*	*Test reps*
180°/s	5	10
300°/s	5	15

Table 8.10 *Isokinetic test protocol for 12 week-post operative anterior cruciate ligament reconstruction*

From the data collected, the individual scores of the player can then be compared to the normative data related to body weight available for this type of injury (Wilk, 1990).

Along with other functional tests, an objective decision can then be made as to whether the individual can start to run.

Direct or indirect **patellofemoral** problems often create problems in determining whether to use open or closed kinetic chain exercises in the rehabilitation phase of recovery. Traditional open kinetic exercises are not as functional as closed kinetic chain, yet weightbearing exercise may aggravate the symptoms. The importance of the knee angle, and the associated symptoms

Table 8.11 *Isokinetic target values for 12 week-post operative anterior cruciate ligament reconstruction*

Isokinetic target values for ACL reconstructed knees, 12 weeks post-op (Wilk, 1990)		
Physical parameter	180°/s	300°/s
Ham./quad. ratio	60–69%	70–79%
QPT to BW ratio	60–65%	45–55%
HPT to BW ratio	40–50%	33–42%
QTW to BW ratio	85–95%	
QAP to BW ratio	170–190%	

created by retropatellar pressure are the key factors to consider. Most functional activities occur with a knee angle of 0–40°, the point at which the patella is at its most unstable due to tibial rotation and raised position in the femoral groove (Van Kampen and Huiskes, 1990). Patellofemoral joint reaction forces have been shown to be greater in open (leg extension) rather than closed kinetic chain (leg press) work in this range (Steinkamp *et al.*, 1993), due to the reduction in patellar tracking created by compensatory movements at the distal and proximal joints and the degree of tibial and femoral rotation in closed chain work (Doucette and Child, 1996). Open chain strengthening may be most beneficial beyond the 40° mark of knee flexion, when patellofemoral forces have been shown to be greater during leg press work than leg extension (Steinkamp *et al.*, 1993).

Case study

In players with patellofemoral problems, whether due to direct injury or as a complication of chronic injury or surgical intervention, the important early factor is to determine the angle at which retropatellar symptoms occur. This can be done by testing the individual on an isokinetic unit, using very slow test velocities (15–60°/s), in concentric and eccentric mode. The normal inverted U-shaped curve will usually demonstrate a 'break' or dent in the curve with such players, which occurs due to pain and associated quadriceps inhibition. The break is only significant when its value exceeds 10% of the magnitude of the pre-break moment (Dvir et al., 1991). From the graphical data produced the degree of break and the angle of knee flexion when the break occurs, concentrically or eccentrically, will provide useful information to the physiotherapist as to the type of work which can be included in the rehabilitation programme. It is very important though to explain to the patient the reasons why such a test should be performed to the maximum, because it is going to aggravate the symptoms for a short time.

Chronic instability of the ankle joint is a common problem for any physiotherapist involved in sports rehabilitation. Integration of all the different joint mechanisms is an important factor in CKC rehabilitation work. The ankle invertors and evertors play important concentric and eccentric roles during

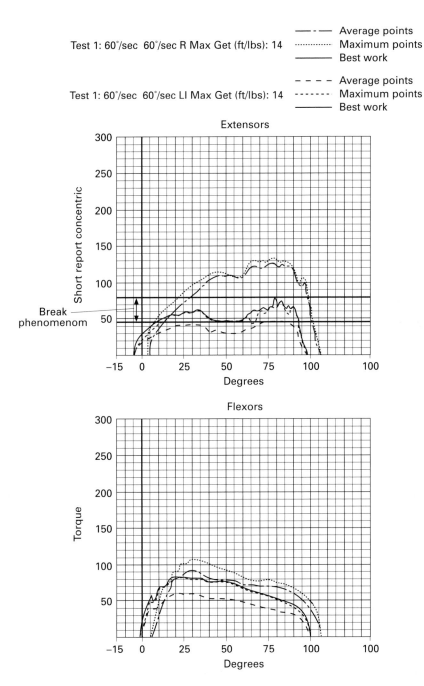

Test 1: 60°/sec 60°/sec R Max Get (ft/lbs): 14
— · — Average points
·········· Maximum points
——— Best work

Test 1: 60°/sec 60°/sec LI Max Get (ft/lbs): 14
— — — Average points
------- Maximum points
——— Best work

Figure 8.30 Break phenomenom, using isokinetic testing, in patellofemoral compression injury.

normal functional movement, responding to the effects of gravity, the ground reaction force and body momentum in various planes of movement.

| Case study | *Rehabilitation of such an injury is usually aimed at increasing ankle evertor muscle strength and reducing proprioceptive response time (Tropp, 1986). It may, however, be worth considering a different approach in some cases, as ankle invertor strength plays an important part in preventing the loss of postural stability that ultimately leads to excessive ankle inversion. When the rear part of the foot is in contact with the ground and weightbearing, lateral displacement of the centre of gravity causes the lower limb to move laterally as well. The medial border of the foot will rise as the rearfoot reaches* |

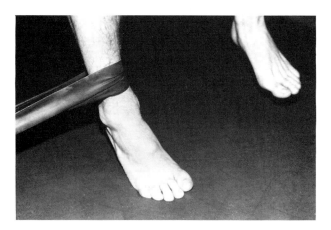

Figure 8.31 Eccentric ankle invertor exercise to prevent unwanted lateral displacement of the centre of gravity.

maximum eversion, producing forefoot inversion. When displacement of the centre of gravity goes beyond the lateral border of the foot, the forefoot reaches maximum inversion, with transference of the inversion torque to the rearfoot to conteract its everted position and prevent lateral tissue damage to the ankle joint. Rehabilitation should therefore include an element of eccentric ankle invertor work to decelerate this lateral displacement of the centre of gravity. This would place less reliance on the concentric capacity of the ankle evertors to maintain medial forefoot contact with the ground.

It should be remembered though that if the heel is in a plantar flexed position and all of the bodyweight is on the forefoot, the only dynamic mechanisms available to prevent excessive inversion are the ankle evertors.

Fitness test

Psychological, physical and functional fitness testing to determine if a player is fit to return to train fully or to play in a particular match is the final stage in the rehabiliation programme.

Testing should incorporate various physical and functional tests, with careful monitoring of the psychological state of the player with regard to the injury. The latter can be influenced tremendously by the relevant success of the rehabilitation programme and the ability of the physiotherapist to communicate

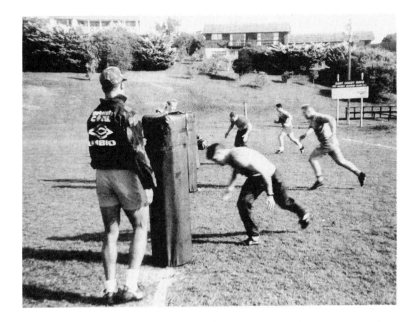

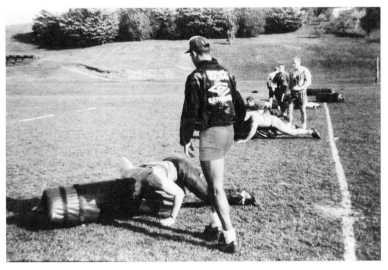

Figure 8.32a,b Collision work using tackle bags to ensure aerobic and physical fitness.

the positive steps that have been made in that time. Realistically, constant monitoring of the fitness levels of the player occurs throughout the recovery period, assessing and reassessing the state of the injury on a daily basis. Areas that should be addressed include:

Healing stage of the injury
Range of movement in relevant joints
Tensile and muscular strength
Proprioception
Functional movement

Functional speed of movement
Positional demands
Anaerobic and aerobic capacity
Psychological state of the player.

Supplementary factors exist, depending on the sport concerned, which may influence performance following injury and those which should also be considered at this stage include:

1. *The player*
   Age – the older player is able to 'read' the game better with experience
   Dominant or standing limb
   External social factors away from the game.
2. *The ball*
   Stationary/moving
   On the ground
   In the air
   Bouncing
   Speed
   Direction.
3. *Mode of functional activity*
   Concentric
   Eccentric
   Isometric
   Rotational.
4. *Environment*
   Surface
   Climate
   Opponent.

Practically, any such progressive testing must be made not on the treatment couch but in the gymnasium or on the playing field, where functional activities which mimic the sporting skills of the game combined with medical knowledge of the player and the injury will allow a measured decision to be made.

In the upper limb, progressive steps of non- to full body weight-bearing plyometric type drills which gradually incorporate a full range of movement need to be included. As the player gains confidence in the injury, then more difficult exercises and drills can be introduced before a final decision is made. Lower limb tests need also to include progressive non- to full weightbearing drills which incorporate hopping, squating, striding, jumping, twisting, cutting, backwards running and plyometric-based exercises.

Some players also have different pain thresholds, a factor which cannot be quantified or analysed without knowing the individual and which must be considered before making a decision on a player's fitness. Experience, which is only gained by active involvement and not solely from academic ability, is the key to act on such variables which exist when making the crucial decision,

Is that player fit to play?

Case study

I remember one of the very first lectures I went to given by a chartered physiotherapist involved in sport. He made a statement that I will never forget, and I believed it to be true until I became involved in sport myself. 'The final decision on a player's fitness must be made by the team physiotherapist. If the player or team manager went against such advice, then I would resign immediately', he said. Personally, I feel that as chartered physiotherapists, we have not got the power or the right to make such a profound statement, particularly when involved in professional sport. I have always worked on the basis that the final decision on a player's fitness is a three-way decision between the physiotherapist, the player and the team manager. The important fact medically is that if you have the respect of the other two individuals and make an appropriate functional and practical case for your decision, then this will have an affect on their thoughts. Communication is the key word in this situation. If both the player (who also has to consider the team and other non-playing factors, such as finances) and the manager (who wants to play his best team) go against your own particular thoughts, then I feel that you can do no more than offer your own professional advice. There is no point in sulking or gloating if you are proved right in the end. The backroom staff must also work as a team, and experience is a great asset in the learning curve of all individuals, no matter who they are.

References

Albert, M. (1991). *Eccentric Muscle Training in Sports and Orthopaedics*. New York: Churchill Livingstone.

Arms, S. W., Pope, M. H., Johnson, R. J. *et al.*, (1984). The biomechanics of anterior cruciate ligament rehabilitation and reconstruction. *Am. J. Sports Med.*, **12**, 8–18.

Astrand, P. O. and Rodahl, K. (1986). *Textbook of Work Physiology*. New York: McGraw-Hill.

Barrack, R. L., Skinner, H. B. and Buckley, S. L. (1989). Proprioception in the anterior cruciate ligament deficient knee. *Am. J. Sports Med.*, **17**, 1–6.

Barrett, D. S. (1991). Proprioception and function after anterior cruciate reconstruction. *J. Bone Joint Surg. (Br.)*, **73B**, 833–837.

Barrett, D. S., Cobb, A. G. and Bentley, G. (1991). Joint proprioception in normal, osteoarthritic and replaced knees. *J. Bone Joint Surg. (Br.)*, **73B**, 53–56.

Baxendale, R. A., Ferrell, W. R. and Wood, L. (1988). Responses of quadriceps motor units to mechanical stimulation of knee joint receptors in the decerebate cat. *Brain Res.*, **453**, 150–156.

Beard, D. J., Kyberd, P. J., Fergusson, C. M. *et al.* (1993). Proprioception after rupture of the anterior cruciate ligament. *J. Bone Joint Surg. (Br.)*, **75B**, 311–315.

Borg, G. A. (1982). Psychophysical basis of perceived exertion. *Med. Sci. Sports Exerc.*, **14**, 377.

Borsa, P. A., Lephart, S. M., Mininder, S. K. *et al.* (1994). Functional assesment and rehabilitation of shoulder proprioception for glenohumeral instability. *J. Sport Rehab.*, **3**, 84–104.

Boyle, M. (1991). Power stride improves lateral movement. *Hi-Tech Coach. Train.*, **1(7)**, 22–23.

Brask, B., Lueke, R. and Soderberg, G. (1984). Electromyographic analysis of selected muscle during the lateral step-up. *Phys. Ther.*, **64(3)**, 324–329.

Brewer, J., Ramsbottom, R. and Williams, C. (1988). *Multistage Fitness Test.* Loughborough: National Coaching Foundation.

Buckley, J. (1997). CKC – an open or shut case?. *Physio. Frntlne.*, **8**, 8–9.

Cabri, J. M. H. (1991). Isokinetic strength aspects of human joints and muscles. *Clin. Rev. Biomed. Eng.*, **19**, 231–259.

Chandler, J. M. and Duncan, P. W. (1988). Eccentric versus concentric force velocity relationships of the quadriceps femoris muscle. *Phys. Ther.*, **68(5)**, 800 (Abstract).

Ciccotti, M. G., Perry, J., Kerian, R. K. *et al.* (1993). An electromyographic analysis of the normal, the rehabilitated ACL deficient, and the ACL reconstructed patient during functional activities. Abstract presented at AOSSM Society's Speciality Day Meeting, San Francisco, CA.

Corrigan, J. P., Cashman, W. F. and Brady, M. P. (1992). Proprioception in the cruciate deficent knee. *J. Bone Joint Surg. (Br.)*, **74B**, 247–250.

Cook, T. M., Zimmermann, C. L., Lux, K. M. *et al.* (1992). EMG comparison of lateral step-up and stepping machine exercise. *J. Sports Phys. Ther.*, **16(3)**, 108–113.

Curwin, S. and Stanish, W. D. (1984). *Tendinitis: Its Etiology and Treatment.* Lexington: Heath and Co.

Davies, G. J. (ed). (1992). *A Compendium of Isokinetics in Clinical Usage.* Onalaska: S. & S. Publishers.

Dean, E. (1988). Physiology and therapeutic implications of negative work. A review. *Phys. Ther.*, **68(2)**, 233–237.

Delorme, T. and Wilkins, A. (1951). *Progressive Resistance Exercise.* New York: Appleton-Century-Crofts.

Doucette, S. A. and Child, D. C. (1996). The effect of open and closed chain exercise and knee joint position on patellar tracking in lateral patellar compression syndrome. *J. Sports Phys. Ther.*, **23(2)**, 104–110.

Duncan, P., Weiner, D., Chandler, J. *et al.* (1990). Functional reach: A new clinical measure of balance. *J. Gerontol.*, **45M**, 192–197.

Dvir, Z. (1995). *Isokinetics.* Edinburgh: Churchill Livingstone.

Dvir, Z, Halperin, N., Shklar, A. *et al.* (1991). Quadriceps function and patellofemoral pain syndrome. Part 2: the break phenomenon during eccentric contractions. *Isok. Ex. Sci.*, **1**, 31–35.

Elftman, H. (1966). Biomechanics of muscle. *J. Bone Joint Surg.*, **48**, 363.

Fitzgerald, G. K., Rothstein, J. M., Mayhew, T. P. *et al.* (1991). Exercise induced muscle soreness after concentric and eccentric exercise. *Phys. Ther.*, **71**, 505–513.

Freeman, M. A. R., Dean, M. R. E. and Hanham, I. W. F. (1965). The etiology and prevention of functional instability of the foot. *J. Bone Joint Surg.*, **47B**, 678–685.

Glousmann, R., Jobe, F. W., Tibone, J. E. *et al.* (1988). Dynamic electromyographic analysis of the throwing shoulder with glenohumeral instability. *J. Bone Joint Surg.*, **70A**, 220–226.

Gryzlo, S. M., Patek, R. M., Pink, M. *et al.* (1994). Electromyographic analysis of knee rehabilitation exercises. *J. Sports Phys. Ther.*, **20(1)**, 36–43.

Hage, P. (1982). Exercise guidelines: which to believe. *Phys. Sports Med.*, **10**, 23.

Henning, C. E., Lynch, M. A. and Glick, K. R. (1985). An *in vivo* strain guage study of elongation of the anterior cruciate ligament. *Am. J. Sports Med.*, **13**, 22–26.

Hettinger, R. (1962). *Physiology of Strength.* Springfield: Charles C. Thomas.

Horak, F. B. and Naschner, L. M. (1986). Central programming of postural movements. Adaption to altered support surface configurations. *J. Neurophysiol.*, **55**, 1369–1381.

Jansen, E., Larsen, R. and Olesen, M. (1982). Quantitative Romberg's test. *Acta Neurol. Scand.*, **66**, 93–99.

Jenkins, W. L., Munns, S. W., Jayaraman, G. *et al.* (1997). A measurement of anterior tibial displacement in the closed and open kinetic chain. *J. Orthop. Sports Phys. Ther.*, **25(1)**, 49–56.

Kaland, S., Sinkjaer, T., Arendt-Neilson, L. *et al.* (1990). Altered timing of hamstring muscle action in anterior cruciate ligament deficent patients. *Am. J. Sports Med.*, **18(3)**, 245–248.

Kennedy, J. C., Alexander, I. J. and Hayes, K. C. (1982). Nerve supply of the human knee and its functional importance. *Am. J. Sports Med.*, **10**, 329–335.

Knight, K. (1979). Knee rehabilitation by the DAPRE technique. *Am. J. Sports Med. Phys. Fitness*, **7**, 336.

Knott, M. and Voss, D. (1968). *Proprioceptive Neuromuscular Facilitation/Patterns and Techniques.* New York: Harper and Row.

Lange, L. (1919). *Über funktionelle Anpassung.* Berlin: Springer Verlag.

Leach, R. E. (1982). Overall view of rehabilitation of the leg for running. Symposium on the Foot and Leg in Running Sports, St Louis: CV Mosby.

Lentell, G. L., Katzman, L. L. and Walters, M. R. (1990). The relationship between muscle function and ankle stability. *J. Orthop. Sport Phys. Ther.*, **11**, 605–611.

Lephart, S. M., Warner, J. P., Borsa, P. A. *et al.* (1994). Proprioception of the shoulder in normal, unstable and post surgical individuals. 1994 American Shoulder and Elbow Surgeons Speciality Day Meeting. American Academy of Orthopaedic Surgeons Annual Meeting, February, New Orleans, LA.

Lutz, G. E., Palmitier, R. A., An, K. A. *et al.* (1993). Comparison of tibiofemoral joint forces during open-kinetic-chain and closed-kinetic-chain exercises. *J. Bone Joint Surg.*, **75A**, 732–739.

MacDougall, J. D., Elder, J. C. B., Sale, D. G. *et al.* (1980). Effects of strength, training and immobilization of human muscle fibres. *Eur. J. Appl. Physiol.*, **43**, 25–34.

MacQueen, I. (1954). Recent advances in the technique of progressive resistance. *Br. Med. J.*, **11**, 11993.

Muller, E. A. (1970). Influence of training and of inactivity on muscle strength. *Arch. Phys. Med. Rehab.*, **51**, 449–462.

Newham, D. J., Mills, K. R., Quigley, B. M. *et al.* (1983). Pain and fatigue after concentric and eccentric muscle contractions. *Clin. Sci.*, **64**, 55.

Noyes, F., Barber, S. and Mangine, R. (1991). Abnormal lower limb symmetry determined by function hop tests after anterior cruciate ligament rupture. *Am. J. Sports Med.*, **19**, 513–518.

Ohkoshi, Y., Yasuda, K., Kaneda, K. *et al.* (1991). Biomechanical analysis of rehabilitation in the standing position. *Am. J. Sports Med.*, **19(6)**, 605–611.

Palmitier, R., Kai-Nan, A., Scott, S. *et al.* (1991). Kinetic chain exercise in knee rehabilitation. *Sports Med.*, **11(6)**, 402–413.

Renstrom, P., Arms, S. W., Stanwyck, T. S., *et al.* (1986). Strain within the anterior cruciate ligament during hamstring and quadriceps activity. *Am. J. Sports Med.*, **14**, 83–87.

Sanders, M. (1990). Weight training and conditioning. In: *Sports Physical Therapy* (B. Sanders, ed.). Norwalk, Conn, Appleton and Lange.

Scott, P. M. (1977). *Clayton Electrotherapy and Actinotherapy.* 7th ed. London: Bailliere Tindall.

Shimba, T. (1984). An estimation of center of gravity from force platform data. *J. Biomech.*, **17**, 53-60.

Skinner, H. B., Barrack, R. L. and Cook. S. D. (1984). Age-related decline in proprioception. *Clin. Orthop.*, **184**, 208–211.

Spurway, N. C. (1992). Aerobic exercise, anaerobic exercise and the lactate threshold. *Br. Med. J.*, **48(3)**, 569–591.

Stanton, P. and Purdham, C. (1989). Hamstring injuries in sprinting: the role of eccentric exercise. *J. Orthop. Sport Phys. Ther.*, **10**, 343–344.

Steindler, A. (1977). *Kinesiology of the Human Body under Normal and Pathological Conditions.* Springfield: Charles C. Thomas.

Steinkamp, L. A., Dillingham, M. F., Markel, M. D. *et al.* (1993). Biomechanical considerations in patello femoral joint rehabilitation. *Am. J. Sports Med.*, **21(3)**, 438–444.

Stone, M. H. and O'Bryant. H. S. (1987). *Weight Training. A Scientific Approach.* Edina: Burgess International Group.

Taber's Cyclopedic Medical Dictionary. (1977). 13th edition, p. 146. Philadelphia: FA Davis.

Tibone, J. E., Antich, T. J., Funton, G. S. *et al.* (1986). Functional analysis of anterior cruciate ligament instability. *Am. J. Sports Med.*, **14(4)**, 276–284.

Townsend, H., Jobe, F. W., Pink, M. *et al.* (1991). Electromyographic analysis of the glenohumeral muscles during a baseball rehabilitation program. *Am. J. Sports Med.*, **19**, 264–272.

Tropp, H. (1985). Functional instability of the ankle joint. Medical dissertation No. 202, p. 7–39. Linkoping University, Sweden.

Tropp, H. (1986). Pronator muscle weakness in functional instability of the ankle joint. *Int. J. Sports Med.*, **7**, 291–294.

Tropp, H., Ekstrand, J. and Gillquist, J. (1984). Factors affecting stabilometry recordings of single limb stance. *Am. J. Sports Med.*, **12**, 185–188.

Van Kampen, A., Huiskes, R. (1990). The three dimensional tracking pattern of the human patella. *J. Orthop. Res.*, **8**, 372–382.

Verkhoshanski, Y. (1969). Perspectives in the improvement of speed-strength preparation of jumpers. *Yessis Rev. Soviet Phys. Ed. Sports*, **4(2)**, 28–29.

Verkhoshanski, Y. (1973). Depth jumping in the training of jumpers. *Track Tech.*, **51**, 1618–1619.

Voight, M. L. and Dravitch, P. (1991). Plyometrics. In: *Eccentric Muscle Training in Sports and Orthopaedics* (M. S. Albert, ed.). New York: Churchill-Livingstone.

Weymans, M. and Reybrouck, T. (1989). Habitual level of physical activity and cardiorespiratory endurance capacity in children. *Eur. J. Appl. Physiol.*, **58(3)**, 803.

Wilk, K. E., Keirns, M. A., Andrews, J. R., Clancy, W. G. *et al.* (1990). Anterior cruciate ligament reconstruction rehabilitation: A six-month follow-up of isokinetic testing in recreational athletes. *Isok. Excse. Sci.*, **1(1)**, 36–43.

Zinovieff, A. (1951). Heavy resistance exercise, the Oxford technique. *Br. J. Physiol. Med.*, **14, 129.**

Index

DRAKE MEMORIAL LIBRARY
WITHDRAWN
THE COLLEGE AT BROCKPORT